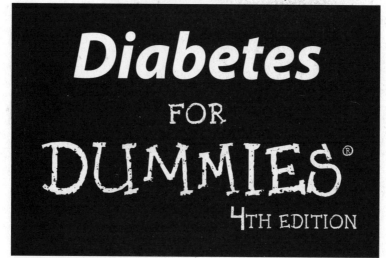

Diabetes

FOR

DUMMIES®

4TH EDITION

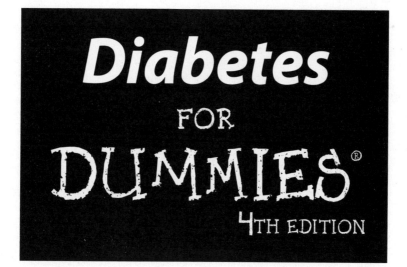

Diabetes FOR DUMMIES® 4TH EDITION

by Alan L. Rubin, MD

WILEY

John Wiley & Sons, Inc.

Diabetes For Dummies®, 4th Edition

Published by
John Wiley & Sons, Inc.
111 River St.
Hoboken, NJ 07030-5774
www.wiley.com

Library of Congress Control Number:

ISBN 978-1-118-29447-5 (pbk); ISBN 978-1-118-41229-9 (ebk); ISBN 978-1-118-41230-5 (ebk); ISBN 978-1-118-41231-2 (ebk)

Manufactured in the United States of America

10 9 8 7 6 5 4 3 2

WILEY

About the Author

Alan L. Rubin, MD, is one of the nation's foremost experts on diabetes. He is a professional member of the American Diabetes Association and the Endocrine Society and has been in private practice specializing in diabetes and thyroid disease for more than 35 years. Dr. Rubin was Assistant Clinical Professor of Medicine at the University of California Medical Center in San Francisco for 20 years. He has spoken about diabetes to professional medical audiences and non-medical audiences around the world. He has been a consultant to many pharmaceutical companies and companies that make diabetes products.

Dr. Rubin was one of the first specialists in his field to recognize the significance of patient self-testing of blood glucose, the major advance in diabetes care since the advent of insulin. As a result, he has been on numerous radio and television programs, talking about the cause, the prevention, and the treatment of diabetes and its complications.

Since publishing *Diabetes For Dummies,* Dr. Rubin has had six other bestselling *For Dummies* books — *Diabetes Cookbook For Dummies, Thyroid For Dummies, High Blood Pressure For Dummies, Type 1 Diabetes For Dummies, Prediabetes For Dummies,* and *Vitamin D For Dummies* — all published by John Wiley & Sons, Inc. His seven books cover the medical problems of 150 million Americans.

Dedication

This book is dedicated to my wife, Enid. She has been the perfect helpmate, always there with a smile and encouragement. There is no question that she promotes all my books better than anyone else. She even listens to my recommendations.

This edition is also dedicated to the thousands of people with diabetes who have written to thank me for helping them to understand what they are dealing with and for telling me where I need to provide more information and emphasis to make this an even better book.

Author's Acknowledgments

For this fourth edition, acquisitions editor Michael Lewis deserves major thanks. I have had the pleasure of working with him for several years. He is supportive, encouraging, and fun, and I look forward to a long association with him. I am also blessed with another great project editor, Chrissy Guthrie, and copy editor, Caitie Copple, who not only made sure that everything was readable and understandable but also offered excellent suggestions to improve the information. My thanks also to Dr. Lori Brame for reviewing the book for scientific accuracy, to Emily Nolan for testing the recipes, and to Patty Santelli, our nutritional analyst.

Ronnie and Michael Goldfield should definitely be considered the godparents of this book.

My friends in the Dawn Patrol, a group of guys with whom I play squash and solve the problems of the world thereafter, kept me laughing throughout the production of this book. Their willingness to follow me convinced me that others would be willing to read what I wrote.

My teachers are too numerous to mention, but one group deserves special attention. They are my patients over the last 35 years, the people whose trials and tribulations caused me to seek the knowledge that you will find in this book.

This book is written on the shoulders of thousands of men and women who made the discoveries and held the committee meetings. Their accomplishments cannot possibly be given adequate acclaim. We owe them big-time.

Publisher's Acknowledgments

We're proud of this book; please send us your comments at `http://dummies.custhelp.com`. For other comments, please contact our Customer Care Department within the U.S. at 877-762-2974, outside the U.S. at 317-572-3993, or fax 317-572-4002.

Some of the people who helped bring this book to market include the following:

Acquisitions, Editorial, and Vertical Websites

Senior Project Editor: Christina Guthrie
(Previous Edition: Jennifer Connolly)

Acquisitions Editor: Michael Lewis

Copy Editor: Caitlin Copple

Assistant Editor: David Lutton

Editorial Program Coordinator: Joe Niesen

Technical Editor: Lori Brame, MD

Editorial Manager: Christine Meloy Beck

Editorial Assistants: Rachelle Amick, Alexa Koschier

Art Coordinator: Alicia B. South

Cover Photos: © iStockphoto.com/ Chris Fertnig

Cartoons: Rich Tennant (`www.the5thwave.com`)

Composition Services

Project Coordinator: Kristie Rees

Layout and Graphics: Carl Byers, Joyce Haughey

Proofreaders: BIM Indexing & Proofreading Services, Jessica Kramer

Indexer: Estalita Slivoskey

Illustrator: Kathryn Born

Recipe Tester: Emily Nolan

Nutritional Analyist: Patty Santelli

Publishing and Editorial for Consumer Dummies

    Kathleen Nebenhaus, Vice President and Executive Publisher

    Kristin Ferguson-Wagstaffe, Product Development Director

    Ensley Eikenburg, Associate Publisher, Travel

    Kelly Regan, Editorial Director, Travel

Publishing for Technology Dummies

    Andy Cummings, Vice President and Publisher

Composition Services

    Debbie Stailey, Director of Composition Services

Contents at a Glance

Table of Contents

Introduction

You're reading the 4th edition of *Diabetes For Dummies,* and you may be wondering why another edition is necessary. The previous edition (published in 2008) had everything you needed to know to reverse the plague of diabetes, yet the problem seems to bc increasing, not decreasing. Following are some of the possible explanations for this situation:

- ✔ Not enough people bought the last edition of the book.
- ✔ Even if they bought it, not enough people followed the recommendations in the book.
- ✔ Too many people aren't even aware that this book exists.
- ✔ No book or books can stop an avalanche after the snow starts rolling downhill.
- ✔ Some new information, not available four years ago, may be able to make a major difference toward reversing diabetes.

The real answer is actually all of the above (and probably several more reasons).

The Centers for Disease Control and Prevention recently suggested that as many as one in three adults in the United States will have diabetes by the year 2050. The International Diabetes Federation reports that 366 million people had diabetes in 2011 and that 552 million will have the disease by 2030 — that's one in every ten people on the Earth. In the last edition of this book, I set this figure at 366 million by 2030, so you can see that today's predictions are even more dire than those of four years ago. This increase is because the population is aging, minority groups who have a higher risk for diabetes are increasing, and, fortunately, people with diabetes are living longer. However, these numbers are based on past trends. The prediction will not turn out to be true if people improve their lifestyle choices through the means discussed in this book.

Over the last decade, a large study was performed in Germany to see if lifestyle change could make a difference. Four major factors were evaluated in over 23,000 Germans. The factors were

- ✔ Never smoking
- ✔ Body-mass index less than 30
- ✔ Exercising for three and a half hours or more a week
- ✔ Following healthy dietary principles: high intake of fruits and vegetables, eating whole-grain bread, and low meat consumption

The happy finding was that the more factors a person followed, the lower the risk of major chronic diseases, including heart disease, diabetes, and cancer. People who followed all four had a 78 percent lower risk of those diseases than people who had no healthy factor. People with three factors were a little less protected, with two a bit less and with one even less but still better than no factors at all.

About This Book

So much has changed in the four years since the third edition of *Diabetes For Dummies* was written that a fourth edition was clearly necessary. I need to tell you about new medicines (see Chapter 10), new glucose meters (Chapter 7), and new ideas about diet and exercise (Chapters 8 and 9). I also need to share new information about diabetes in children (Chapter 13) and the occupational and insurance problems of people with diabetes (Chapter 15). Just about every chapter has something new, especially (obviously) Chapter 16, which deals specifically with what's new in diabetes care.

A new edition also gives me the opportunity to thank the thousands of people who have thanked me for *Diabetes For Dummies.* You have given me a sense of enormous gratification for writing this book. You have shared your stories with me, permitting me to laugh and cry with you. One of the best is the following from Andrea in Canada:

> *My 3-year-old daughter was recently diagnosed with diabetes type one. It has been a rough time. To help us out, my brother and his wife bought us your book,* Diabetes For Dummies. *One day my daughter saw this bright yellow book and asked what I was reading. I told her Diabetes For Dummies. As soon as the words came out of my mouth, I regretted it. I didn't want her to think that dummies got diabetes so I quickly added, "I am the dummy." Without missing a beat, she then asked, "Am I the diabetes?"*
>
> *The story doesn't just end there. The other day she was relaxing on the couch. She looked at me and said, "I don't want to have diabetes anymore." Feeling terrible, I responded, "I know sweetie; I don't want you to have it anymore either." I then explained that she would have diabetes for the rest of her life. With a very concerned look she then asked, "Will you be the dummy for the rest of your life?"*
>
> *As sad as it is, I guess you're right,* **one must look for humor in every-thing,** *otherwise we would have broken down by now.*

You're not required to read this book from cover to cover, although if you know nothing about diabetes, reading straight through may be a good approach. This book is designed to serve as a source for information about the problems that arise over the years. You can find the latest facts about diabetes and the best sources to discover any information that comes out after the publication of this edition.

Conventions Used in This Book

Throughout this book I use some specific conventions to make the text clearer, to highlight information, and to make your read as effortless as possible. These conventions are important to know, so I list them here:

- ✔ **Sugar versus glucose:** Diabetes, as you may know, is all about sugar. But sugars come in many types. So doctors avoid using the words *sugar* and *glucose* interchangeably. In this book (unless I slip up), I use the word *glucose* rather than *sugar.* (You may as well get used to it.)

- ✔ **Emphasis on type 2 diabetes:** There are a number of different types of diabetes (see my explanation in Chapter 3), and the most common are type 1 diabetes and type 2 diabetes. Because I recently published *Type 1 Diabetes For Dummies* (Wiley), most of what you read here is about type 2 diabetes.

- ✔ **Abbreviations:** To save time, I use the following abbreviations:

   - **T1DM:** Type 1 diabetes mellitus (formal name of type 1 diabetes)

   - **T2DM:** Type 2 diabetes mellitus (formal name of type 2 diabetes)

- ✔ **Pharmaceutical drug names:** When I mention a drug used in the treatment of diabetes, I give the generic name. I provide the trade name in parentheses if relevant.

What You're Not to Read

Throughout the book, you find shaded areas called *sidebars.* These sidebars contain material that is interesting but not essential. I hereby give you permission to skip them if the material inside them is of no particular interest to you. You will still understand everything else.

In addition, I've marked some paragraphs that have a more technical nature with the Technical Stuff icon (see the section "Icons Used in This Book," later in this Introduction for more information on icons). Although these paragraphs deepen your knowledge of diabetes as well as broaden your vocabulary, you can still understand the text without reading them.

Foolish Assumptions

The book assumes that you know nothing about diabetes. So you will not suddenly have to face a term that you've never heard of before and that is not explained. For those who already know a lot about diabetes, you can find more in-depth explanations in this book as well. You can pick and choose how much you want to know about a subject, but the key points are clearly marked.

How This Book Is Organized

This book is divided into six parts to help you find out all you can about the topic of diabetes.

Part I: Dealing with the Onset of Diabetes

To slay the dragon, you have to be able to identify it. This part explains the different types of diabetes, how you get them, and whether you can give them to others.

In this part, you find out how to deal with the emotional and psychological consequences of the diagnosis and what all those big words mean. You also find out how to prevent the complications of diabetes.

Part II: How Diabetes Affects Your Body

Some diseases seem to affect every part of the body. Diabetes is one of them. If you understand diabetes, you will have a pretty good grasp of how other illnesses can change the state of your health.

In this part, you find out what you need to know about both the short- and long-term complications of diabetes. You also find out about some sexual problems related to diabetes and the problems of a diabetic pregnancy.

Part III: Managing Diabetes: The "Thriving with Diabetes" Lifestyle Plan

In this part, you discover all the tools available to treat diabetes. You find out about the kinds of tests that you should be doing on your own as well as the tests your doctor should order to get a clear picture of the severity of your diabetes. I also show you what to do about your specific condition and how to follow the success of therapy.

In these chapters, you also discover the dietary changes that you need to make to control your blood glucose and how to get the most out of your exercise routine and medications. Finally, you find out about the huge amount of help available to you and your family. It is yours for the taking, and you definitely should take advantage of it.

Part IV: Special Considerations for Living with Diabetes

The way that diabetes develops is different for each age group. In this part, you discover those differences and how to manage them. I have a lot more to say in these chapters about children and the elderly with type 2 diabetes mellitus (T2DM). You also find out about some of the special economic problems of people with diabetes, which relate to jobs and insurance.

Lastly, this part covers all the new developments in diagnosing, monitoring, and treating diabetes and helps correct a lot of misinformation about diabetes treatment.

Part V: The Part of Tens

This part presents some key suggestions: the stuff you most need to know as well as the stuff you least *want* to know.

You discover the ten commandments of diabetes care and the myths that confuse many diabetic patients. You also find out how to get others to help you in your efforts to control your diabetes.

Part VI: Appendixes

Three special appendixes help you help yourself. One appendix points out hot spots to visit on the Internet to find info about diabetes, another provides you with a handy glossary in case you forget what a diabetes-related term means, and the third appendix helps you improve your diet by giving you some delicious diabetic-friendly recipes to try.

Icons Used in This Book

The icons alert you to information you must know, information you should know, and information you may find interesting but can live without.

When you see this icon, it means the information is essential and you should be aware of it.

This icon points out when you should see your doctor (for example, if your blood glucose level is too high or you need a particular test done).

This icon marks important information that can save you time and energy.

I use this icon whenever I tell a story about patients.

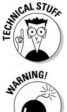

This icon gives you technical information or terminology that may be helpful, but not necessary, to your understanding of the topic.

This icon warns against potential problems (for example, if you don't treat a complication of diabetes properly).

Where to Go from Here

Where you go from here depends on your needs. If you already have basic knowledge of diabetes and want to know more about complications, go to Chapter 3. If you are a novice, start at Chapter 1. If you want to know more about the medications you are taking, go to Chapter 10. Each chapter title clearly tells you what you can find there, so check the table of contents to find what you need rapidly.

You're ready to get started on this trip we're taking together. Welcome! I hope it will be as much fun and as enlightening for you as it was for me.

As you will find out, keeping a positive attitude and finding some humor in your diabetes can help you a great deal. At times you will feel like doing anything but laughing. But scientific studies are clear about the benefits of a positive attitude. In a very few words: He who laughs, lasts. Another point is that people learn more and retain more when humor is part of the process.

Part I
Dealing with the Onset of Diabetes

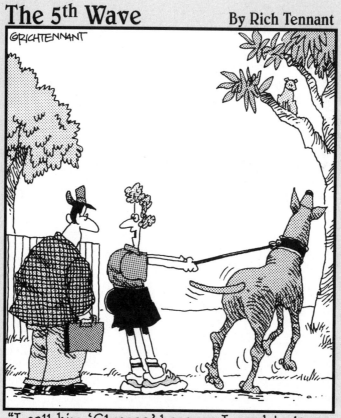

The 5th Wave — By Rich Tennant

"I call him 'Glucose,' because I need to keep him under control every day."

In this part . . .

You have found out that you or a loved one has diabetes. What do you do now? This part tells you about the emotional crisis that you may go through and emerge prepared to live with this chronic disease. I walk you through stages from wondering whether the diagnosis is correct to avoiding the complications associated with diabetes. You will discover the different kinds of diabetes and where you fit in. I also explain the concept of *prediabetes* and discuss how you can actually prevent diabetes.

Chapter 1

Dealing with Diabetes

*I*f you have diabetes, in the course of a year you live with that diagnosis for about 8,760 hours. During that time, you spend perhaps one hour with a physician. In Chapter 11, I introduce you to many of the other people who may help you to manage your disease. Clearly, however, the ball is in your hands alone practically all the time. How you deal with your diabetes determines whether you score or are shut out.

One of my patients told me about working at her first job out of college, where each employee birthday was celebrated with cake. She came to the first celebration and was urged to eat a slice. She refused and refused, until finally she had to say, "I can't eat the cake because I am diabetic." The woman urging her said, "Thank God. I thought you just had incredible willpower." Twenty years later, my patient clearly remembers being told that having diabetes is better than having willpower. Another patient told me the following: "The hardest thing about having diabetes is having to deal with doctors who do not respect me." Several times over the years, she had followed her doctor's recommendations exactly, but her glucose control hadn't been satisfactory. The doctor blamed her for this "failure."

Unless you live alone on a desert island (in which case I'm impressed that you got your hands on this book), your diabetes doesn't affect just you. How you deal with your diabetes affects your family, friends, and co-workers. This chapter shows you how to cope with diabetes and how to understand its impact on your important relationships.

Achieving Anything . . . Or Everything!

Carol Channing, Broadway's "first lady of musical comedy," is 91 and has type 1 diabetes. You could hardly say that her diabetes has been an impediment in her life. She has been a star on Broadway and in film and received the Oscar Hammerstein Award for Lifetime Achievement in Musical Theater. Now, I can't guarantee that your lovely singing voice and flair for comedy will let you become the next Carol Channing. But I can promise you that if you follow the advice in this book, your diabetes will never prevent you from accomplishing your goals. In fact, your success in managing diabetes may lead to success in other areas of your life.

Keeping good company

Diabetes is becoming more and more common. The list of people with diabetes is long, and you may be amazed at the caliber of the company you keep. The point is that every one of these people lives or lived with this chronic illness, and every one of them was able to do something special with his or her life.

Among the movie stars with diabetes is Halle Berry. She developed type 1 diabetes in 1989 and has been in numerous films and TV shows since that time, winning just about every award an actor can receive, including an Academy Award, an Emmy, a Golden Globe, a Screen Actors' Guild award, and a British Academy of Film and Television Arts award. She also found time to have a baby.

Drew Carey is another award-winning star of stage and screen who has lived and thrived with diabetes. In addition to performing, he has written for many of the hundreds of shows in which he has performed, including *The Drew Carey Show, Whose Line Is It Anyway?,* and *The Price Is Right.* He is also involved in sports and has been very generous in building and supporting libraries. He has shown by example that a person with type 2 diabetes can almost eliminate the diabetes with diet and exercise.

Aida Turturro, whom you may know as the sister of mobster Tony Soprano in the HBO series *The Sopranos,* has had type 2 diabetes for more than ten years, developing it during the run of the show. She continued to act on the show until it ended, seven years after her diagnosis.

Diabetes doesn't prevent the achievement of great records in sports. Athletes tend to develop T2DM (type 2 diabetes mellitus) when they are no longer in great physical shape, but exceptions exist. Diabetes didn't stop Mike Sinclair from becoming a three-time Pro-Bowl player in the National Football League during 11 seasons. Few others could box like Joe Frazier despite his diabetes mellitus. Billie Jean King put women's tennis on the map when she beat Bobby Riggs; diabetes certainly didn't slow her serve. Gary Hall is a swimmer with diabetes who won a total of ten Olympic medals in 2000 and 2004. Adam Morrison is a professional basketball player with diabetes. Diabetes didn't stop these and other professional athletes from becoming topflight examples of the potential skills that a person with diabetes can attain. (To read about the role of sports and exercise in your life, see Chapter 9.)

What about brain power? The list of scientists with diabetes is long and notable, headed by Thomas Alva Edison, who invented the light bulb, the phonograph, and numerous other major inventions. George Minot, who did pivotal research on vitamin B12, was the first person with diabetes to win the Nobel Prize for Physiology or Medicine. His work saved the lives of thousands of people. Albert Ellis did key work in psychology as the founder of cognitive-behavior therapy, which has effectively treated stuttering, anxiety disorders, mood disorders, and severe mental disorders including after a stroke.

Realizing your potential

The names in the preceding paragraphs are just a few examples of people with diabetes who have achieved greatness. Here is my point: *Diabetes shouldn't stop you from doing what you want to do with your life.* If you follow the rules of good diabetic care, as I describe in Chapters 7 through 12, you will actually be healthier than people without diabetes who smoke, overeat, and/or don't exercise enough.

Reacting to Your Diagnosis

Do you remember what you were doing when you found out that you had diabetes? Unless you were too young to understand, the news was quite a shock. Suddenly you had a condition from which people can die. In fact, many of the feelings that you went through were exactly those of a person learning that he or she is dying. The following sections describe the normal stages of reacting to a diagnosis of a major medical condition such as diabetes.

Experiencing denial

Your first response was probably to deny that you had diabetes, despite all of the evidence. Your denial mindset may have begun when your doctor tried to sugarcoat (forgive the pun) the news of your condition by telling you that you had just "a touch of diabetes," (an impossibility equivalent to "a touch of pregnancy"). You probably looked for any evidence that the whole thing was a mistake. Perhaps you even neglected to take your medication, follow your diet, or perform the exercise that is so important to maintaining your body. But ultimately, you had to accept the diagnosis and begin to gather the information you needed to help yourself.

When you accepted the diabetes diagnosis, I hope you also shared the news with your family, friends, and people close to you. Having diabetes isn't something to be ashamed of, and you shouldn't hide it from anyone. You need the help of everyone in your community: your co-workers who need to know not to tempt you with treats that you can't eat, your friends who need to know how to give you *glucagon* (a treatment for low blood glucose) if you become unconscious from a severe insulin reaction (see Chapter 4), and your family who needs to know how to support and encourage you to keep going.

Your diabetes isn't your fault — nor is it a form of leprosy or some other disease that carries a social stigma. Diabetes also isn't contagious; no one can catch it from you.

Feeling anger

When you pass the stage of denying that you have diabetes, you may become angry that you're saddled with this "terrible" diagnosis. But you'll quickly find that diabetes isn't so terrible and that you can't do anything to rid yourself of the disease. Anger only worsens your situation, and being angry about your diagnosis is detrimental in the following ways:

- ✔ If your anger becomes targeted at a person, he or she is hurt.
- ✔ You may feel guilty that your anger is harming you and those close to you.
- ✔ Anger can prevent you from successfully managing your diabetes.

As long as you're angry, you are not in a problem-solving mode. Diabetes requires your focus and attention. Use your energy positively to find creative ways to manage your diabetes. (For help managing your diabetes, see Part III.)

Bargaining for more time and feeling depressed

The stage of anger often transitions into a stage when you become increasingly aware of your mortality and bargain for more time. Even though you probably realize that you have plenty of life ahead of you, you may feel overwhelmed by the talk of complications, blood tests, and pills or insulin. When you realize that bargaining doesn't work, you may even experience depression, which makes good diabetic care all the more difficult.

Studies have shown that people with diabetes suffer from depression at a rate that is two to four times higher than the rate for the general population. People with diabetes also experience anxiety at a rate three to five times higher than people without diabetes.

If you suffer from depression, you may feel that your diabetic situation creates problems for you that justify being depressed. You may rationalize your depression in the following ways:

✔ You can't make friends as easily because diabetes hinders you.

✔ You don't have the freedom to choose your leisure activities.

✔ You're too tired to overcome difficulties.

✔ You dread the future and possible diabetic complications.

✔ You don't have the freedom to eat what you want.

✔ You're constantly annoyed by all of the minor inconveniences of dealing with diabetes.

All of the preceding concerns are legitimate, but they also are all surmountable. How do you handle your many concerns and fend off depression? Following are a few important methods:

✔ Try to achieve excellent blood glucose control (see Part III).

✔ Begin a regular exercise program (Chapter 9).

✔ Tell a friend or relative how you are feeling; get it off your chest (Chapter 20).

✔ Recognize that every abnormal blip in your blood glucose is not your fault (Chapter 7).

If you can't overcome the depression brought on by your diabetic concerns, you may need to consider therapy or antidepressant drugs. But you probably won't reach that point.

Moving on

You may experience the various stages of reacting to your diabetes in a different order than I describe in the previous sections. Some stages may be more prominent for you, and others may be hardly noticeable.

Don't think that any anger, denial, and depression are wrong. These feelings are natural coping mechanisms that serve a psychological purpose for a brief time. Allow yourself to have these feelings — and then drop them. Move on and learn to live normally with your diabetes.

Here are some key steps you can take to manage the emotional side of diabetes:

✔ **Focus on your successes.** Some things may go wrong as you find out how to manage diabetes, but most things will go right. As you concentrate on your successes, you will realize that you can cope with diabetes and not let it overwhelm you.

✔ **Involve the whole family in your diabetes.** A diabetic lifestyle is a healthy lifestyle for everyone. For instance, the exercise you do is good for the whole family. By doing it together, you strengthen the family ties while everyone gets the health benefits. Also, should you need your family to help you, for instance, during a particularly severe case of low blood glucose, their early involvement in learning about diabetes will give them the peace of mind to know they are helping you, not hurting you. (See Chapter 20 for ways to enlist help from people around you.)

✔ **Develop a positive attitude.** A positive attitude gives you a can-do mind-set, whereas a negative attitude leads to low motivation preventing you from doing all that is necessary to manage your diabetes.

✔ **Find a great team, pinpoint problems, and set goals.** Determine the most difficult problems that you have with your diabetes and then consider how you can solve them by yourself or with a great team of supporting players like a diabetes specialist, a diabetes educator, a dietitian, an eye doctor, a foot doctor, and so forth. Set realistic goals to get past your problems. (Chapter 11 tells you everything you need to know about getting help from the supporting players.)

✔ **Don't expect perfection.** Although you may feel that you're doing everything right, you may experience blood glucose levels that are too high or too low. This uncontrollable situation happens to every person with diabetes, and it's one of the biggest frustrations of the disease. Don't beat yourself up over something you can't control. Keep doing the things I suggest in the treatment section, and you will be very gratified at the end.

Maintaining a High Quality of Life

You may assume that a chronic disease like diabetes leads to a diminished quality of life, but you don't have to settle for anything less than a full and fulfilling life.

Many studies have evaluated the quality-of-life question, and the following sections not only describe what these studies found but also describe my hope that you can take control and ensure that you maintain a high quality of life.

Exercising regularly

People who do regular exercise often describe it as addictive. They find it so pleasurable that they look forward to the next session. And the benefits for the person with diabetes are enormous.

In one long-term study on quality of life for people with diabetes, a factor that contributed to a lower quality of life rating was a lack of physical activity, which is one negative factor that you can alter immediately. Physical activity is a habit that you must maintain on a lifelong basis. (See Chapter 9 for advice on exercise.) The problem is that making a long-term change to a more physically active lifestyle is difficult; most people become more active for a time but eventually fall back into inactive routines.

Another study demonstrated the tendency for people with diabetes (and for people in general) to abandon exercise programs after a certain period of time. This information was reported in the *New England Journal of Medicine* in July 1991. In this study, a group of people with diabetes received professional support for two years to encourage them to increase physical activity. For the first six months, the study participants responded well and exercised regularly, resulting in improved blood glucose, weight management, and overall health. After that, participants began to drop out and not come to training sessions. At the end of the two-year study, most participants had regained their weight and slipped back into poor glucose control. However, the few people who didn't stop their exercise maintained the benefits and continued to report an improved quality of life.

Factoring in the (minimal) impact of insulin treatments

Perhaps you're afraid that intensified insulin treatment, which involves three or four daily shots of insulin and frequent testing of blood glucose, will keep you from doing the things that you want to do and will diminish your daily quality of life. (See Chapter 10 for more information about intensified insulin treatment.) Your fears are not justified by the facts.

A study published in *Diabetes Care* in 1998 explored whether the extra effort and time consumed by such diabetes treatments had an adverse effect on people's quality of life. The study compared people with diabetes to people with other chronic diseases, such as gastrointestinal disease and hepatitis (liver infection). The diabetic group reported a higher quality of life than the other chronic illness groups. Interestingly, the people in the diabetic group were not so much concerned with the physical problems of diabetes, such as intense and time-consuming tests and treatments, as they were concerned with the social and psychological difficulties.

Another report in *Diabetes Care* in 1998 stated that insulin injections don't reduce the quality of life; the person's sense of physical and emotional well-being remains the same after beginning insulin injections as it was before injections were necessary.

Teenagers who require insulin injections don't always accept the treatment as well as adults do, so teenagers more often experience a diminished quality of life. However, a study of more than 2,000 such teenagers, published in *Diabetes Care* in 2001, showed that as their diabetic control improved, teens felt like they were in better health, experienced greater satisfaction with their lives, and therefore believed themselves to be less of a burden to their families.

Managing stress

A study described in *Diabetes Care* in January 2002 showed that lowering stress lowers blood glucose. Patients were divided into two groups, one of which received diabetes education alone and the other of which received diabetes education plus five sessions of stress management. The latter group showed significant improvement in diabetic control versus the former group.

Whether stress raises the blood glucose directly by causing the release of stress hormones or raises it indirectly by causing overeating, under-exercising, and failure to take medications, managing stress certainly helps to manage your diabetes. Here are some of the things you can do to help manage stress in your life:

- **Identify the source of the stress.** Are you adding to stress yourself by accepting it as an unchanging part of your life or blaming others or outside events that you can't control?

- **Examine the way that you cope with stress now.** Do you smoke, drink too much, overeat, spend too much time in front of screens, sleep too much, or overschedule yourself so you have no time?

- **Replace unhealthy coping mechanisms with healthy ones.** Avoid the stress you've identified or make a change in your life. Adapt to the stress or accept it. You can't avoid your diabetes, but you can make it less stressful by following my recommendations in Part III.

- **Take time out for fun and relaxation.** Here are some of the things you might do:

    - Have a picnic lunch

    - Get a massage

    - Take a long bath

    - Work in a garden

    - Play with a pet or go to the zoo

    - Listen to your favorite music

    - Go to a comedy show or rent a funny movie

    - Stay in bed with your significant other

Considering other key quality-of-life factors

Many other studies have examined the different aspects of diabetes that affect quality of life. These studies show some useful information on the following topics:

- **Family support:** People with diabetes greatly benefit from their family's help in dealing with their disease. But does having a close family help people with diabetes maintain better diabetic control? One study in *Diabetes Care* in February 1998 addressed this question and found some unexpected results. Having a supportive family didn't necessarily mean that the person with diabetes would maintain better glucose control. But a supportive family did make the person with diabetes feel more physically capable in general and much more comfortable with his or her place in society.

- **Quality of life over the long term:** How does a person's perception of quality of life change over time? As they age, do most people with diabetes feel that their quality of life increases, decreases, or persists at a steady level? The consensus of several studies is that most people with diabetes experience an increasing quality of life as they get older. People feel better about themselves and their diabetes after dealing with the disease for a decade or more. This report shows the healing property of time.

Following are some other factors that improve quality of life for people with diabetes. Though I can't cite any particular studies here, doctors and patients alike can vouch for their importance.

- **Blood glucose levels:** Keep your blood glucose as normal as possible (see Part III for tips).

- **Continuing education:** Stay aware of the latest developments in diabetes care.

- **Your attitude:** Maintain a healthy attitude. Remember that someday you will laugh about things that bug you now, so why wait?

When you're having trouble coping

You wouldn't hesitate to seek help for your physical ailments associated with diabetes, but you may be reluctant to seek help when you can't adjust psychologically to diabetes. The problem is that sooner or later your psychological maladjustment will ruin any control that you have over your diabetes. And, of course, you won't lead a very pleasant life if you're in a depressed or anxious state all the time. The following symptoms are indicators that you're past the point of handling your diabetes on your own and may be suffering from depression:

✔ You can't sleep or you sleep too much.

✔ You have no energy when you're awake.

✔ You can't think clearly.

✔ You can't find activities that interest or amuse you.

✔ You feel worthless.

✔ You have frequent thoughts of suicide.

✔ You have no appetite.

✔ You find no humor in anything.

If you recognize several of these symptoms in your daily life, you need to get some help. Your sense of hopelessness may include the feeling that no one else can help you — but that's simply not true. First, go to your primary physician or endocrinologist (diabetes specialist) for advice. He or she may help you to see the need for some short-term or long-term therapy. Well-trained therapists — especially therapists trained to take care of people with diabetes — can see solutions that you can't see in your current state. You need to find a therapist whom you can trust so that when you're feeling low you can talk to this person and feel assured that he or she is very interested in your welfare.

Your therapist may decide that you would benefit from medication to treat the anxiety or depression. Currently, many drugs are available that are proven safe and free of side effects. Sometimes a brief period of medication is enough to help you adjust to your diabetes.

You can also find help in a support group. The huge and continually growing number of support groups shows that positive things are happening in these groups. In most support groups, participants share their stories and problems, helping everyone involved cope with their own feelings of isolation, futility, or depression.

Chapter 2

It's the Glucose and the Hemoglobin A1c

*T*he Greeks and Romans knew about diabetes. The way they tested for the condition was — prepare yourself — by tasting people's urine. In this way, the Romans discovered that the urine of certain people was *mellitus,* the Latin word for *sweet.* (They got their honey from the island of Malta, which they called *Mellita.*) In addition, the Greeks noticed that when people with sweet urine drank, the fluids came out in the urine almost as fast as they went in the mouth, like a siphon. The Greek word for *siphon* is *diabetes.* Thus we have the origins of the modern name for the disease, *diabetes mellitus.*

In this chapter, I cover some not-so-fun stuff about diabetes — the big words, the definitions, and so on. If you really want to understand what's happening to your body when you have diabetes — and I know I would — then you won't want to skip this chapter.

Realizing the Role of Glucose

The body has three sources of energy: protein, fat, and carbohydrates. I discuss the first two sources in greater detail in Chapter 8, but I tackle the third one now. Sugar is a carbohydrate. Many different kinds of sugars exist in nature, but glucose, the sugar that has the starring role in the body, provides a source of instant energy so that muscles can move and important chemical reactions can take place. Table sugar, or *sucrose,* is actually two different kinds of sugar — glucose and fructose — linked together. Fructose is the type of sugar found in fruits and vegetables. Because fructose is sweeter than glucose, sucrose (the combination of fructose and glucose) is sweeter than glucose alone as well. Therefore, your taste buds don't need as much sucrose or fructose to get the same sweet taste of glucose.

In order to understand the symptoms of diabetes, you need to know a little about the way the body normally handles glucose and what happens when things go wrong. A hormone called *insulin* finely controls the level of glucose in your blood. A *hormone* is a chemical substance made in one part of the body that travels (usually through the bloodstream) to a distant part of the body where it performs its work. In the case of insulin, that work is to act like a key to open a cell (such as a muscle, fat, or liver cell) so that glucose can enter. If glucose can't enter the cell, it can provide no energy to the body.

Insulin is essential for growth. In addition to providing the key to entry of glucose into the cell, insulin is considered the *builder hormone* because it enables fat and muscle to form. It promotes the storage of glucose in a form called *glycogen* for use when fuel is not coming in. It also blocks the breakdown of protein. Without insulin, you do not survive for long.

With this fine-tuning, your body keeps the level of glucose pretty steady at about 60 to 100 mg/dl (3.3 to 6.4 mmol/L) all the time.

Your glucose starts to rise in your blood when you don't have a sufficient amount of insulin or when your insulin is not working effectively (see Chapter 3). When your glucose rises above 180 mg/dl (10.0 mmol/L), glucose begins to spill into the urine and make it sweet. Up to that point, the kidneys, the filters for the blood, are able to extract the glucose before it enters your urine. The loss of glucose into the urine leads to many of the short-term complications of diabetes. (See Chapter 4 for more on short-term complications.)

Understanding the Hemoglobin A1c

Your *blood glucose level* is the level of sugar in your blood, a key measure of diabetes. Individual blood glucose tests are great for deciding how you're doing at that moment and what to do to make it better, but they do not give the big picture. They are just a moment in time. Glucose can change a great deal even in 30 minutes. What you need is a test that gives an integrated picture of many days, weeks, or even months of blood glucose levels. The test that accomplishes this important task is called the *hemoglobin A1c.*

Hemoglobin is a protein that carries oxygen around the body and drops it off wherever it's needed to help in all the chemical reactions that are constantly taking place. The hemoglobin is packaged within red blood cells that live in the bloodstream for 60 to 90 days. As the blood circulates, glucose in the blood attaches to the hemoglobin and stays attached. It attaches in several different ways to the hemoglobin, and the total of all the hemoglobin attached to glucose is called *glycohemoglobin.* Glycohemoglobin normally makes up about 6 percent of the hemoglobin in the blood. The largest fraction, two-thirds of the glycohemoglobin, is in the form called *hemoglobin A1c,* making it easiest to measure. The rest of the hemoglobin is made up of hemoglobin A1a and A1b.

The more glucose in the blood, the more glycohemoglobins form. Because red blood cells carrying glycohemoglobin remain in the blood for two to three months, glycohemoglobin is a reflection of the glucose control over the entire time period and not just the second that a single glucose test reflects.

Hemoglobin A1c has a number of advantages over the variety of glucose tests for diagnosing diabetes, which I discuss in the later section "Diagnosing diabetes through testing." Hemoglobin A1c is now as well standardized as glucose testing, and it has the following benefits:

- A1c reflects chronic high blood glucose rather than a few seconds in time.
- A1c has been found to reflect future complications (see Chapter 5) better than fasting glucose.
- Fasting isn't necessary, and acute changes like diet and exercise don't affect A1c.
- A1c is not as affected by sample delays on the way to or in the lab.
- A1c is also used to follow the course of diabetes, so the level of treatment needed is immediately understood.
- A1c is cost-effective, because no further testing is immediately necessary when results are abnormal (whereas an abnormal glucose test requires another glucose or A1c as the next test).

Following are some disadvantages of hemoglobin A1c:

- Abnormal glucose after eating is a better predictor of heart disease than A1c.
- Some subjects with anemia, a recent blood transfusion, and abnormal hemoglobin types (there are several types of hemoglobin) produce an unreliable A1c result.
- Different ethnic groups have different levels for their abnormal A1c.

According to one study, in the United States, hemoglobin A1c detects that diabetes is present in one in every five people admitted to a hospital for any reason without a diagnosis of diabetes.

Getting a Wake-Up Call from Prediabetes

Diabetes doesn't suddenly appear one day without previous notification from your body. For a period of time, which may last up to ten years, you may not quite achieve the criteria for a diagnosis of diabetes but not be quite normal either. During this time, you have what's called *prediabetes.*

A person with prediabetes doesn't usually develop eye disease, kidney disease, or nerve damage (all potential complications of diabetes, which I discuss in Chapter 5). However, a person with prediabetes has a much greater risk of developing heart disease and brain attacks than someone with entirely normal blood glucose levels. Prediabetes has a lot in common with insulin-resistance syndrome, also known as the *metabolic syndrome,* which I discuss in Chapter 5. The following two sections take the mystery out of whether you may have prediabetes by giving you some guidelines on when to get tested as well as explaining what testing for prediabetes involves.

Knowing whether you should get tested

Approximately 80 million people in the United States have prediabetes, although most of them don't know it. Testing for prediabetes is a good idea for everyone over the age of 45. I also recommend getting tested if you're under 45 and overweight and have one or more of the following risk factors:

✔ A high-risk ethnic group: African American, Hispanic, Asian, or Native American

✔ High blood pressure

✔ Low HDL ("good") cholesterol

✔ High triglycerides

✔ A family history of diabetes

✔ Diabetes during a pregnancy or giving birth to a baby weighing more than 9 pounds

A study in the journal *Diabetes Care* in November 2007 showed that testing for prediabetes in overweight or obese people over age 45 is highly cost effective if they then undergo lifestyle modification (see Chapters 7 through 12) or take medication if necessary.

Testing for prediabetes

Testing for prediabetes involves finding out your blood glucose level, the level of sugar in your blood. Prediabetes exists when the body's blood glucose level is higher than normal but not high enough to meet the standard definition of diabetes mellitus (which I discuss in the section "Diagnosing diabetes through testing," later in this chapter). Testing is done by measuring a random capillary blood glucose. If the level is greater than 100 milligrams per deciliter (mg/dl), a fasting plasma glucose or oral glucose tolerance test is performed. As of 2010, the American Diabetes Association recommends that the hemoglobin A1c (see the next section) can also be used for the definition. Table 2-1 shows the hemoglobin A1c and glucose levels that indicate prediabetes:

- ✔ If the glucose before the test (the fasting plasma glucose) is between 100 and 125 mg/dl, the person has impaired (abnormally high) *fasting glucose,* the glucose before eating (see Table 2-1). The glucose in the fasting state (no food for eight hours) is not normal, but it's not high enough to diagnose diabetes.

- ✔ If the glucose is between 140 and 199 mg/dl at two hours after eating 75 grams of glucose, the person has impaired glucose tolerance. Both impaired fasting glucose and impaired glucose tolerance may be present.

- ✔ A hemoglobin A1c between 5.7 and 6.4 percent suggests prediabetes.

Table 2-1	Diagnosing Prediabetes		
Condition	*Glucose Before Eating*	*Glucose Two Hours After Eating 75 gm Glucose*	*Hemoglobin A1c*
Normal	Less than 100 mg/dl (5.5 mmol/L)	Less than 140 mg/dl (7.8 mmol/L)	Less than 5.7 percent
Prediabetes	100–125 mg/dl (5.5–7 mmol/L)	140–199 mg/dl (7.8–11.1 mmol/L)	5.7–6.4 percent

Mg/dl, or *milligrams per deciliter,* is the unit of measurement commonly used in the United States. The rest of the world uses the International System (SI), where the units are mmol/L, which means *millimoles per liter.* To get mmol/L, you divide mg/dl by 18. Therefore, 200 mg/dl equals 11.1 mmol/L.

Diagnosing prediabetes can be the best thing that ever happened to a person! It could be the wake-up call that he or she needs. The diagnosis may motivate a person to make crucial lifestyle changes, especially in diet and exercise, which have been shown to prevent the onset of diabetes in people with prediabetes. And for people whose prediabetes doesn't respond to lifestyle changes, medication may accomplish the same thing.

After a diagnosis of prediabetes is made, all the techniques described in Chapters 7 through 12 can help prevent the onset of clinical diabetes. If patients with prediabetes are left untreated, large numbers of these patients will develop diabetes over time. Preventing diabetes saves a person almost $10,000 in costs for the treatment of diabetes. And properly responding to a diagnosis of prediabetes prevented almost 20 percent of people with prediabetes from becoming diabetic.

Detecting Diabetes

When prediabetes becomes diabetes, the body's blood glucose level registers even higher. In this section, I discuss the evidence for diabetes and the symptoms you may experience with diabetes.

Diagnosing diabetes through testing

The standard definition of diabetes mellitus is *excessive glucose in a blood sample.* For years, doctors set this level fairly high. The standard level for normal glucose was lowered in 1997 because too many people were experiencing complications of diabetes even though they did not have the disease by the then-current standard. In November 2003, the standard level was modified again. In 2009, the International Expert Committee on Diagnosis and Classification of Diabetes Mellitus recommended using the hemoglobin A1c as a diagnostic criterion for diabetes, and the American Diabetes Association subsequently accepted the recommendation.

After much discussion, many meetings, and the usual deliberations that surround a momentous decision, the American Diabetes Association published the new standard for diagnosis, which includes any *one* of the following four criteria:

- **Hemoglobin A1c equal to or greater than 6.5 percent.**

- **Casual plasma glucose concentration greater than or equal to 200 mg/dl, along with symptoms of diabetes.** *Casual plasma glucose* refers to the glucose level when the patient eats normally prior to the test. I discuss symptoms in the section "Examining the symptoms of diabetes" later in this chapter.

- **Fasting plasma glucose (FPG) of greater than or equal to 126 mg/dl or 7 mmol/L.** *Fasting* means that the patient has consumed no food for eight hours prior to the test.

✔ **Blood glucose of greater than or equal to 200 mg/dl (11.1 mmol/L) when tested two hours (2-h PG) after ingesting 75 grams of glucose by mouth.** This test has long been known as the oral glucose tolerance test. Although this time-consuming, cumbersome test is rarely done, it remains the gold standard for the diagnosis of diabetes.

Following is another way to look at the criteria for diagnosis:

✔ FPG less than 100 mg/dl (5.5 mmol/L) is a normal fasting glucose.

FPG greater than or equal to 100 mg/dl but less than 126 mg/dl (7.0 mmol/L) is impaired fasting glucose (indicating prediabetes).

FPG equal to or greater than 126 mg/dl (7.0 mmol/L) gives a provisional diagnosis of diabetes.

✔ 2-h PG less than 140 mg/dl (7.8 mmol/L) is normal glucose tolerance.

2-h PG greater than or equal to 140 mg/dl but less than 200 mg/dl (11.1 mmol/L) is impaired glucose tolerance.

2-h PG equal to or greater than 200 mg/dl gives a provisional diagnosis of diabetes.

✔ Hemoglobin A1c equal to or greater than 6.5 percent gives a provisional diagnosis of diabetes. As the hemoglobin A1c rises from normal, the occurrence of diabetes rises with it. If the hemoglobin A1c is equal to or greater than 5.6, the patient has a threefold chance of developing diabetes in the next six years.

Testing positive for diabetes one time isn't enough to confirm a diagnosis. Any one of the tests must be positive on another occasion to make a diagnosis of diabetes. I've had patients come to me with a diagnosis of diabetes after being tested only once, and a second test has shown the initial diagnosis to be incorrect.

Examining the symptoms of diabetes

The following list contains the most common early symptoms of diabetes and how they occur. One or more of the following symptoms may be present when diabetes is diagnosed:

✔ **Frequent urination and thirst:** The glucose in the urine draws more water out of your blood, so more urine forms, making you feel the need to urinate more frequently. As the amount of water in your blood declines, you feel thirsty and drink much more frequently.

✔ **Blurry vision:** As the glucose level shifts from normal to very high, the lens of the eye swells due to water intake. This swelling prevents the eye from focusing light at the correct place, and blurring occurs.

- **Extreme hunger:** Inability to get energy in the form of glucose into the muscle cells that need it leads to a feeling of hunger despite all the glucose that is floating in the bloodstream. Such hunger is called "starvation in the midst of plenty."

- **Fatigue:** Without sufficient insulin, or with ineffective insulin, glucose can't enter cells (such as muscle and fat cells) that depend on insulin to act as a key. (The most important exception here is the brain, which does not need insulin to extract glucose from the blood.) As a result, glucose can't be used as a fuel to move muscles or to facilitate the many other chemical reactions that have to take place to produce energy. A person with diabetes often complains of fatigue and feels much stronger after treatment allows glucose to enter his or her cells again.

- **Weight loss:** Weight loss occurs among some people with diabetes because they lack insulin, the builder hormone. When the body lacks insulin for any reason, the body begins to break down. You lose muscle tissue. Some of the muscle converts into glucose even though the glucose can't get into cells. It passes out of your body in the urine. Fat tissue breaks down into small fat particles that can provide an alternate source of energy. As your body breaks down and you lose glucose in the urine, you often experience weight loss. However, most people with diabetes are heavy rather than skinny. (I explain why in Chapter 3.)

- **Persistent vaginal infection among women:** As blood glucose rises, all the fluids in your body contain higher levels of glucose, including the sweat and body secretions such as semen in men and vaginal secretions in women. Many bugs, such as bacteria and yeast, thrive in the high-glucose environment. Women begin to complain of itching or burning, an abnormal discharge from the vagina, and sometimes an odor.

Similar symptoms; different diseases

Frequent thirst and urination are the most commonly recognized symptoms of diabetes, but diabetes mellitus is not the only condition that causes these symptoms. Another condition in which fluids go in and out of the body like a siphon is called *diabetes insipidus*. With this condition, the urine is not sweet. Diabetes insipidus is an entirely different disease that you should not mistake for diabetes mellitus.

Diabetes insipidus results when a hormone in the brain called *antidiuretic hormone* is missing or when the kidneys can't properly respond to antidiuretic hormone. This hormone normally helps the kidneys prevent the loss of a lot of water in the body. Other than the name *diabetes,* this condition has nothing to do with diabetes mellitus.

A study in the November 2007 issue of *Diabetes Care,* however, showed that in a group of over 15,000 people being treated for diabetes, 44 percent of people with type 2 diabetes reported not one of the symptoms above in the previous year when given a questionnaire. It is no wonder that a third of people with diabetes don't know they have it.

Tracing the History of Diabetes Treatment

More than 2,000 years ago, people writing in China and India described a condition that must have been diabetes mellitus. The description is the same one that the Greeks and Romans reported — urine that tasted sweet. Scholars from India and China were the first to describe frequent urination. But not until 1776 did researchers discover the cause of the sweetness — glucose. And it wasn't until the 19th century that doctors developed a new chemical test to actually measure glucose in the urine.

Later discoveries showed that the pancreas produces a crucial substance that controls the glucose in the blood: insulin. Since that discovery was made, scientists have found ways to extract insulin and purify it so it can be given to people whose insulin levels are too low.

After insulin was discovered, diabetes specialists, led by Elliot Joslin and others, recommended three basic treatments for diabetes that are as valuable today as they were in 1921:

- Diet (see Chapter 8)
- Exercise (see Chapter 9)
- Medication (see Chapter 10)

Although the discovery of insulin immediately saved the lives of thousands of very sick individuals for whom the only treatment had been starvation, it did not solve the problem of diabetes. As these people aged, they were found to have unexpected complications in the eyes, the kidneys, and the nervous system (see Chapter 5). And insulin didn't address the problem of the much larger group of people with diabetes now known as type 2 (see Chapter 3). Their problem was not lack of insulin but resistance to its actions. (Fortunately, doctors do have the tools now to bring the disease under control.)

Tracking diabetes around the world

Diabetes is a global health problem. Type 2 diabetes is especially prevalent where obesity is common. In 2008, more than 1.5 billion people were overweight (body-mass index greater than 25 kilograms/meter squared — see Chapter 7) and 500 million people were obese (body-mass index greater than 30) in the world. Currently 366 million people have diabetes. Diabetes is most concentrated in areas where large food supplies allow people to eat more calories than they need, causing them to develop excessive fat. Several different types of diabetes exist, but the type usually associated with obesity, called *type 2 diabetes* (see Chapter 3), is far more prevalent than the other types.

Another reason diabetes cases have continued to grow in number throughout the world is that the life span of the population is increasing. What's the connection? Well, as a person ages, his or her chances of developing diabetes increases greatly. Along with obesity, age is a major risk factor for diabetes. (See Chapter 3 for more risk factors.) So as other diseases are controlled and the population in general gets older, more diabetes is being diagnosed.

One very interesting study traced people of Japanese ancestry as they went from living in Japan to living in Hawaii to living in the United States mainland. In Japan, where people customarily maintain a normal weight, they tended to have a very low incidence of diabetes. As they moved to Hawaii, the incidence of diabetes began to rise along with their average weight. On the U.S. mainland, where food is most available, these Japanese had the highest rate of diabetes of all.

In general, as people migrate to areas of the world consuming a Western diet, not only the number of calories they consume but also the composition of their diets changes. Before they migrate, they tend to consume a low-fat, high-fiber diet. After they reach their destination, they adopt the local diet, which tends to be higher in fat and lower in fiber. The carbohydrates in the new diet are from high-energy foods, which do not tend to be filling, which in turn promotes more caloric intake.

The next major leap in the effort to treat diabetes, occurring in 1955, was the discovery of the group of drugs called *sulfonylureas* (see Chapter 10), the first drugs that could be taken by mouth to lower blood glucose levels. But even while those drugs were improving patient care, the only way to know if someone's blood glucose level was high was to test the urine, which was entirely inadequate for good diabetic control (see Chapter 7).

Around 1980, the first portable meters for blood glucose testing became available. For the first time, doctors and patients could relate treatment to a measurable outcome. This development has led, in turn, to the discovery of other great drugs for diabetes, such as metformin, exenatide, and others yet to come.

If you are not using these wonderful tools for your diabetes, you are missing the boat. You can find out exactly how to use portable meters in Part III.

Explaining the Obesity (and Diabetes) Epidemic

Many changes explain the epidemic of obesity and diabetes that began to explode in the 1950s and '60s. Here are some of them:

✔ The availability of fast-food restaurants and vending machines

✔ The frequency of television commercials for foods filled with fats and sugar

✔ The large number of screens watched passively all day, from TVs to smartphones

✔ The larger, higher-calorie meals that tend to be eaten, both at home and at restaurants

✔ The dependence on vehicles for much movement

✔ The huge increase in mass-produced, high-calorie convenience foods

What steps can people take to reverse this trend? Some of the ideas developed to reverse the high rate of cigarette smoking can be recycled, but the process takes years for the whole population. What you can do immediately is contained in Part III. Some of the population-wide measures include the following strategies:

✔ A tax on low-nutrition foods like sweetened beverages

✔ Better labeling of foods; for example, a red label for low-nutrition, high-calorie foods; a yellow label for intermediate foods; and a green label for low-calorie, high-nutrition foods

✔ A ban on or reduction of advertising of junk foods

✔ School-based programs promoting healthier eating and elimination of soft drinks and sugared juices

✔ A low, fixed amount of screen time for children

Putting Faces to the Numbers: Sharing Some Real Patient Stories

The numbers that are used to diagnose diabetes don't begin to reflect the human dimensions of the disease. People end up with test results after days, months, or even years of minor discomforts that reach the point where they can no longer be tolerated. The next few stories of real (though renamed) patients can help you understand that diabetes is a disease that happens to real people — people who are working, relaxing, traveling, sleeping, and doing many other things that make life so complex.

Sal Renolo was a 46-year-old black-belt judo instructor. Despite his very active lifestyle, he was not careful about his diet and had gained 16 pounds in the last few years. He was more fatigued than he had been in the past but blamed this fatigue on his increasing age. His mother had diabetes, but he assumed that his physical fitness would protect him from this condition. However, he could barely get through a one-hour class without excusing himself for a bathroom break. One of his new students had diabetes, and he suggested to Sal that he ought to have the problem checked, but Sal insisted that he could not possibly have diabetes with all his activity. The symptoms of fatigue and frequent urination got worse, and Sal finally made an appointment with the doctor. Blood tests revealed a random blood glucose level of 264 mg/dl (14.7 mmol/L). The following week, another random blood glucose was 289 (16.0 mmol/L). The doctor told Sal he had diabetes, but Sal refused to believe it. He left the doctor's office angry but vowed to lose weight and did so successfully. On a repeat visit to the doctor, a random glucose was 167 mg/dl (9.3 mmol/L). Sal told the doctor that he knew he didn't have diabetes, but his resolve to eat carefully didn't last, and he was back six weeks later with a glucose of 302 mg/dl (16.8 mmol/L). Finally, Sal accepted the diagnosis and started treatment. He rapidly returned to his usual state of health, and the fatigue disappeared.

Debby O'Leary's active sex life with her husband was continually being interrupted by vaginal yeast infections, which resulted in an unpleasant odor, redness, itching. Over-the-counter preparations promptly cured the condition, but it always rapidly returned. Finally, after three of these infections in two months, she decided to see her gynecologist. The gynecologist told her she needed a prescription drug. The cure lasted a little longer this time, but the infection promptly returned. On a return visit, the gynecologist did a urinalysis and found glucose in her urine. A random blood test showed a glucose of 243 mg/dl (13.5 mmol/L). He sent her to an internist, who ordered a variety of tests including a fasting blood glucose, which was 149 mg/dl (8.3 mmol/L). The doctor told her she had diabetes and recommended exercise and diet change to start with. She followed his advice, and as a result she not only lowered her blood glucose to the point that she no longer developed yeast infections but also lost weight and increased her energy, making her sex life with her husband even more satisfying.

Chapter 3

Defining the Various Types of Diabetes

In This Chapter

▶ Paying attention to your pancreas

▶ Comparing type 1 and type 2 diabetes

▶ Being aware of other types of diabetes

Ladies and gentlemen, I'd like to introduce you to your pancreas. This shy little organ — to which you've probably never given any attention — can rear its lovely head at entirely unexpected moments. (You probably didn't even know that your pancreas has a head and a tail, but it does. Now you've broken the ice!) Most of the time, your pancreas hides behind your stomach, quietly doing its work by assisting with digestion first and then helping to make use of the digested food. The information in this chapter should put you on closer terms with your pancreas, which is good, because you need your pancreas as much as it needs you. In one way or another, the pancreas plays a role in all of the various types of diabetes.

Here's the good news: You can prevent diabetes. Here's the bad news: You can't do so quite as easily as you may like. Your best method for preventing diabetes is to pick your parents carefully, but that method is slightly impractical, even with modern technology.

In general, you can prevent a disease if it meets two requirements. First, you have to be able to identify if you are at high risk for getting the disease. Second, some treatments or actions must exist that can definitely reduce the occurrence of the disease. This chapter shows you how to identify whether you're at risk for type 1 or type 2 diabetes, and it covers definite actions that you can take to prevent both of these types of diabetes.

This chapter helps you get a clear understanding of your type of diabetes, how it relates to the other types of diabetes, and how the failure of your friendly pancreas to do its assigned job can lead to a host of unfortunate consequences. (I cover these consequences in detail in Part II.)

Getting to Know Your Pancreas and Its Role in Diabetes

You don't see your pancreas very often, but you hear from it all the time. It has two major functions. One is to produce *digestive enzymes,* which are the chemicals in your small intestine that help to break down food. The digestive enzymes don't have much relation to diabetes. Your pancreas's other function is to produce a hormone of major importance, *insulin,* and to secrete it directly into the blood. The following sections explore the ins and outs of your pancreas and insulin so that you're well acquainted with both.

Examining your pancreas

Figure 3-1 shows the microscopic appearance of the pancreas. The following list explains the different cells found in the pancreas as well as their functions:

- **B cells:** The insulin-producing pancreas cells (also called *beta* cells) are found in groups called *Islets of Langerhans.*

- **A cells:** These cells produce *glucagon,* a hormone that's very important to people with diabetes because it raises blood glucose when the glucose level gets too low. A cells are present in the Islets of Langerhans.

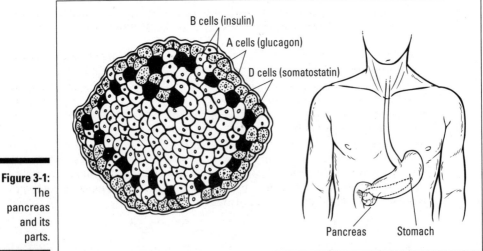

Figure 3-1: The pancreas and its parts.

Illustration by Kathryn Born

> ✔ **D cells:** These cells make *somatostatin* (a hormone that blocks the secretion
> of other hormones but doesn't have a use in diabetes because it causes
> high blood sugar and increased ketones by blocking insulin as well). Like
> the cells described above, D cells are also found in the Islets of Langerhans.

Understanding insulin

REMEMBER

If you understand only one hormone in your body, insulin should be that hormone (especially if you want to understand diabetes). Over the course of your
life, the insulin that your body produces or the insulin that you inject into
your body (as I describe in Chapter 10) affects whether or not you control the
glucose levels in your blood and avoid the complications of the disease.

Think of your insulin as an insurance agent who lives in San Francisco (which
is your pancreas) but travels from there to do business in Seattle (your
muscles), Denver (your fat tissue), Los Angeles (your liver), and other places.
This insulin insurance agent is insuring your good health.

Wherever insulin travels in your body, it opens up the cells so that glucose
can enter them. After glucose enters, the cells can immediately use it for
energy, store it in a storage form of glucose (called *glycogen*) for rapid use
later on, or convert it to fat for use even later as energy.

After glucose leaves your blood and enters your cells, your blood glucose
level falls. Your pancreas can tell when your glucose is falling, and it turns
off the release of insulin to prevent *hypoglycemia,* an unhealthy low level of
blood glucose (see Chapter 4). At the same time, your liver begins to release
glucose from storage and makes new glucose from amino acids in your blood.

If your insurance agent (insulin, remember? — stick with me here!) doesn't
show up when you need him (meaning that you have an absence of insulin,
as in type 1 diabetes) or he does a poor job when he shows up (such as when
you have a resistance to insulin, as in type 2 diabetes), your insurance coverage may be very poor (in which case your blood glucose starts to climb).
High blood glucose is the beginning of all your problems.

Doctors have proven that high blood glucose is bad for you and that keeping
the blood glucose as normal as possible prevents the complications of diabetes (which I explain in Part II). Most treatments for diabetes are directed at
restoring the blood glucose to normal.

Type 1 Diabetes and You

John Phillips, a 6-year-old boy, was always very active, and his parents became concerned when the counselors at summer camp told them that he seemed to not have much energy. When he got home from camp, John's parents noticed that he was thirsty all the time and running to the bathroom. He was very hungry but seemed to be losing weight, despite eating more than enough. John's parents took him to the pediatrician, who did several blood glucose tests and diagnosed their son with *type 1 diabetes mellitus* (T1DM), which used to be called *juvenile diabetes* or *insulin-dependent diabetes.*

This story has a happy ending because John's parents were willing to do the necessary things to bring John's glucose under control. John is just as energetic as ever, but he has had to get used to a few inconveniences in his daily routine. (I cover such daily lifestyle changes in Part III.) The following sections touch on the symptoms and causes of this type of diabetes.

Note: Type 1 diabetes is covered extensively in my book *Type 1 Diabetes For Dummies* (Wiley). Because this book is mainly about type 2 diabetes, I simply point out where the two types are the same and where they differ.

Identifying symptoms of type 1 diabetes

Following are some of the major signs and symptoms of type 1 diabetes. If you find you have any of these symptoms and haven't already been diagnosed with diabetes, call your doctor.

- Frequent urination
- Increase in thirst
- Weight loss
- Increase in hunger
- Weakness

Type 1 diabetes used to be called *juvenile diabetes* because it occurs most frequently in children. However, so many cases are found in adults that doctors don't use the term *juvenile* any more. Some children are diagnosed early in life, and other children have a more severe onset of the disease as they get a little older.

With children over age 10 and adults, the early signs and symptoms of diabetes may have been missed. These people have a great deal of fat breakdown in their bodies to provide energy, and this fat breakdown creates other problems. *Ketone bodies,* products of the breakdown of fats, begin to accumulate in the blood and spill into the urine. Ketone bodies are acidic and lead to nausea, abdominal pain, and sometimes vomiting.

At the same time as fat is breaking down, the child's blood glucose rises higher. From a normal level of 80 mg/dl (4.4 mmol/L), blood glucose can rise to the unhealthy level of 300 mg/dl (16 mmol/L) and even up to the dangerously high levels of 400 to 600 mg/dl (22.2 to 33.3 mmol/L). At high levels, the child's blood is like thick maple syrup and doesn't circulate as freely as normal. The large amount of water leaving the body with the glucose depletes important substances such as sodium and potassium. Vomiting causes the child to lose more fluids and body substances. All these abnormalities cause the child to become very drowsy and possibly lose consciousness. This situation is called *diabetic ketoacidosis,* and if it isn't identified and corrected quickly, the child can die. (See Chapter 4 for more details on the symptoms, causes, and treatments of ketoacidosis.)

A few special circumstances affect the symptoms that you may see in persons with type 1 diabetes. Remember the following factors:

- ✓ **The "honeymoon" period, a natural occurrence, is a time after the diagnosis of diabetes when the person's insulin needs decline for one to six months and the disease seems to get milder.** The honeymoon period is longer when a child is older at the time of diagnosis, but the apparent diminishing of the disease is always temporary.

- ✓ **Males and females get type 1 diabetes to an equal degree.**

- ✓ **Warm summer months are associated with a decrease in the occurrence of diabetes compared to the winter months, particularly in children over 10.** The probable reason for this occurrence is that a virus is involved in bringing on diabetes (which I discuss in "Getting type 1 diabetes"), and viruses spread much more when children are learning and playing together inside in the winter.

Investigating the causes of type 1 diabetes

When your doctor diagnoses you with type 1 diabetes, you almost certainly will wonder what could have caused you to acquire the disease. Did someone with diabetes sneeze on you? Did you eat so much sugary food that your body reacted by giving you diabetes? Rest assured that the causes of diabetes aren't so simple.

Type 1 diabetes is an *autoimmune disease,* meaning that your body is unkind enough to react against — and in this case, destroy — a vital part of itself, namely the insulin-producing *beta (B) cells* of the pancreas. One way that doctors discovered that type 1 diabetes is an autoimmune disease is by measuring proteins in the blood, called *antibodies,* which are literally substances directed against your body — in particular, against your islet cells. Another clue that type 1 diabetes is an autoimmune disease is that drugs that reduce autoimmunity also delay the onset of type 1 diabetes. Also, type 1 diabetes tends to occur in people who have other known autoimmune diseases.

You may wonder how doctors can know in advance that certain people will develop type 1 diabetes. The method of prediction isn't 100 percent accurate, but people who get type 1 diabetes more often have certain abnormal characteristics on their genetic material, their *chromosomes,* that are not present in people who don't get type 1 diabetes. Doctors can look for these abnormal characteristics on your DNA. But having these abnormal characteristics doesn't guarantee that you'll get diabetes.

Another essential factor in predicting whether you will develop type 1 diabetes is your exposure to something in the environment, most likely a virus. I discuss this factor in detail in the next section.

Getting type 1 diabetes

To develop diabetes, most people also have to come in contact with something in the environment that triggers the destruction of their beta cells, the cells that make insulin. Doctors think that this environmental trigger is probably a virus. This type of virus can cause diabetes by attacking your pancreas directly and diminishing your ability to produce insulin, which quickly creates the diabetic condition in your body. The virus can also cause diabetes if it is made up of a substance that is also naturally present in your pancreas. If the virus and your pancreas possess the same substance, the antibodies that your body produces to fight off the virus will also attack the shared substance in your pancreas, leaving you in the same condition as if the virus itself attacked your pancreas.

A small number (about 10 percent) of patients who develop type 1 diabetes don't seem to need an environmental factor to trigger the diabetes. In them, the disease is entirely an autoimmune destruction of the beta cells. If you fall into this category of people with diabetes, you may have other autoimmune diseases, such as autoimmune thyroid disease.

Although genetics plays a role in developing type 1 diabetes, the connection is relatively minor. An identical twin has only a 20 percent chance of developing type 1 diabetes if his identical twin (who has the exact same genetic material) has it.

Preventing type 1 diabetes

The most important study of prevention of diabetes complications ever done for type 1 diabetes is called the Diabetes Control and Complications Trial (DCCT), published in 1993. The DCCT showed that keeping very tight control over your blood glucose is possible but difficult. The difficult part of keeping your blood glucose close to normal is that you increase your risk of having low blood glucose, or hypoglycemia (see Chapter 4). The DCCT study showed that you can prevent the complications of diabetes — including eye, kidney, and nerve disease — by keeping your blood glucose as close to normal as possible. If you already suffer from such complications, improving your blood glucose control very significantly slows the progression of the complications. Since the DCCT, doctors generally treat type 1 diabetes by keeping the patient's blood glucose as close to normal as is possible and practical.

If you would like to read much more on the subject of type 1 diabetes, please see my book *Type 1 Diabetes For Dummies* (Wiley).

Having Type 2 Diabetes

Edythe Fokel, a 46-year-old woman, has gained about 10 pounds in the last year, so that her 5-foot 5-inch body now weighs about 155 pounds. Edythe doesn't do much exercise. She has felt somewhat fatigued recently, but she blames her age and approaching menopause. She also blames the fact that she now gets up several times a night to urinate, which she didn't used to do. She is disturbed because her vision is blurry and her job requires working on a computer. Finally, Edythe goes to her gynecologist after developing a rash and discharge in her vagina. When Edythe describes her symptoms, her gynecologist decides to do a blood glucose test. He refers her back to her primary physician when Edythe's blood glucose level registers at 220 mg/dl (12.2 mmol/L).

Edythe's primary doctor asks her whether other members of her family have had diabetes, and she replies that her mother and a sister are both being treated for it. The doctor also asks Edythe about any tingling in her feet, and she admits that she has noticed some tingling for the past few months but didn't think it was important. The primary doctor repeats the random blood glucose test, which comes back at 260 mg/dl (14.4 mmol/L). He informs Edythe that she has type 2 diabetes (T2DM).

The signs and symptoms that Edythe manifests in this scenario, along with the results of the two blood glucose tests, provide a textbook picture of type 2 diabetes. (Type 2 diabetes used to be known as *adult-onset diabetes* or *non-insulin-dependent diabetes*.) But be aware that people with type 2 diabetes may have few or none of these symptoms. Because of the varying symptoms, your doctor needs to check your blood glucose level on a regular basis. (I discuss how often you should do this test in Chapter 7.)

Most people with type 2 diabetes are over the age of 40, but I am seeing more and more cases in children and young adults. Your chances of getting type 2 diabetes increase as you get older. Type 2 diabetes is a disease of gradual onset rather than the severe emergency that can herald type 1 diabetes. Because the symptoms are so mild at first, you may not notice them.

You may ignore these symptoms for years before they become bothersome enough to consult your doctor. No autoimmunity is involved in type 2 diabetes, so no antibodies are found. Doctors believe that no virus is involved in the onset of type 2 diabetes.

Recent statistics show that ten times more people worldwide have type 2 diabetes than type 1 diabetes. Although type 2 is much more prevalent, those with type 2 diabetes seem to have milder severity of complications (such as eye disease and kidney disease) from diabetes. (See Part II for details about the possible complications of diabetes. See Part III for treatments that can help you prevent these complications.)

Identifying symptoms of type 2 diabetes

A fairly large percentage of the U.S. population (approximately 26 million people) has type 2 diabetes. The numbers are on the rise, and one reason is an increase in the incidence of obesity, a major risk factor for T2DM. If you're obese, you are considerably more likely to acquire T2DM than you would be if you maintained your ideal weight. (See Chapter 8 for the details on how to figure out your weight classification.)

The following signs and symptoms are good indicators that you have type 2 diabetes. If you experience two or more of these symptoms and haven't already been diagnosed with diabetes, call your doctor:

- **Fatigue:** Type 2 diabetes makes you tired because your body's cells aren't getting the glucose fuel that they need. Even though your blood has plenty of insulin, your body is resistant to its actions. (See the "Getting to Know Your Pancreas and Its Role in Diabetes" section for more explanation.)

- **Frequent urination and thirst:** As with type 1 diabetes, you find yourself urinating more frequently than usual, which dehydrates your body and leaves you thirsty.

- **Blurred vision:** The lenses of your eyes swell and shrink as your blood glucose levels rise and fall. Your vision blurs because your eyes can't adjust quickly enough to these lens changes.

- **Slow healing of skin, gum, and urinary infections:** Your white blood cells, which help with healing and defend your body against infections, don't function correctly in the high-glucose environment present in your body when it has diabetes. Unfortunately, the bugs that cause infections thrive in the same high-glucose environment. So diabetes leaves your body especially susceptible to infections.

- **Genital itching:** Yeast infections also love a high-glucose environment, so diabetes is often accompanied by the itching and discomfort of yeast infections.

✔ **Numbness in the feet or legs:** You experience numbness because of a common long-term complication of diabetes called *neuropathy.* (I explain the details of neuropathy in Chapter 5.) If you notice numbness and neuropathy along with the other symptoms of diabetes, you probably have had the disease for quite a while, because neuropathy takes more than five years to develop in a diabetic environment. Occasionally numbness occurs earlier when extreme elevations of the glucose happen.

✔ **Heart disease, stroke, and peripheral vascular disease:** Heart disease, stroke, and peripheral vascular disease (blockage of arteries in the legs) occur much more often in type 2s than in the nondiabetic population. But these complications may appear when you are merely glucose-intolerant (which I explain in the next section), before you actually have diagnosable diabetes.

The signs and symptoms of type 2 diabetes are similar in some cases to the symptoms of type 1 diabetes (which I cover in the "Identifying symptoms of type 1 diabetes" section, earlier in this chapter), but in many ways they are different. The following list shows some of the differences between symptoms in type 1 and type 2 diabetes:

✔ **Age of onset:** People with type 1 diabetes are usually younger than those with type 2 diabetes. However, the increasing incidence of type 2 diabetes in overweight children is making this difference less useful for separating type 1 and type 2 diabetes.

✔ **Body weight:** Those with type 1 diabetes are usually thin or normal in weight, but obesity is a common characteristic of people with type 2 diabetes.

✔ **Level of glucose:** People with type 1 diabetes have higher glucose levels at the onset of the disease. Type 1 diabetics usually have blood glucose levels of 300 to 400 mg/dl (16.6 to 22.2 mmol/L), and people with type 2 diabetes usually have blood glucose levels of 200 to 250 mg/dl (11.1 to 13.9 mmol/L).

✔ **Severity of onset:** Type 1 diabetes usually has a much more severe onset, but type 2 diabetes gradually shows its symptoms.

Investigating what causes (and what doesn't cause) type 2 diabetes

If you've been diagnosed with type 2 diabetes, you're probably shocked and curious about why you developed the disease. Doctors have learned quite a bit about the causes of type 2 diabetes. For example, they know that T2DM runs in families.

Usually, people with type 2 diabetes can find a relative who has had the disease. Therefore, doctors consider T2DM to be much more of a genetic disease than T1DM. In studies of identical twins, when one twin has type 2 diabetes, the likelihood that it will develop in the other twin is nearly 100 percent.

Insulin resistance

People with type 2 diabetes have plenty of insulin in their bodies (unlike people with type 1 diabetes), but their bodies respond to the insulin in abnormal ways. Type 2 diabetics are *insulin-resistant,* meaning that their bodies resist the normal, healthy functioning of insulin. This resistance, combined with not having enough insulin to overcome the insulin resistance, causes the disease.

Most people who develop type 2 diabetes are born with the genes for insulin resistance. Before diabetes is present, future T2DM patients already show signs of insulin resistance. First, the amount of insulin in their blood is elevated compared to normal people. Second, a shot of insulin doesn't reduce the blood glucose in these insulin-resistant people nearly as much as it does in people without insulin resistance. (See Chapter 10 to find out more about insulin shots in diabetes.)

When your body needs to make extra insulin just to keep your blood glucose normal, your insulin is, obviously, less effective than it should be — which means that you have insulin resistance. If your insulin resistance worsens to the point that your body can't produce enough insulin to keep your blood glucose normal, or if your pancreas starts to get "tired" of making so much extra insulin, your blood sugars become abnormal. This condition is prediabetes, because your blood glucose is still lower than the levels needed for a diagnosis of diabetes (see Chapter 2). When you add other factors such as weight gain, a sedentary lifestyle, certain medications, and aging, your pancreas can't keep up with your insulin demands, and you develop prediabetes, followed by diabetes.

Another factor that comes into play when doctors make a diagnosis of type 2 diabetes is the release of sugar from the glycogen stored in your liver, known as your *hepatic glucose output.* People with T2DM have high glucose levels in the morning after having fasted all night. You would think that your glucose would be low in the morning if you haven't eaten any sugar. But your liver is a storage bank for a lot of glucose, and it can make even more from other substances in the body. As your insulin resistance increases, your liver begins to release glucose inappropriately, and your fasting blood glucose level rises.

Mistaken beliefs about type 2

People often think that the following factors cause type 2 diabetes, but they actually have nothing to do with the onset of the disease:

✔ **Sugar:** Eating excessive amounts of sugar does not cause diabetes, but it may bring out the disease to the extent that it makes you fat. Eating too much protein or fat will do the same thing.

✔ **Emotions:** Changes in your emotions do not play a large role in the development of type 2 diabetes, but they may be very important in dealing with diabetes mellitus and subsequent control.

✔ **Stress:** Too much stress isn't a major factor that causes diabetes.

✔ **Antibodies:** Antibodies against islet cells are not a major factor in type 2 diabetes (see the section "Investigating the causes of type 1 diabetes," earlier in this chapter). Type 2 diabetes isn't an autoimmune disease like type 1.

✔ **Gender:** Males and females are equally as likely to develop type 2 diabetes. Gender doesn't play a role in the onset of this disease.

✔ **Diabetic ketoacidosis:** Type 2 diabetes isn't generally associated with diabetic ketoacidosis (see Chapter 4). People with type 2 diabetes are ketosis resistant, except under extremely severe stress caused by infections or trauma. (See Chapter 4 for a discussion of *hyperosmolar syndrome,* a related condition in which people with type 2 diabetes have extremely high glucose but don't have the fat breakdown that leads to ketoacidosis.)

Getting type 2 diabetes

Genetic inheritance is necessary in type 2 diabetes, but environmental factors such as obesity and lack of exercise trigger the disease. People with type 2 diabetes are insulin-resistant before they become obese or sedentary. Aging, poor eating habits, obesity, and failure to exercise combine to worsen insulin resistance and bring out the disease.

Inheritance seems to be a much stronger factor in type 2 diabetes than in type 1 diabetes. Consider the following facts:

✔ If your father has type 2 diabetes but your mother doesn't, you have about a 4 percent chance of getting the disease.

✔ If your mother has type 2 diabetes but your father doesn't, your chances of getting it leap to about 10 percent.

✔ If your identical twin has type 2 diabetes, you have a nearly 100 percent chance of eventually getting the disease.

✔ If your brother or sister (*not* an identical twin) gets type 2, you have about a 40 percent chance of doing the same.

Here's an interesting fact: Spouses of people with type 2 diabetes are at higher risk of developing diabetes and should be screened just like relatives of people with diabetes. Why? Because they share the environmental risk factors for diabetes, such as poor diet and a sedentary lifestyle. If your wife is a good cook and you have a big-screen TV, watch out!

Preventing the causes of type 2 diabetes

Doctors can predict type 2 diabetes years in advance of its actual diagnosis by studying the close relatives of people who have the condition. This early-warning period offers plenty of time to try techniques of primary prevention. After a doctor discovers that someone's blood glucose levels are high and diagnoses type 2 diabetes, complications such as eye disease and kidney disease (see Chapter 5) usually take ten or more years to develop in that person. During this time, doctors can apply secondary prevention techniques (the various treatments I discuss in Part III).

Because so many people suffer from type 2 diabetes, doctors have had a wealth of people to study in order to determine the most important environmental factors that turn a genetic predisposition to type 2 diabetes into a clinical disease. Following are the major environmental factors:

✔ **High body-mass index:** The *body-mass index (BMI)* is the way that doctors look at weight in relation to height. BMI is a better indicator of a healthy weight than just weight alone, because taller people tend to weigh more. For instance, a person who weighs 150 pounds and is 62 inches tall is overweight, but a person who weighs 150 pounds and is 70 inches tall is thin.

You can easily determine your BMI by using the following formula: Multiply your weight (in pounds) by 703, and then divide that number by your height (in inches). Divide that result by your height (in inches) again. If you use the metric system, divide your weight in kilograms by your height in meters and divide that result by your height in meters again. Using this formula, the 150-pound person with a height of 62 inches has a BMI of 27.5, whereas the person with the height of 70 inches has a BMI of 21.6.

Current guidelines state that a person with a BMI from 25 to 29.9 is overweight, and a person with a BMI of 30 or greater is obese. A BMI between 18.5 and 25 is considered normal. A person with a BMI of 40 or higher has morbid obesity.

Many studies have verified the great importance of the BMI level in determining who gets diabetes. For example, a large study of thousands of nurses in the United States showed that nurses with a BMI greater than 35 had diabetes almost 100 times more often than nurses with a BMI less than 22. Even among the women in this study considered to be lean, those with the higher BMI, though still in the category of normal, had three times the prevalence of diabetes compared to those with lower BMI. Another large study of U.S. physicians found the same relationship of high BMI to high levels of type 2 diabetes. The same study showed that the length of time that you're obese is important; participants who were obese for ten years were more likely to have diabetes than those who had become obese more recently.

✔ **Physical inactivity:** Physical inactivity has a high association with diabetes, as evidenced in many studies. Former athletes have diabetes less often than nonathletes. The same study of nurses' health that I cite in the preceding bullet showed that women who were physically active on a regular basis had diabetes only two-thirds as often as the couch potatoes. A study conducted in Hawaii, which did not include any obese people, showed that the occurrence of diabetes was greatest for people who don't exercise.

✔ **Central distribution of fat:** When people with diabetes become fat, they tend to carry the extra weight as centrally distributed fat, also known as *visceral fat.* You check your visceral fat when you measure your waistline, because this type of fat stays around your midsection. So a person with visceral fat is more apple-shaped than pear-shaped. Visceral fat also happens to be the type of fat that probably comes and goes most easily on your body, and it is relatively easy to lose when you diet. Visceral fat seems to cause more insulin resistance than fat in other areas, and it is also correlated with the occurrence of coronary artery disease. If you have a lot of visceral fat, losing just 5 to 10 percent of your weight may very dramatically reduce your chance of diabetes or a heart attack.

Even when the BMI is within the normal range (less than 25), people with a greater waist circumference have an increased mortality. If you are 40 or younger and your waistline measures 39.5 inches (100 centimeters) or greater, or you are between the ages of 40 and 60 and your waistline measures 35.5 inches (90 centimeters) or more, you have a significantly increased risk of a heart attack. Try to shrink your waistline as well as your weight.

Asians tend to develop visceral fat at a lower weight than non-Asians and are therefore more prone to type 2 diabetes at a lower weight. Asian Indians are particularly susceptible, developing diabetes up to ten years earlier than Chinese and Japanese.

✔ **Low intake of dietary fiber:** Populations with a high prevalence of diabetes tend to eat a diet that is low in fiber. Dietary fiber seems to be protective against diabetes because it slows down the rate at which glucose enters the bloodstream.

If you recognize any of the preceding factors in your body or lifestyle, you can correct them in time to prevent diabetes. Type 2 diabetes allows the high-risk individual or the diagnosed person the time to work toward prevention or control of the disease. In Part III, I show you specific ways to reduce your weight, increase your exercise, improve your diet, and prevent or reverse diabetes and diabetic complications.

Type 2 diabetes begins with insulin resistance and worsens with reduced beta-cell function. An ideal agent that prevents type 2 diabetes would have to

✔ Be effective in treating type 2 diabetes

✔ Improve sensitivity to glucose or beta-cell function

✔ Promote weight loss

✔ Improve risk factors for heart disease

✔ Not cause low blood glucose

✔ Be required only once a day or even once a week

✔ Not cause unacceptable side effects

A drug that fulfills all of these requirements has been available for some time. It's called a glucagon-like peptide-1 agonist, and I discuss it extensively in Chapter 10.

Recognizing variants of type 1 and 2 diabetes

Certain groups of patients with diabetes do not follow the classic description of type 1 or 2. They make up a sizable portion of type 2 patients and require individualized treatment (and you could be among them), so I briefly explain their characteristics in this section.

LADA

As many as 10 percent of people diagnosed with type 2 diabetes do not respond well to medications that stimulate the pancreas to release more insulin like the sulfonylurea class of drugs (see Chapter 10). When they are tested, they are found to have GAD antibodies similar to those found in

T1DM. This condition, called *latent autoimmune diabetes in adults* (LADA), is really adult-onset T1DM rather than T2DM. It is generally more mild than type 1 diabetes, with lower blood glucose levels, and presents without ketosis or weight loss. The treatment is similar to that for T1DM.

If you are having trouble controlling your diabetes with oral drugs that work by causing more insulin release, ask your doctor to test you for GAD antibodies.

Possibilities for future prevention of diabetes

Researchers have performed many valuable studies on the prevention of type 2 diabetes. The results of these studies suggest that you can prevent diabetes, but probably only by making major lifestyle changes and sticking to them over a long period of time. Here are some important conclusions based on prevention research:

✔ Taking drugs that don't treat your insulin resistance doesn't help to prevent your diabetes or its complications.

✔ Exercising regularly may delay the onset of diabetes.

✔ Maintaining a proper diet can delay the onset of diabetes and slow the complications that may occur.

✔ Controlling both your blood pressure and your blood glucose has substantial benefits for preventing the complications of diabetes.

The results of the Diabetes Prevention Program, a study of more than 3,000 people, were published in the *New England Journal of Medicine* in February 2002. They clearly showed that diet and exercise are effective in preventing type 2 diabetes. Participants who successfully modified their diet and exercise routines reduced their chances of developing type 2 diabetes by 58 percent. They generally did 30 minutes of moderate exercise (like walking) every day and lost between 5 and 7 percent of their body weight during the three-year study period. In contrast, patients who used a drug called *metformin* (see Chapter 10) without modifying their diet and exercise reduced their risk of developing type 2 diabetes by only 31 percent.

Another study, the Finnish Diabetes Prevention Study (reported in *Diabetes Care* in December 2003), shows that lifestyle changes can be accomplished and sustained not only in a research setting (like that of the Diabetes Prevention Program) but in a community setting as well, where patients are taken care of by their own doctors. Study participants worked with a nutritionist to improve their diets and received some advice on exercise. They continue to be successful after three years, with the same 58 percent reduction in the onset of diabetes.

Restoring insulin sensitivity in people at risk for prediabetes (see Chapter 2) was the focus of another study, published in *Diabetes Care* in March 2002. This study compared intensive lifestyle change, both diet and exercise, with moderate lifestyle change. The intensive group ate less fat and did more vigorous exercise than the moderate group, and every member of the intensive group increased his or her insulin sensitivity, which resulted in holding off the development of diabetes.

MODY

One to five percent of all patients with type 2 diabetes have a condition called *maturity onset of diabetes of the young* (MODY). Although most cases of type 2 diabetes result from abnormalities in multiple genes, MODY results from an abnormality in a single gene of that patient. If one parent has MODY, his or her children have a 50 percent chance of inheriting the disease.

MODY can be diagnosed in any family with a high degree of inheritance of diabetes by doing genetic studies. Clinically, the disease looks like a mild form of type 2 diabetes that begins in early adolescence or early adulthood but is not diagnosed until later in life (unless it is suspected in the family and a glucose tolerance test and genetic testing are done). It generally does not require insulin, and it responds to oral agents (see Chapter 10).

Having Gestational Diabetes

If you're pregnant (yes, that excludes you men) and you've never had diabetes before, during your pregnancy you could acquire a form of diabetes called *gestational diabetes*. If you already have diabetes when you become pregnant, it's called *pregestational diabetes*. As I discuss in Chapter 6, the difference between pregestational diabetes and gestational diabetes is very important in terms of the consequences for both mother and baby. Gestational diabetes occurs in about 2 percent of all pregnancies. (I discuss diabetes in pregnancy extensively in Chapter 6.)

During your pregnancy, you can acquire gestational diabetes because the growing fetus and the placenta create various hormones to help the fetus grow and develop properly. Some of these hormones have other characteristics, such as anti-insulin properties, that decrease your body's sensitivity to insulin, increase glucose production, and can cause diabetes.

Recognizing Other Types of Diabetes

Cases of diabetes other than type 1 and type 2 are rare and usually don't cause severe diabetes in the people who have them. But occasionally one of these other types is responsible for a more severe case of diabetes, so you should know that they exist. The following list gives you a brief rundown of the symptoms and causes of other types of diabetes:

✔ **Diabetes due to loss or disease of pancreatic tissue:** If you have a disease, such as cancer, that necessitates the removal of some of your pancreas, you lose your pancreas's valuable insulin-producing beta cells and your body becomes diabetic. This form of diabetes isn't always severe, because you lose glucagon, another hormone found in your pancreas, after your pancreatic surgery. Glucagon blocks insulin action in your body, so when your body has less glucagon, it can function with less insulin, leaving you with a milder case of diabetes.

✔ **Diabetes due to iron overload:** Another disease that damages the pancreas, as well as the liver, the heart, the joints, and the nervous system, is *hemochromatosis.* This condition results from excessive absorption of iron into the blood. When the blood deposits too much iron into these organs, damage can occur. This hereditary condition is present in 1 of every 200 people in the United States; half of those who have it develop a clinical disease, sometimes diabetes.

Hemochromatosis is less common in younger women, who are protected by the monthly loss of iron that occurs with menstrual bleeding. This finding has led to the current treatment for hemochromatosis, which is removing blood from the patient regularly until the blood iron returns to normal; then repeating the procedure occasionally to keep iron levels normal. If treatment is done early enough (before organs are damaged), complications such as diabetes are avoidable.

✔ **Diabetes due to other diseases:** Your body contains a number of hormones that block insulin action or have actions that are opposed to insulin's actions. You produce these hormones in glands other than your pancreas. If you get a tumor on one of these hormone-producing glands, the gland sometimes produces excessive levels of the hormones that act in opposition to insulin. Usually, this condition gives you simple glucose intolerance rather than diabetes, because your pancreas makes extra insulin to combat the hormones. But if you have a genetic tendency to develop diabetes, you may develop diabetes in this case.

✔ **Diabetes due to hormone treatments for other diseases:** If you take hormones to treat a disease other than diabetes, those hormones could cause diabetes in your body. The hormone that is most likely to cause diabetes in this situation is *hydrocortisone,* an anti-inflammatory agent used in diseases of inflammation, such as arthritis. (Similar drugs are prednisone and dexamethasone.) If you take hydrocortisone and you have the symptoms of diabetes listed in earlier sections of this chapter, talk to your doctor.

✔ **Diabetes due to other drugs**: If you're taking other commonly used drugs, be aware that some of them raise your blood glucose as a side effect. Some antihypertensive drugs, especially hydrochlorothiazide, raise your blood glucose level. Niacin, a drug commonly used for lowering cholesterol, also raises your blood glucose. Even the wonder drugs for lowering cholesterol, the statins, have been implicated. If you have a genetic tendency toward diabetes, taking these drugs may be enough to give you the disease.

Conditions and hormones that can lead to diabetes

Excess hormones can be caused by tumors and their associated conditions. Following is a partial list of the common culprits:

✔ Excessive adrenal gland hormone (hydrocortisone) is present in Cushing's syndrome. Hydrocortisone stimulates the liver to put out more glucose while it blocks the uptake of glucose by muscle tissue.

✔ Excessive prolactin is present in a prolactin-secreting tumor of the pituitary gland. It blocks insulin action, and glucose intolerance results.

✔ Excessive growth hormone is made by a tumor of the pituitary gland resulting in acromegaly. Growth hormone reduces insulin sensitivity and forces the pancreas to make much more insulin.

✔ Excessive epinephrine is made by a pheochromocytoma (a tumor of another part of the adrenal gland). It causes increased liver production of glucose and blocks insulin secretion.

✔ Excessive aldosterone is made by still another part of the adrenal gland in a condition called *primary hyperaldosteronism*. This condition causes glucose intolerance in a different way — by facilitating the loss of body potassium, which has a negative effect on insulin production.

✔ Excessive thyroid hormone found in hyperthyroidism causes the liver and other organs to produce excessive quantities of glucose and destroy insulin more rapidly. Hyperthyroidism is also a disease of autoimmunity, which may play a role in the loss of glucose tolerance.

✔ A glucagon-secreting tumor of the pancreas can create excessive glucagon. Glucagon has many properties that are opposite to insulin. This condition is rare; only around 100 cases of it have been described in medical literature, so don't lose sleep over this one.

✔ A somatostatin-secreting tumor of the pancreas can create excessive somatostatin. Somatostatin is another hormone made in a cell present in the Islets of Langerhans. Somatostatin actually blocks insulin from leaving the beta cell, but it also blocks glucagon and other hormones, so the diabetes is very mild. This condition occurs even less often than the glucagon-secreting tumor.

✔ Cystic fibrosis, a genetic disease diagnosed in children that causes the body to produce thick mucus that clogs the lungs and obstructs the pancreas, may lead to diabetes.

Part II
How Diabetes Affects Your Body

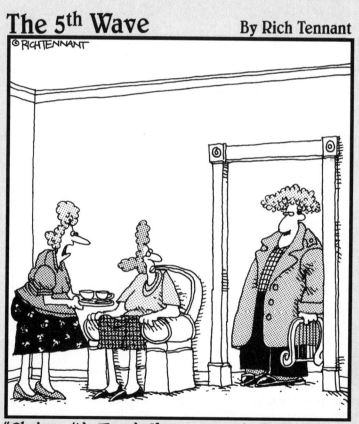

The 5th Wave   By Rich Tennant

"Oh dear, it's Troy's Harpo-glycemia. I can always tell — fatigue, confusion, the compulsion to play the harp in a trench coat and fright-wig...."

In this part . . .

Diabetes can affect every part of your body but especially the eyes, the kidneys, the nervous system, and the heart. However, none of these potential problems need ever happen. This part explains these effects, how they occur, the kinds of symptoms they produce, and what you and your doctor need to do to treat them. Remember that everything I describe in this part is preventable, and even if you have not been able to prevent them, they're very treatable.

The effects mentioned above are due to hyperglycemia, or high blood glucose, and occur only after years. This part has lots of information about hypoglycemia, or low blood glucose, that often occurs at the beginning of treatment and is usually due to overtreatment. I discuss at length a condition called the *metabolic syndrome* that predates diabetes but can cause heart disease. And speaking of length, I also describe in detail the new drugs available to treat erection problems resulting from diabetes. It is important that you know about the effects and respond to them appropriately.

Chapter 4

Battling Short-Term Complications

. . . .

In This Chapter

▶ Defining short-term complications

▶ Dealing with low blood glucose

▶ Handling very high blood glucose

. . . .

After receiving a diagnosis of type 2 diabetes, you need to understand how the disease can affect you. The previous chapters cover some of the signs and symptoms of diabetes, which you could consider to be the shortest of the short-term complications of the disease because they're generally mild and begin to subside when you start treatment. This chapter covers the more serious forms of short-term complications, which occur when your blood glucose is out of control, reaching dangerously high or low levels.

With the exception of mild *hypoglycemia* (low blood glucose that you can manage it yourself), you should treat all the complications in this chapter as medical emergencies. Keep in touch with your doctor and go to the hospital promptly if your blood glucose is uncontrollably high or you're unable to hold down food. You may need a few hours in the emergency room or a day or two in the hospital to reverse your problems.

Solving (and Avoiding) Short-Term Complications

Although the complications that I cover in this chapter are called *short-term*, you may experience them at any time during the course of your diabetes. *Short-term* simply means that these complications arise rapidly in your body, as opposed to the long-term complications (discussed in Chapter 5) that take ten or more years to develop. Short-term complications develop in days or even hours, and fortunately they respond to treatment just as rapidly.

Generally, you experience the severe short-term complications associated with high blood glucose when you aren't monitoring your blood glucose levels. Small children and older folks who live alone or have illnesses are most susceptible to lapses in glucose monitoring and, therefore, to short-term complications. If you suffer an acute illness or trauma, you should monitor your glucose even more frequently than usual because you're more vulnerable to short-term complications.

The short-term complications of diabetes affect your ability to function normally. For example, if you're a student, you may have difficulty studying or taking tests. Or you may have trouble driving your car properly. For this reason, you may find that the Bureau of Motor Vehicles and the Federal Aviation Association are extra careful about giving people with diabetes a driver's license or pilot's license. Potential employers may question your ability to perform certain jobs. But most companies and government agencies are very enlightened about diabetes and do everything possible to accommodate you in these situations.

You can control your diabetes, and all the short-term complications are avoidable. If you take your medication at the appropriate time, eat the proper foods at the proper times, and monitor your blood glucose regularly, you're unlikely to suffer from any severe short-term complications. Your blood glucose may drop to lower than normal levels, but closely monitoring it quickly alerts you to the drop so you can treat it before it affects your mental and physical functioning. (See Chapter 7 for all the details on glucose monitoring and other testing.)

Dropping Too Low: Hypoglycemia

The condition of having low blood glucose is known as *hypoglycemia*. If you have diabetes, you can get hypoglycemia only as a consequence of your diabetes treatment.

One of the readers who wrote to thank me for the first edition of this book told me how her son had once gone on a blind date. He and his date went to a bar where they had a drink before dinner. As he sat there, he began to say, "Sugar, baby, sugar, baby, sugar, baby." At first his date was offended until she realized that he had a glazed look in his eyes and found that he was wearing a bracelet identifying him as a person with diabetes. He was suffering from hypoglycemia and needed glucose.

This story is amusing, but the subject is very serious. Hypoglycemia can ruin your day and leave you feeling dazed and exhausted afterwards. You also run the risk of overtreating it, leaving yourself with very high blood glucose.

Hypoglycemia is a barrier that prevents most patients with diabetes from achieving normal blood glucose levels. They can lower their blood glucose enough to prevent long-term complications such as eye disease, kidney disease, and nerve disease, but preventing heart disease requires a lower glucose level that is difficult to sustain because of the threat of hypoglycemia, particularly for people with type 1 diabetes. A normal blood glucose is between 80 and 140 mg/dl. Hypoglycemia begins below 80 mg/dl, but you may not feel symptoms until it goes below 60 mg/dl.

The positive news is that most patients experience complete recovery from the effects of hypoglycemia.

Identifying the signs of hypoglycemia

Your body doesn't function well when you have too little glucose in your blood. Your brain needs glucose to run the rest of your body, as well as to function intellectually. Your muscles need the energy that glucose provides in much the same way that your car needs gasoline. So when your body detects that it has low blood glucose, it sends out a group of hormones that rapidly raise your glucose. But those hormones have to fight the strength of the diabetes medication that has been pushing down your glucose levels.

At what level of blood glucose do you develop hypoglycemia? Unfortunately, the level varies for different individuals, particularly depending on the length of time that the person has had diabetes. But most experts agree that a blood glucose of 60 mg/dl (3.3 mmol/L) or less is associated with signs and symptoms of hypoglycemia in most people.

Doctors usually put the symptoms of hypoglycemia into two categories:

✔ **Symptoms due to the side effects of the hormones (especially epinephrine) that your body sends out to counter the glucose-lowering effect of insulin:** This category of symptoms is called *adrenergic* symptoms, because epinephrine comes from your adrenal gland. They occur most often when your blood glucose falls rapidly.

   • Whiteness, or pallor, of your skin

   • Sweating

   • Rapid heartbeat

   • Palpitations, or the feeling that your heart is beating too fast

   • Anxiety

   • Numbness in the lips, fingers, or toes

   • Irritability

   • Sensation of hunger

✔ **Symptoms due to your brain not receiving enough fuel, causing your intellectual function to suffer:** This category of symptoms is called *neuroglycopenic* symptoms, which is medicalese for "not enough *(penic)* glucose *(glyco)* in the brain *(neuro)*." (If your brain could speak, it would just say, "Whew, I'm ready for a meal!") These symptoms occur most often when your hypoglycemia takes longer to develop, and they become more severe as your blood glucose drops lower.

- Headache
- Loss of concentration
- Visual disorders, such as double vision or blurred vision
- Fatigue
- Confusion and trouble concentrating
- Trouble hearing
- Poor color vision
- Feeling of warmth
- Slurred speech
- Convulsions
- Coma, or an inability to be awakened

People lose their ability to think clearly when they become hypoglycemic. They make simple mistakes, and other people often assume that they are drunk.

 If you take insulin or a *sulfonylurea drug,* which squeezes more insulin out of your reluctant pancreas, you should wear or carry with you some form of identification, in case you unexpectedly develop hypoglycemia. (See Chapter 10 for a full explanation of insulin and the sulfonylurea medications.) You can find a simple bracelet at the Medicalert Foundation at www.medicalert.org. If you prefer something a little sexier that you will be proud to wear as jewelry, try www.mylifewear.com.

Categorizing levels of hypoglycemia

The severity of hypoglycemia falls into three categories, defined by the level of the blood glucose:

- **Mild hypoglycemia:** This level, corresponding to blood glucose of around 75 mg/dl, is easily treated by the patients themselves. It doesn't cause the patients to change their routine, other than taking a little glucose, and in fact is discovered not so much by symptoms as by routine testing of the blood.

- **Moderate hypoglycemia:** This level is achieved when the blood glucose is around 65 mg/dl. Patients begin to feel the adrenergic symptoms described earlier, especially anxiety and a rapid heartbeat. Patients who have moderate hypoglycemia may not recognize that they need glucose and may have to be helped by someone else.

✔ **Severe hypoglycemia:** This level, at which blood glucose is less than 55 mg/dl, leaves patients severely impaired and thus requiring outside assistance to restore their glucose. An emergency injection of glucagon or intravenous glucose solution is necessary.

The level of glucose that causes you to have mild, moderate, or severe hypoglycemia may differ from these numbers. They are only approximate. If you are alert with a blood glucose level of 55 mg/dl, taking glucose by mouth will reverse the hypoglycemia.

Managing the causes of hypoglycemia

Hypoglycemia results from elevated amounts of insulin driving down your blood glucose to low levels, but an extra high dose of insulin or sulfonylurea medication isn't always the culprit. Your blood glucose level is also affected by the amount of food you take in, the amount of fuel (glucose) that you burn for energy, the amount of insulin circulating in your body, and your body's ability to raise glucose by releasing it from the liver or making it from other bodily substances.

On average, hypoglycemia occurs about 10 percent of the time in people with type 1 diabetes, but it causes noticeable symptoms only about twice a week and is severe perhaps once a year. In people with type 2 diabetes, severe hypoglycemia occurs only one-tenth as often. (The medications described in the next section are part of the reason that people with type 1 diabetes have to deal with hypoglycemia more often.) The following sections cover the causes of hypoglycemia and the ways you can manage those factors to keep your blood glucose level in check.

Insulin and sulfonylurea medications

All people with type 1 diabetes (and some with type 2) rely on insulin injections to control the disease. When you take insulin shots, you have to time your food intake to raise your blood glucose as the insulin is taking effect. Chapter 10 explains the different kinds of insulin and the proper methods for administering them. But remember that the different types of insulin are most potent at differing amounts of time (minutes or hours) after you inject them. If you skip a meal or take your insulin too early or too late, your glucose and insulin levels won't be in sync and you'll develop hypoglycemia. If you go on a diet and don't adjust your medication, the same thing happens.

If you take sulfonylurea drugs, you need to follow similar restrictions. You and your doctor must adjust your dosage when your calorie intake falls. Other drugs don't cause hypoglycemia by themselves, but when combined with sulfonylureas they may lower your glucose enough to reach hypoglycemic levels. (Chapter 10 discusses these other drugs.)

Diet

Your diet plays a major role in helping you avoid hypoglycemia if you take medication. You should try to have a snack in the middle of the morning and in the afternoon — in addition to your usual breakfast, lunch, and dinner — especially if you take insulin. A properly timed snack provides you with a steady source of glucose to balance the insulin that you're taking.

You can use your blood glucose level to determine whether to have a snack at bedtime. If your glucose is greater than 180 mg/dL (10 mmol/L), you probably don't need a snack. If your glucose is between 126 and 180 mg/dL (7 to 10 mmol/L), a couple slices of bread and an ounce of cheese will prevent hypoglycemia. If your glucose is less than 126 mg/dL (7 mmol/L), a couple ounces of meat plus a slice of bread will do the trick.

Exercise

Exercise burns your body's fuel, which is glucose, so it generally lowers your blood glucose level. Some people with diabetes use exercise in place of extra insulin to get their high blood glucose down to a normal level. But if you don't adjust your insulin dose or food intake to match your exercise level, exercise can result in hypoglycemia.

One of my patients is dedicated to exercise. He has taken insulin shots for years but requires very little insulin to control his glucose because he burns so much glucose through exercise. He avoids hypoglycemia by measuring his blood glucose level many times a day — especially before vigorous exercise. If his level is low at the beginning of exercise, he eats extra carbohydrates before he starts. Chapter 8 tells you which foods to eat (and when) to achieve the intended effect on your glucose levels.

People who exercise regularly require much less medication and generally can manage their diabetes more easily than nonexercisers can. Chapter 9 covers much more about the benefits of exercise.

Non-diabetes drugs

Several drugs that you may take unrelated to your diabetes can lower your blood glucose. One of the most widely used, which you may not even think of as a drug, is alcohol, which can block your liver's ability to release glucose. It also blocks hormones that raise blood glucose and increases the glucose-lowering effect of insulin. If you're malnourished or you simply haven't eaten in a while and you drink alcohol before going to bed, you may experience severe fasting hypoglycemia the next morning. As well, if you take insulin or sulfonylurea drugs, don't drink alcohol without eating some food at the same time. Food counteracts some of the glucose-lowering effects of alcohol.

Also, be aware that aspirin (and all of the drugs related to aspirin, called *salicylates*) can lead to hypoglycemia. In adults who have diabetes, aspirin can increase the effects of other drugs that you're taking to lower your blood glucose. In children with diabetes, aspirin has an especially profound effect on lowering blood glucose to hypoglycemia levels. However, the low dose of aspirin taken daily to reduce the risk of heart attacks does not cause hypoglycemia.

More than 160 drugs have been associated with severe hypoglycemia. Usually it is found in a person taking insulin or a drug that works by increasing the body's own insulin. Following are the major drugs that cause hypoglycemia:

- **Angiotensin-converting enzyme inhibitors:** Blood pressure drugs, most of which end in *-pril*

- **Beta blockers:** Blood pressure drugs, most of which end in *-olol* (which also block the warning symptoms of hypoglycemia)

- **Pentamidine:** An antibiotic

- **Quinine:** Used to treat malaria

- **Quinolones:** A group of drugs that are antibiotics, most of which end in *-floxacin*

Hormonal changes

As type 1 diabetes progresses, your body produces fewer and fewer hormones that counteract insulin when hypoglycemia is present. This situation leads to more severe hypoglycemia later in type 1 diabetes, especially if you and your doctor don't adjust your insulin injections in response to your lower glucose levels. People with type 2 diabetes who take insulin also develop this loss of protective hormones.

These same hormones also play the role of giving you warning signs when your blood glucose drops, such as sweating, a rapid heartbeat, and anxiety, so you are prompted to eat. When the hormone levels drop, these warning signs don't occur, so you aren't signaled that you need to eat. This situation is called *hypoglycemia unawareness.*

Understanding the risks of hypoglycemia in special situations

Hypoglycemia is also present in a few special situations. They are discussed in this section.

Hypoglycemia with fasting

When you fast, your body doesn't permit the glucose to fall to hypoglycemic levels. If you take no insulin or oral drug that raises insulin and you become hypoglycemic during fasting anyway, you may have an internal source of excessive insulin, such as a tumor of the beta cells of the pancreas, an *insulinoma.* Insulinoma is easily diagnosed by fasting a person and checking the blood glucose over 72 hours. If it falls, the patient shows symptoms of hypo-glycemia, and the insulin is elevated, a tumor of the pancreas is likely.

Hypoglycemia in the critically ill

On the basis of one small study, some doctors believed that keeping the blood glucose of a critically ill person as normal as possible would decrease the possibility of death. The trouble is that in making the blood glucose normal, these patients often suffer severe hypoglycemia. More recent stud-ies have shown that keeping blood glucose normal in certain populations is not only not associated with decreased mortality but also is associated with increased risk of death.

Hypoglycemia and intellectual changes

Occasional severe hypoglycemia in younger people doesn't seem to have long-term consequences. The same is not true for the elderly. An increasing incidence of loss of mental function (dementia) occurs as elderly patients have one, two, or three episodes of severe hypoglycemia. That's all the more reason for frequently checking blood glucose levels (at least once or twice daily with type 2 diabetes and four or more times daily with type 1 or type 2 on multiple shots of insulin per day).

Hypoglycemia and the heart

Recent evidence suggests that hypoglycemia may be the cause of sudden unexplained death in young people with type 1 diabetes. Death may be caused by changes in the electrical rhythm of the heart. Hypoglycemia is often associated with low potassium, which can stop the heart. In patients with known heart disease, the highest death rate due to heart problems occurs at the lowest and highest blood glucose levels.

Treating hypoglycemia

Although hypoglycemia is preventable, you may still experience it at some point. Fortunately, the vast majority of cases are mild. You can treat hypogly-cemia with a small quantity of glucose in the form of:

- Two sugar cubes
- Three or four glucose tablets (available in any drugstore, and any person with diabetes who may develop hypoglycemia should carry them)
- A small amount (6 ounces) of a sugary soft drink
- 8 ounces of milk or 4 ounces of orange juice
- Anything that has about 15 grams of pure glucose in it

Sometimes you may need a second treatment. Approximately 20 minutes after you try one of these solutions, measure your blood glucose to find out whether your level has risen sufficiently. If it is still low, give a second treatment.

Keep the following in mind to aid in your treatment of hypoglycemia:

✔ **You can easily overtreat hypoglycemia,** causing your blood glucose to rise higher than you'd like. However, the high blood glucose resulting from overtreatment of hypoglycemia usually doesn't last long. You're better off not using a drug or insulin to bring it down, because doing so can result in alternate highs and lows.

✔ **Make sure that your friends or relatives know in advance what hypoglycemia is and what to do about it,** because your mental state may be mildly confused when you have it. Inform people about your diabetes and about how to recognize hypoglycemia. Don't keep your diabetes a secret. The people close to you will be glad to know how to help you.

✔ **Try to eat a snack of carbohydrates and protein every hour if you are doing prolonged exercise,** such as playing a baseball or soccer game that lasts several hours. (For example, half a turkey sandwich would work well.) And carry jelly beans (or any source of pure glucose) at all times, just in case — six or seven are all you need to combat mild symptoms of hypoglycemia.

If you are losing consciousness and can't sit up and swallow properly when you have hypoglycemia, no one should try to feed you. One of the following options should be used:

✔ **Someone helping you can use an emergency kit, such as the kit called "Glucagon for Emergencies."** This kit includes a syringe with 1 mg of *glucagon,* one of the major hormones that raises glucose, which your helper should inject under your skin or into your muscle. The injection of glucagon raises your blood glucose so that you regain consciousness within 20 minutes. Glucagon corrects your hypoglycemic condition for about an hour after you receive an injection.

You need to get a prescription from your doctor for this type of glucagon kit. If you don't use your kit for a long time, make sure the date on the kit indicates that it's still active.

✔ **If your hypoglycemia recurs shortly after you receive glucagon or doesn't respond to the glucagon, the person helping you should call 911.** (Sulfonylurea drugs are most often the cause of such a severe prolonged case of hypoglycemia.) The emergency crew checks your blood glucose and gives you an intravenous (IV) dose of high-concentration glucose. Most likely, you will continue the IV in the emergency room until you show stable and normal blood glucose levels.

Combating Ketoacidosis

In Chapter 3, I talk about the tendency of people with type 1 diabetes to suffer from a severe diabetic complication called *ketoacidosis,* or very high blood glucose with large amounts of acid in the blood. This section explains the symptoms, causes, and treatments of ketoacidosis.

The prefix *keto* refers to *ketones* — substances that your body makes when fat breaks down during ketoacidosis. *Acid* is part of the name because your blood becomes acidic from the presence of ketones.

Occasionally, ketoacidosis is the symptom that alerts doctors that you have type 1 diabetes, but more frequently it occurs after you already know that you have the disease. Although ketoacidosis occurs mostly in people with type 1 diabetes (who develop diabetes at an early age), the person is usually 40 or more years old when ketoacidosis actually begins.

Ketoacidosis occurs mostly in people with type 1 diabetes because they have no insulin in their bodies except what they inject as medication. People with type 2 diabetes (or with other forms of the disease) rarely get ketoacidosis, because they have some insulin in their bodies. People with type 2 diabetes get ketoacidosis mainly when they have severe infections or traumas that put their bodies under great physical stress. Because ketoacidosis is a complication of type 1 diabetes and only very rarely type 2 diabetes, I provide only a short discussion of ketoacidosis here. For a much more complete explanation, see my book *Type 1 Diabetes For Dummies* (Wiley).

Spotting symptoms of ketoacidosis

The symptoms of ketoacidosis regularly alert doctors to type 1 diabetes in children. But ketoacidosis more often occurs in adults with type 1 diabetes, so they should also keep an eye out for the following symptoms:

- Nausea and vomiting
- Rapid breathing (also known as *Kussmaul breathing,* after the man who first described it)
- Extreme tiredness and drowsiness
- Weakness

In this age of self-monitoring for blood glucose levels, ketoacidosis is becoming more rare, but it still occurs. (See Chapter 7 for more on self-monitoring.)

You may notice that you have some symptoms of ketoacidosis and begin to suspect that you have this complication. But that diagnosis is best made by a doctor — preferably in the hospital, where you can begin treatment immediately. Doctors make a diagnosis of ketoacidosis when they see the following abnormalities:

- High blood glucose, usually more than 300 mg/dl (16.6 mmol/L)
- Acid condition of your blood
- Excessive levels of ketones in your blood and urine
- Dry skin and tongue, indicating dehydration
- Deficiency of potassium in your body
- An acetone smell on your breath

When your doctor finds these abnormalities, he or she will want to begin treatment immediately.

Clarifying the causes of ketoacidosis

The two most common causes of ketoacidosis are the interruption of your insulin treatment and an infection. Your body can't go for many hours without insulin activity before it begins to burn fat for energy and begins to make extra glucose that it can't use.

Whether you have diabetes or not, if you go on a strict diet to lose weight, your body burns some of its fat stores and produces ketones, similar to how it burns fat when you lack insulin. But in this case, your glucose remains low and (unless you have type 1 diabetes) you have sufficient insulin to prevent the excessive production of new glucose or the release of large amounts of glucose from your liver. So a strict diet doesn't generally lead to ketoacidosis but rather a benign condition called *ketosis*.

Treating ketoacidosis

Ketoacidosis is a serious condition that requires professional treatment. But even though you leave the treatment to a professional rather than trying to manage it yourself, you should know the treatment processes so that you understand what's happening to you or to your loved one.

The basis of ketoacidosis treatment is to restore the proper amount of water to your body, reduce the acid condition of your blood by getting rid of the ketones, restore substances such as potassium that you've lost, and return your blood glucose to its normal level of around 80 to 120. All these improvements should happen simultaneously after you begin treatment. For an in-depth discussion of the treatment of ketoacidosis, see my book *Type 1 Diabetes For Dummies* (Wiley).

Most of the time, your doctor can control ketoacidosis with little or no risk to you. But be aware that ketoacidosis is fatal for 10 percent of people with diabetes who get it — mostly elderly people with diabetes and those with other illnesses that complicate treatment. Recognizing the symptoms early and seeking treatment quickly greatly enhance your chances of an uneventful recovery from ketoacidosis.

Managing Hyperosmolar Syndrome

The highest blood glucose condition that you may find yourself in is called *hyperosmolar syndrome.* Like ketoacidosis, hyperosmolar syndrome, referring to the excessive levels of glucose in the blood, is a medical emergency that needs to be treated in a hospital.

Hyperosmolar syndrome is also like ketoacidosis in its effects on your body. It creates ketones in your blood, but it doesn't make your blood as acidic as ketoacidosis does. However, it raises your blood glucose levels considerably higher than ketoacidosis does. (See the "Combating Ketoacidosis" section earlier in this chapter for more information.)

Hyper means "larger than normal," and *osmolar* has to do with concentrations of substances in the blood. So hyperosmolar, in this situation, means that the blood is simply too concentrated with glucose. Other hyperosmolar syndromes occur when other substances are at fault.

The following sections explain hyperosmolar syndrome's symptoms, causes, and treatments.

Heeding the symptoms of hyperosmolar syndrome

Because hyperosmolar syndrome is so similar to ketoacidosis, it has many of the same symptoms as ketoacidosis. The main difference is that with hyperosmolar syndrome, you don't experience the rapid Kussmaul breathing, because your blood isn't overly acidic as a part of this complication. Also, the symptoms of hyperosmolar syndrome develop over many days or weeks, unlike the quick and acute development of ketoacidosis in your body.

If you measure your blood glucose on a daily basis, you should never develop hyperosmolar syndrome because you'll notice that your blood glucose is getting high before it reaches the critical complication level.

Following are the most important signs and symptoms of hyperosmolar syndrome:

✔ Frequent urination

✔ Thirst

✔ Weakness

✔ Leg cramps

✔ Sunken eyeballs

✔ Rapid pulse

✔ Decreased mental awareness or (if you delay treatment) coma

✔ Blood glucose of 600 or even higher if you delay seeing a doctor

You may also develop more threatening symptoms with this complication. Your blood pressure may be low. Your nervous system may be affected with paralysis of the arms and legs, but these problems respond to treatment.

Finding the cause

Hyperosmolar syndrome afflicts mostly elderly diabetes patients who live alone or in nursing homes where they're not carefully monitored. Age and usually some neglect combine to increase the likelihood that a person with diabetes will lose large quantities of fluids through vomiting or diarrhea and then not replace those fluids. These people tend to have mild type 2 diabetes, which is sometimes undiagnosed and untreated.

Another reason why age is a contributing cause of hyperosmolar syndrome is that your kidneys gradually become less efficient as you age. When your kidneys are in their prime, your blood glucose level needs to reach only 180 mg/dl before your kidneys begin to remove some excess glucose through your urine. But as your kidneys grow older and slower, they require a gradually higher blood glucose level before they start to send excess glucose to your urine. If you're at an age (usually 70 or older for people in average health) when your kidneys are really laboring to remove the excess glucose from your body and you happen to lose a large amount of fluids from sickness or neglect, your blood volume decreases, which makes it even harder for your kidneys to remove glucose. At this point, your blood glucose level begins to skyrocket. If you don't replace some of the lost fluids quickly, your glucose rises even higher.

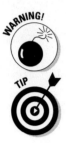

If you allow your blood glucose to rise and don't get the fluids that you need, your blood pressure starts to fall and you get weaker and weaker. As the concentration of glucose in your blood continues to rise, you become increasingly confused, and your mental state diminishes until you eventually fall into a coma.

Other factors — such as infection, failure to take your insulin, and taking certain medications — can raise your blood glucose to the hyperosmolar syndrome levels, but not replacing lost body fluids is the most frequent cause.

Treating hyperosmolar syndrome

Hyperosmolar syndrome requires immediate and skilled treatment from a doctor. By no means should you try to treat yourself. In fact, you should avoid doctors who are not experienced in treatment of this condition. You need the proper treatment from an experienced doctor — and you need it fast. The death rate for hyperosmolar syndrome is high because most people who suffer from it are elderly and often have other serious illnesses that complicate treatment.

When you arrive at your doctor's office or emergency room with hyperosmolar syndrome, your doctor must accomplish the following tasks fairly rapidly:

✔ Restore large volumes of water to your body

✔ Lower your blood glucose level

✔ Restore other substances that your body has lost, such as potassium, sodium, chloride, and so on

Chapter 5

Preventing Long-Term Complications

*F*irst, the good news: Between the years 1998 and 2006, lower-limb amputations (which are mostly due to diabetes) dropped 37 percent in the United States. At the same time a striking reduction in other long-term complications, including nerve disease, eye disease, and kidney disease, also occurred. Doctors believe that this reduction is due to improved testing of the blood glucose (see Chapter 7) and more use of insulin and other medications to lower the glucose (see Chapter 10). Furthermore, benefits in terms of reduction in complications persist for years after a period of tight control of the blood glucose.

Now the bad news: The incidence of type 2 diabetes is increasing so rapidly that it will overwhelm improvements in treatment over the next 20 years unless some major improvement in diabetes prevention takes place. Complications will start to rise again.

The complications detailed in this chapter are the problems that occur if you permit your blood glucose to rise and remain high over many years. The point that I stress throughout this book is that you have a choice. Working with your doctor and other helpers, you can keep your blood glucose near normal so that you never have to deal with these long-term complications.

Knowing How Long-Term Complications Develop and How to Avoid Them

For most long-term complications — such as kidney disease, eye disease, and nerve disease — doctors believe that years of high blood glucose levels initiate the complications. (Heart disease is an exception. In that case, high blood glucose levels may make the disease worse or more complicated but not actually cause it.) Most long-term complications require ten or more years to develop, which seems like a long time until you consider that many people with type 2 diabetes have it for five or more years before a doctor diagnoses it.

Often the long-term complication itself (rather than a high blood glucose level) is the clue that leads a doctor to diagnose diabetes in a patient. Therefore, doctors need to look for long-term complications immediately after diagnosing diabetes, because the diabetes and any long-term complications may have been with the patient for quite some time already.

If you're preventing short-term complications (see Chapter 4), you're also preventing long-term complications. But here are the differences you need to remember between short-term and long-term complications:

✔ Short-term complications result from the immediate effects of very high and very low blood glucose levels, and they're reversible.

✔ Long-term complications result from damage done by high blood glucose levels as well as abnormal fat levels and abnormal blood pressure. After a while, long-term complications aren't reversible.

The struggle to live an uncomplicated life with diabetes reminds me of a commercial airplane pilot who took the airplane down for a rough landing. As was his custom, after the plane landed the pilot stood at the exit while passengers departed. A little old lady walked to the exit with her cane and said to the pilot, "Tell me, did we land, or were we shot down?" The choice is yours: You can have a smooth landing, free of complications, that goes relatively unnoticed by you and those around you. Or you can have the feeling that you have been shot down.

Kidney Disease

Your kidneys rid your body of many harmful chemicals and other compounds produced during the process of normal metabolism. Your kidneys act like a filter through which your blood pours, trapping the waste and sending it out in your urine while the normal contents of the blood go back into your bloodstream. They also regulate the salt and water content of your body. When kidney disease (also known as *nephropathy*) causes your kidneys to fail, you must either use artificial means, called *dialysis,* to cleanse your blood and control the salt and water or receive a new working donor kidney, called a *transplant.*

Chronic kidney disease is more prevalent now than it has been in the past, and the major source of all these new cases is diabetes. In the United States today, half the patients who require long-term dialysis require it because of diabetes. Fortunately, the number requiring dialysis is on the decline because of the increasing awareness among people that they need to control their blood glucose. The incidence of kidney disease is only about 5 percent among people with type 2 diabetes, compared to 30 percent among people with type 1 diabetes; however, the absolute number of patients with kidney disease is about the same for the two groups because type 2 diabetes is so much more common than type 1.

How high glucose leads to complications

Although doctors aren't certain about the causes of most long-term complications of diabetes, I mention the current theories about the causes of the complications as I explain each complication in this chapter. However, all long-term complications share some common characteristics.

Advanced glycated end-products (AGEs) are one of the substances that damage tissues. AGEs can damage the eyes, the kidneys, the nervous system, and other organs in your body. You always have glucose in your blood, and some of that glucose attaches to other substances in your bloodstream to form *glycated* (glucose-attached) products. In this way, hemoglobin, which carries oxygen through your blood to cells and tissues throughout your body, attaches to glucose to form hemoglobin A1c. Albumin, a protein in blood, forms glycated albumin. Glucose can attach to red blood cells and white blood cells, as well as to other cells and molecules in the bloodstream. When these normal body substances attach to glucose, they no longer work normally.

Your body handles a certain level of glycated substances. But when your blood glucose is elevated for prolonged periods of time, the level of glycated cells and substances becomes excessive, and the complications I describe in this chapter result.

The Polyol Pathway is another major source of damage to the body in diabetes. *Polyol Pathway* refers to one direction that glucose can take as it is *metabolized* (broken down).

When you have a lot of glucose in your blood, an abnormal amount is metabolized to become a product called *sorbitol,* which accumulates in many tissues where it can damage them in the following ways:

- ✔ **Damage from swelling:** Sorbitol causes body water to enter cells, which causes damage and destruction of cells.

- ✔ **Damage from chemical reactions:** During the production of sorbitol, other compounds are produced that chemically damage the cells and tissues.

- ✔ **Autoantibodies:** Autoantibodies to autonomic nerves are present in patients with diabetes. Autoimmunity may be yet another mechanism by which diabetes causes long-term complications.

This section tells you what you need to know to prevent and manage diabetic kidney disease. I tell you how diabetes affects your kidneys, what changes are occurring in your body, and how you can both check for them while they are still reversible and prevent them from getting any worse.

The impact of diabetes on your kidneys

Your kidneys consist of about a million units called nephrons. Each nephron contains a structure called the *glomerulous* (the plural is *glomeruli*) (see Figure 5-1) that filters blood and separates out waste products and some water. Glomeruli cleanse your blood through the following process:

1. Your blood passes from incoming arterioles through tiny glomerular capillaries within the Bowman's capsule.

2. Your filtered blood travels through tubules connected to the glomerular capillaries.

3. As your filtered blood passes through the tubules:

   a. Your body reabsorbs most of the water and the normal contents of the blood.

   b. A small amount of water and waste passes from the kidney into the ureter and then into the bladder and out through the urethra.

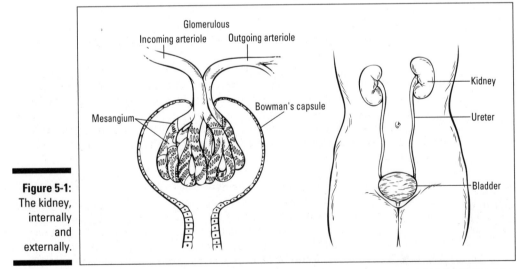

Figure 5-1:
The kidney, internally and externally.

Illustration by Kathryn Born

When you first get diabetes, your kidneys are enlarged and seem to function abnormally well, judging by how fast they clear wastes from your body. Your kidneys seem to function so well because you have a large amount of glucose entering your kidneys, which draws a lot of water with it and causes an increase in the pressure inside each glomerulous. This more-rapid transit of blood through the kidneys is known as an increased *glomerular filtration rate* (GFR). Early in the development of your diabetes, the membrane surrounding your glomeruli, called the *glomerular basement membrane,* thickens, as do other adjacent structures. These expanding membranes and structures begin to take up the space occupied by the capillaries inside the glomeruli, so the capillaries are unable to filter as much blood.

Fortunately, you have many more glomeruli than you really need. In fact, you can lose the equivalent of a whole kidney (half of each kidney) and still have plenty of reserve to clean your blood. If your kidney disease goes undetected for about 15 years, damage may become so severe that your blood shows measurable signs of the beginning of kidney failure, called *azotemia.* If the neglect of the disease reaches 20 years, both kidneys may fail entirely.

Not every person with diabetes is at equal risk for kidney disease and kidney failure. This complication seems to be more common in certain families and among certain racial groups, especially African Americans, Mexican Americans, and Native Americans. It is certainly more common when high blood pressure is present. Although doctors and researchers believe that high blood glucose is the major factor leading to nephropathy, only half of the people whose blood glucose has been poorly controlled go on to develop nephropathy.

Early indications of kidney disease

A healthy kidney permits only a tiny amount of *albumin,* a protein in the blood, to enter the urine. However, a kidney being damaged by nephropathy is unable to hold back as much albumin, and the level in the urine increases, causing *microalbuminuria* (the presence of tiny but abnormally high amounts of albumin in your urine). If your kidneys are on their way to being damaged by *diabetic nephropathy* (kidney disease caused by diabetes), doctors can detect microalbuminuria in your urine.

For three-quarters of the patients in the early stages of kidney disease, however, the amount of albumin in your urine is so small that it won't trigger a positive result when the traditional urine dipstick test is used. Therefore, your doctor should perform a more sophisticated test for microalbuminuria. This test can be done by collecting a 24-hour urine specimen (meaning you save all the urine you produce in 24 hours and have it tested), by taking a random urine sample. or by collecting a specimen over a certain time period, usually four hours. If the level of albumin is abnormally high, it needs to be checked once again to be certain, because some factors (such as exercise) can trigger a false positive test. A second positive test should lead to action to protect your kidneys.

Because microalbuminuria can be detected about five years before a urine dipstick would test positive for albumin, you have time to treat the onset. Furthermore, treatment during the stage of microalbuminuria can reverse the kidney disease. After macroalbuminuria is found using the dipstick method, the disease can be slowed but not stopped.

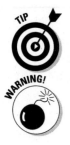

If you have had type 1 diabetes for five years or more, or if you've recently been diagnosed with type 2 diabetes, *your doctor must check for microalbuminuria* unless you've already tested positive for albumin with a urine dipstick. If your test comes back negative, you should have it rechecked annually.

As many as 25 percent of patients with no microalbuminuria still have kidney disease, so treatment with drugs that protect your kidneys makes sense.

In June 2003 in the *New England Journal of Medicine,* researchers showed that microalbuminuria does not always lead to kidney failure. Patients with type 1 diabetes who improved their blood glucose levels, blood pressure, and abnormal blood fats (which I discuss in the next section) experienced a decline in microalbuminuria and, therefore, a decline in kidney damage. The levels of improvement indicated by this study are as follows:

- ✔ Lowered blood glucose as indicated by a hemoglobin A1c of less than 8 percent (see Chapter 7)

- ✔ Lowered blood pressure, with the upper number (the *systolic blood pressure*) kept under 115 mm mercury

- ✔ Cholesterol kept under 198 mg/dl (5.12 mmol/L)

- ✔ Triglycerides kept below 145 mg/dl (1.64 mmol/L)

Progressive changes in the kidneys

If diabetes is poorly controlled for five years or more, your kidney experiences a significant expansion of the *mesangial tissue,* the cells between the capillaries in the kidneys. The amount of microalbuminuria (discussed in the preceding section) correlates to the amount of mesangial expansion. Thickening of the glomerular basement membrane is taking place at the same time but does not correlate as well with the amount of microalbuminuria.

Over the next 15 to 20 years, the open capillaries and tubules are squeezed shut by the encroaching tissues. Less and less filtration of the blood can take place, ultimately ending in *uremia,* a condition in which the kidneys are not doing any cleansing.

Other factors besides high blood glucose contribute to the continuing destruction of the kidneys. They include the following:

- ✔ **High blood pressure (hypertension):** This factor may be almost as important as the glucose level. If your blood pressure is controlled by drugs, the damage to your kidneys slows very significantly.

- ✔ **Factors of inheritance:** Certain families and ethnic groups have a higher incidence of diabetic nephropathy, as I discuss in the section "The impact of diabetes on your kidneys," earlier in this chapter.

- ✔ **Abnormal blood fats:** Research shows that elevated levels of certain cholesterol-containing fats promote enlargement of the mesangium.

Diabetic nephropathy does not occur alone. If you experience kidney disease, you need to be aware that the following complications are associated with it:

- ✔ **Diabetic eye disease:** When someone experiences complete failure of the kidneys, called *end-stage renal disease,* diabetic retinopathy (eye disease) is almost always present (see the section "Eye Disease," later in this chapter). As kidney disease gets worse, retinopathy accelerates. But only half the people with retinopathy also have nephropathy.

    If you test positive for microalbuminuria, you will likely also have some retinopathy if diabetes is the cause of your kidney problems. If you have diabetes and have microalbuminuria but retinopathy is not present, your doctor should look for another cause of kidney disease besides diabetes.

- ✔ **Diabetic nerve disease (neuropathy):** Fewer than 50 percent of patients with nephropathy also experience diabetic nerve disease, or neuropathy. Neuropathy gets worse as kidney disease gets worse, but after dialysis has begun, some of the neuropathy disappears. This situation indicates that part of the neuropathy may be due to wastes that are retained because of the failing kidney rather than true damage to the nervous system. (For more on this condition, see the section "Nerve Disease, or Neuropathy" later in this chapter.)

- ✔ **High blood pressure (hypertension):** Hypertension plays an important role in accelerating kidney damage. One-third of patients who have urine dipstick tests that are positive for albumin also have high blood pressure. As the blood tests for kidney failure begin to rise, two-thirds of patients are hypertensive. With end-stage renal disease, almost all have high blood pressure.

- ✔ **Edema:** Edema, or water accumulation, in the feet and legs occurs as the amount of protein in the urine exceeds one or two grams a day.

Treatment for diabetic nephropathy

If the information in the previous section is making your blood pressure rise, take a deep breath. I'm happy to report that all the inconvenience and discomfort associated with diabetic nephropathy can be avoided. Following are a few key treatments that you can do to prevent the disease or significantly slow it down after it begins:

- **Control your blood glucose.** This crucial step has been shown to avoid the onset of nephropathy and to slow it down after it starts. Both the Diabetes Control and Complications Trial (DCCT) in the United States, which studied glucose control in type 1 diabetes, and the United Kingdom Prospective Diabetes Study Groups in type 2 diabetes have proved this point. If you keep your blood glucose close to normal, you will not develop diabetic nephropathy. (For information on controlling your blood glucose, see Part III.)

  One of the best findings from the DCCT is that even eight years after the trial ended, participants experienced persistent benefits of reduced blood pressure and reduced albumin excretion (a marker for kidney damage). Controlling your blood glucose now will pay off years in the future.

- **Control your blood pressure.** This step protects the kidneys from rapid deterioration. Treatment begins with a low-salt diet, but drugs are usually needed. High blood pressure can be controlled by a variety of drugs, but one class of drugs seems particularly valuable in nephropathy. This class is called the *angiotensin converting enzyme inhibitors,* or ACE inhibitors. (For more on ACE inhibitors, see the sidebar "ACE inhibitors to the rescue.") If ACE inhibitors can't be used for any reason, a similar class of drugs called *angiotensin II receptor blockers* are equally or more effective. Be especially alert for kidney damage if you have *white-coat high blood pressure* (WCH). This condition occurs in patients who have normal blood pressure at home but high blood pressure in the doctor's office. WCH has a high correlation with both kidney damage and eye damage.

- **Control the blood fats.** Because abnormalities of blood fats seem to make kidney disease worse, you must lower your bad, or LDL, cholesterol and raise your good, or HDL, cholesterol while lowering the other fat that is damaging — the triglycerides. A number of excellent drugs, in a class called *statins,* can accomplish this task. The ACE inhibitors also seem to help the levels of fats. (See the sidebar on ACE inhibitors for more information.)

- **Avoid other damage to the kidneys.** People with diabetes tend to have more urinary-tract infections, which damage the kidneys. Urinary tract infections must be looked for and treated. People with diabetes also have damage to the nerves that control the bladder, producing a neurogenic bladder. (See the section "Disorders of automatic [autonomic] nerves," later in this chapter.) When the nerves that detect a full bladder fail, proper emptying of the bladder is inhibited, which can lead to infections.

✔ **Discuss the possibility of taking aliskiren (Tekturna) with your doctor.** Aliskiren is a drug that was originally used to lower blood pressure but has been found to promote significant reduction in protein loss in the urine. However, a new warning is out not to use aliskiren in combination with ACE inhibitors or ARBs.

If you have disease in the urinary system, your doctor may want to do an *intravenous pyelogram* (IVP), a study to observe the appearance and function of your kidneys and the rest of your urinary tract. But people with diabetes with some kidney failure are at high risk for complete failure of the kidneys as a result of an IVP. Your doctor should use another type of study that does not put your kidneys at risk.

If these preventative treatments fail, the patient undergoes dialysis or a kidney transplant.

When the kidneys fail, a main source for the breakdown of insulin is gone, and the patient requires much less or no insulin, so control of the blood glucose may actually get easier. Drugs like the sulfonylureas are also reduced or stopped because the failed kidneys no longer break them down.

✔ **Dialysis:** Two dialysis techniques are currently in use.

- **Hemodialysis:** The patient's artery is hooked into a tube that runs through a filtering machine that cleanses the blood and then sends it back into the patient's bloodstream. When the patient is moderately well, hemodialysis is done three times a week in a hospital setting. The potential exists for many complications, including infection and low blood pressure.

- **Peritoneal dialysis:** A tube is inserted into the body cavity that contains the stomach, liver, and intestines, called the peritoneal cavity. A large quantity of fluid is dripped into the cavity, and it draws out the wastes, which are then removed as the fluid drains out of the cavity. Peritoneal dialysis is done at home, often on a daily basis. Peritoneal dialysis requires the use of sugar in the fluid, so people with diabetes have very high blood glucose levels (which is undesirable) unless insulin is added to the bags of dialysis fluid. Alternatively, the patient's subcutaneous insulin doses are increased. Peritoneal dialysis is also associated with a high rate of infection where the tube enters the peritoneal cavity.

Poor control of the blood glucose during any form of dialysis is associated with a higher death rate. Make sure you control your glucose!

Little difference exists in the long-term survival of patients treated with hemodialysis compared with peritoneal dialysis, so the choice becomes one of convenience and whether insurance covers one procedure more than the other. People with diabetes do not tolerate kidney failure well, so dialysis tends to be started earlier in them than in people without diabetes.

ACE inhibitors to the rescue

The class of drugs called *angiotensin converting enzyme inhibitors,* or ACE inhibitors, has long been known to lower blood pressure. Recent studies show that these drugs also lower the pressure inside the *glomeruli* (the structures inside your kidneys that cleanse your blood). The result is a 50 percent reduction in death due to diabetic nephropathy and an equal reduction in the need for dialysis or a kidney transplant.

Your doctor should prescribe one of these medications if your blood pressure is 140/90 or higher. The target blood pressure is 120/80 in people with kidney disease and even lower in younger people. ACE inhibitors can even be used to reverse early kidney disease if you have microalbuminuria without hypertension, because the microalbuminuria suggests that there is increased pressure within the kidney. When ACE inhibitors are used, the excretion of albumin begins to fall; if you are leaking albumin into the urine, your urine albumin level can be used to monitor the drugs' effectiveness if your blood pressure is normal.

ACE inhibitors aren't perfect: They cause a cough in some patients, which some people find hard to tolerate, but the choice of a particular ACE inhibitor may solve this problem. In addition, ACE inhibitors tend to raise the potassium level in the blood. The potassium level is already an issue with failing kidneys, so a higher potassium level may add to the problem. A very high potassium level can cause abnormalities in the heart. Angiotensin II receptor blockers (ARBs) can replace ACE inhibitors when necessary. They're not associated with the cough but do raise potassium.

Other drugs used for high blood pressure include the calcium channel blockers, which may be as useful as ACE inhibitors. Other antihypertensives that have been standards in the past for hypertension may cause unacceptable side effects. Water pills (diuretics such as hydrochlorothiazide) raise the blood glucose. Beta blockers like propranolol make the abnormal fats worse. They also cause a difficulty in recognizing when the blood glucose has gone down to very low levels.

  ✔ **Kidney transplant:** Patients who receive a kidney transplant seem to do better than dialysis patients, but in the United States, because of a lack of kidneys, 80 percent of patients have dialysis and 20 percent have a transplant. Obviously, a transplanted kidney is foreign to the person who receives it, and the body tries to reject it. To avoid this result, the patient is given antirejection drugs, some of which make diabetic control more complicated. The kidney that is least rejected is the one from a donor who is most closely related to the patient.

  When a healthy kidney enters the body of a person with diabetes, it is subject to the damage done by elevated glucose levels. After a transplant, controlling your blood glucose is crucial.

Diabetes-related end-stage kidney disease (total kidney failure) is declining in all age groups thanks to better control of glucose, blood pressure, and fat.

Eye Disease

The eyes are the second major organ of the body affected by diabetes over the long term. Blurred vision, often present at diagnosis, is reversible with control of the glucose. Some eye diseases, such as glaucoma and cataracts, also occur in the nondiabetic population, though they appear at a higher rate and earlier in people with diabetes. Glaucoma and cataracts respond to treatment very well. Diabetic retinopathy, however — which I explain in the next section — is limited to the diabetic population and may lead to blindness. In the past, blindness was inevitable, but that is not the case today. In fact, after 20 years of diabetes, eye disease occurred in 30 percent of patients with type 1 diabetes before 1979, in 18 percent between 1980 and 1984, and in only 6 percent after 1984.

In the following sections you find out about the normal function of the eye and how diabetes can damage or even eliminate that function. You also discover the importance of early diagnosis by regular eye exams and how you can stop the progress of eye disease should it occur.

Common eye problems in diabetics

In order to help you understand how diabetes affects the eyes, Figure 5-2 shows you the different parts of the eye.

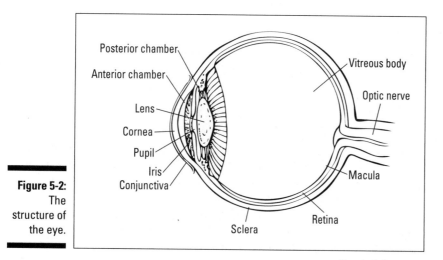

Figure 5-2: The structure of the eye.

Posterior chamber
Anterior chamber
Lens
Cornea
Pupil
Iris
Conjunctiva
Vitreous body
Optic nerve
Macula
Retina
Sclera

Illustration by Kathryn Born

Light enters the eye through the lens, where it is bent and focused on the retina. The place in the retina where the lens focuses is called the *macula*. The retina collects an image and transfers it to the optic nerve, which carries it to the brain, where the image is interpreted. Between the lens and the retina is a transparent material called the *vitreous body*. Many more structures exist within the eye, but they're not important for my purposes in this chapter. The eye muscles surround the eye on all sides and are attached to it. These muscles permit you to look up, down, and sideways without moving your head. These eye muscles are important in the discussion of diabetic nerve damage, called *neuropathy*. (For more on this condition, see the section "Nerve Disease, or Neuropathy," later in this chapter.)

Following is a list of common eye diseases found in people with diabetes:

- ✔ **Cataracts:** These opaque areas of the lens can block vision if they're large enough. Cataracts tend to be more common in people with diabetes, even at a young age, both as a result of advanced glycated end-products (AGEs) that form within the lens and as a result of the increased concentration of sorbitol in the lens. (I discuss AGEs and sorbitol in the sidebar "How high glucose leads to complications," earlier in this chapter.) Cataracts can be surgically removed by a fairly routine operation. The entire lens is removed, and an artificial lens is put in its place. With removal, you have an excellent chance for the restoration of your vision.

- ✔ **Glaucoma:** This condition, high pressure inside the eye, is enough to do damage to the optic nerve. Glaucoma is found more often in people with diabetes than in the nondiabetic population. If left unchecked, the high pressure can destroy the optic nerve and destroy your vision. Fortunately, medical treatment can lower the eye pressure and save the eye. Eye doctors check for glaucoma on a routine basis.

- ✔ **Retinopathy:** Diabetic retinopathy refers to a number of changes that are seen on the retina of the eye. These changes indicate that the patient has been exposed to high levels of blood glucose over time. If untreated at the appropriate time, retinopathy can lead to blindness. The first changes are seen after ten years of diabetes in both type 1 and 2. Because retinopathy is much more complicated and less treatable than the other two conditions, I discuss it in detail in the next section.

If you have diabetes, you must get an annual eye examination by an ophthalmologist or optometrist to preserve your vision. This situation is one where an expert is definitely needed. Doctors who are not ophthalmologists or optometrists diagnose retinopathy correctly only 50 percent of the time, while ophthalmologists and optometrists are correct more than 90 percent of the time. You need to get an eye examination as soon as you are diagnosed with type 2 diabetes or five years after the diagnosis of type 1 diabetes, and you need to be rechecked every year after that.

The risks of retinopathy

Ophthalmologists break down retinopathy, damage to the retina caused by high blood glucose, into two major types according to their potential to cause visual loss:

- ✔ **Background retinopathy:** This type is usually benign but can be a predictor of worse problems. The first changes noted by the ophthalmologist are *retinal aneurysms,* which are the result of weakening of the capillaries of the eye; they produce outpocketing of the capillaries, which look like tiny balloons. These aneurysms appear as small red dots on the back of the eye. They are benign and disappear over time.

  The weakened capillaries also rupture sometimes and release blood to form *retinal hemorrhages* and *hard exudates.* The hard exudates, which are yellowish and appear round and sharp, are scars from the hemorrhage. If they extend into the macular area, they reduce vision. If the capillaries in the retina allow fluid to flow into the macula, you get *macular edema,* which also causes loss of vision. These exudates and hemorrhages can last for years. As the capillaries close, you have a decreased blood supply to the retina, and *cotton wool spots* or *soft exudates* appear. These spots represent destruction of the nerve fiber layer because of the lack of blood.

  These changes usually do not cause complete loss of vision, but in about 50 percent of cases, they go on to the more serious proliferative retinopathy.

- ✔ **Proliferative retinopathy:** This condition results in vision loss if untreated. Just as in many other parts of the body, when the blood supply in the eye is reduced, new blood vessels form to carry more blood to the retina. This is the stage of proliferative retinopathy. This condition is when some visual loss becomes more certain. The growth of blood vessels takes place into the vitreous body. Hemorrhage into the vitreous body blocks vision. As the hemorrhage forms a clot and contracts, it may pull up the retina to produce retinal detachment. Because the lens can no longer focus the light onto the macula, you have a complete loss of vision.

Like diabetic nephropathy, retinopathy has a number of important associations:

- ✔ Certain ethnic groups are at very high risk for retinopathy, including certain American Indian groups, like the Pima Indians, and Mexican Americans. Researchers aren't yet certain if African Americans are at higher risk.

- ✔ Specific genetic material, if found in a person with diabetes, increases the incidence of retinopathy. This material can be found by doing a chemical analysis of a person's *chromosomes,* the material in each cell that holds the genes. If the genetic material is found, that person has a higher likelihood of developing retinopathy.

✔ Males and females get retinopathy equally.

✔ Greater duration of diabetes results in more eye disease.

✔ High blood pressure may worsen the eye disease.

✔ Nephropathy occurs along with the eye disease. (See the "Progressive changes in the kidneys" section, earlier in this chapter.)

✔ Smoking worsens retinopathy, and alcohol abuse causes reduced visual acuity but not increased retinopathy.

✔ Patients with severe diabetic retinopathy are at increased risk for heart attacks. An article in Diabetes Care in July 2007 strongly confirmed this relationship. People with diabetic retinopathy are twice as likely to have a heart attack as people with diabetes who don't have retinopathy. If they have a heart attack, it's three times as likely to be fatal.

In recent clinical studies, ranibizumab (Lucentis) has been highly effective in treating diabetic retinopathy. It is injected directly into the eye but is not as painful as it sounds. It may become the treatment of choice. Up to now laser surgery is has been an excellent treatment option. And the use of laser surgery to create many burns in the retina has been shown to save many eyes. Only 5 percent of diabetics with proliferative retinopathy who undergo laser treatment develop severe visual loss. Because the retina is being burned, you have some minor loss of vision. You also have a mild decrease in night vision and a minor decrease in the size of the field that your eye can take in at one time. The procedure is done outside the hospital. It is used for treating macular edema with success as well.

Tight control of the blood glucose (maintaining a hemoglobin A1c under 7 percent) is associated with a much better response to laser surgery than loose control.

Laser surgery can't treat a retinal detachment that has already occurred. To do so, a surgical procedure called *vitrectomy* is used. This operation, done under general anesthesia, involves removing the vitreous body and replacing it with a sterile solution. Attachments to the retina are cut, and the retina returns to its place. Any hemorrhages in the vitreous body are removed at the same time. Vitrectomy is successful in restoring some vision about 80 to 90 percent of the time. If a retinal detachment is present in addition to hemorrhage, the amount of improvement depends on the extent and duration of the retinal detachment, with restoration of vision occurring about 50 to 60 percent of the time.

Resources for the blind and visually impaired

A search for resources for the blind and visually impaired must begin with the World Wide Web. One helpful site is the Blindness Resource Center (www.nyise.org/text/blindness.htm), sponsored by the New York Institute for Special Education, which contains a huge list of other sources of information. The site itself uses large print, so a person with impaired vision can easily read it.

Here are some other useful sites regarding blindness (and which you can link to from the Blindness Resource Center's site):

- ✔ Blind Net (www.blind.net) provides useful information about blindness.

- ✔ New York Institute for Special Education's Blindness Resource Center, www.nyise.org/blind.htm, provides programs for children who are blind or visually disabled.

- ✔ *Dialogue* magazine (www.blindskills.com) is written specifically for the blind.

- ✔ Guide Dogs for the Blind (www.guidedogs.com) explains everything you want to know about these amazing animals.

 Undoubtedly, one of the best resources is the American Foundation for the Blind (AFB) at www.afb.org. It would take a good part of a lifetime to read all of the resource materials that the AFB provides on thousands of web pages. The AFB is the organization that Helen Keller devoted her life to, and it has every imaginable resource — and some that are unimaginable.

The web is a tremendous resource for the visually handicapped and should be utilized by friends, relatives, or the impaired person if that is possible. You have no reason to feel alone with your visual problem.

Nerve Disease, or Neuropathy

The third major part of the body that's attacked by poorly controlled diabetes is the nervous system. Sixty percent of people with diabetes have some abnormality of the nervous system. These patients usually don't realize it, because the disease doesn't have any early symptoms. These patients usually have poor glucose control, smoke, and are over age 40. Nerve disease is found most often in the people who have diabetes the longest. Diabetic neuropathy often leads to foot infections, foot ulcerations, and amputation — complications that are all entirely preventable (see the section "Diabetic Foot Disease," later in this chapter). The sections that follow describe the basics of nerve disease as well as disorders associated with nerve disease.

Basics of neuropathy

How high glucose levels damage nerves remains uncertain. Doctors do know that the *axon,* the part of the nerve that connects to other nerves or to muscle, becomes degenerated. The damage may be *vascular* in some cases, resulting from a cut-off of blood to the nerve, and *metabolic* in others, resulting from chemical toxins produced by the metabolism of too much glucose.

Diabetic neuropathy occurs in any situation where the blood glucose is abnormally elevated, usually for ten years or more. It is therefore not limited to type 1 or type 2 diabetes, although it's most commonly paired with these diseases. When the elevated blood glucose is brought down to normal, the signs and symptoms improve. In some cases, the neuropathy disappears.

The fact that intensive control of the blood glucose improves the neuropathy suggests that the disease is a consequence of abnormal metabolism that damages the nerves.

The speed with which a nervous impulse travels down a nerve fiber is called the *nerve conduction velocity*. In diabetic neuropathy, the nerve conduction velocity (NCV) is slowed. This slowing may not be accompanied by any symptoms at first; testing the NCV provides a way of diagnosing neuropathy in people without symptoms. If a patient who has very mild symptoms takes medication to control neuropathy, the improvement that follows may be hard to detect except by doing a nerve conduction velocity study. Medication that helps the neuropathy is expected to speed up the NCV.

In addition to a persistently high blood glucose level, neuropathy is made worse by the following conditions:

- ✔ **Age:** Neuropathy is most common in people over 40.
- ✔ **Height:** Neuropathy is more common in taller individuals, who have longer nerve fibers to damage.
- ✔ **Alcohol consumption:** Even small quantities of alcohol can make neuropathy worse.

Doctors can test nerve function in a variety of ways because different nerve fibers seem to be responsible for different kinds of sensation, such as light touch, vibration, and temperature. The connection between the kind of test and the fiber it tests for is as follows:

- ✔ **Vibration testing:** Using a tuning fork, for example, can bring out abnormalities of large nerve fibers.
- ✔ **Temperature testing:** Uses a warm or cold item tests for damage to small fibers, which are very important in diabetes. When small fibers are damaged, the patient can lose the ability to feel that he is entering a burning hot bath, for instance.

✔ **Light touch testing:** Perhaps the most important test that is done reflects the large fibers, which sense anything touching the skin. This test is done using a filament that looks like a hair. The thickness of the filament determines how much force is needed to bend the filament so that it is felt. For example, a filament that bends with 1 gram of force can be felt by normal feet. If a patient can feel a filament that bends with 10 grams of force, the person is unlikely to suffer damage to the foot without feeling it. If the patient cannot feel any sensation with a filament that requires 75 grams of force to bend, that area is considered to have lost all sensation.

Either you or your doctor can use the 10-gram filament to discover whether you are at risk for damage to your feet because you cannot feel the pain. This test takes a minute to do and can save your feet from amputation. (See the section about the diabetic foot, later in this chapter.)

Disorders of sensation

Disorders of sensation are the most common and bothersome disorders of nerves in diabetes, because they are often associated with pain. They occur where the sensory nerves are damaged, and they include a number of different conditions that break down into two categories:

✔ **Diffuse neuropathies:** Involve many nerves

✔ **Focal neuropathies:** Involve one or several nerves

This section focuses on the diffuse neuropathies affecting sensation.

Distal polyneuropathy

Distal polyneuropathy is the most frequent form of diabetic neuropathy. *Distal* means far away from the center of the body — in other words, the feet and hands. *Poly* means many, and *neuropathy* is disease in nerves. So this disease concerns many nerves and is noticed in the feet and hands.

Physicians believe that distal polyneuropathy is a metabolic disease (a problem of too much glucose in the blood, specifically) because patients who have other diseases with a general abnormality of metabolism, such as kidney failure or vitamin deficiency, experience a distal polyneuropathy as well.

The signs and symptoms of distal polyneuropathy are

✔ Diminished ability to feel light touch (numbness) or feel the position of a foot, whether bent back or forward, resulting from the loss of the large fibers

✔ Diminished ability to feel pain and temperature from loss of small fibers

  ✔ Insignificant weakness

  ✔ Tingling and burning

  ✔ Extreme sensitivity to touch

  ✔ Loss of balance or coordination

  ✔ Worsening of symptoms at night

The danger of this kind of neuropathy is that the patient doesn't know, without looking, whether he has trauma to his feet, such as a burn or stepping on a tack. When the small fibers are lost, the symptoms are uncomfortable but not as serious. The patient may feel pain when the bed covers are on his feet or other uncomfortable sensations. The majority of patients with this condition are unaware of the loss of nerve fibers, and the disease is detected by nerve-conduction studies.

The complications of this loss of sensation are preventable. If you can't feel your feet, you must look at them. In the section on feet, later in this chapter, I offer specific techniques to preserve your feet when neuropathy is present.

The most serious complication of loss of sensation in the feet is the neuropathic foot ulcer. A person with normal nerve function feels pains when pressure mounts on an area of the foot. However, a person with diabetic neuropathy doesn't feel this pressure. A callus forms and, with continued pressure, the callus softens and liquefies, finally falling off to leave an ulcer. This ulcer becomes infected. If it isn't promptly treated, it spreads, and amputation may be the only way of saving the patient. In this situation, loss of blood supply to the feet is not an important contributing factor to the ulceration — in fact, the blood supply may be very good.

A less common complication in distal polyneuropathy is *neuroarthropathy,* or Charcot's Joint. In this condition, trauma, which isn't felt, occurs to the joints of the foot or ankle. The bones in the foot get out of line, and many painless fractures may occur. The patient has redness and painless swelling of the foot and ankle. The foot becomes unusable and is described as a bag of bones.

Treatment of distal polyneuropathy starts with the best glucose control possible and extremely good foot care. Your doctor should look at your feet during each visit, particularly if you have any evidence of loss of feeling.

Some drugs can help in various ways:

  ✔ Nonsteroidal anti-inflammatory agents, like ibuprofen and sulindac, can reduce the inflammation.

  ✔ Antidepressants, such as amitriptyline and imipramine, reduce the pain and other discomfort.

✔ Topical capsaicin creams reduce pain as well. The results of these treatments are variable and seem to work about 60 percent of the time. However, the longer the pain has been present and the worse the pain, the less likely these drugs are to work.

✔ A drug called *gabapentin* has been found to work more often than many of the older drugs, but it causes dizziness and sleepiness, which may make treatment more complicated.

✔ A spray of isosobide dinitrate may be helpful. According to a study in *Diabetes Care* in October 2002, the spray was effective in half of the patients treated for painful diabetic neuropathy.

✔ Alpha lipoic acid, which has to be injected into a vein, was very successful in improving pain and other symptoms in a large trial study. (The results were reported in *Diabetes Care* in March 2003.)

✔ Duloxetine (Cymbalta) has been effective for diabetic peripheral neuropathy in several clinical trials when compared to a placebo.

An even newer and apparently successful therapy called *Anodyne therapy* involves the placement of pads that emit an infrared light that increases circulation under the pad. In a study reported in *Diabetes Care* in January 2004, the treatment improved sensation in the feet, improved balance, and reduced pain in the treated foot compared to the untreated foot. Those patients who had the greatest impairment did not improve, however.

Polyradiculopathy-diabetic amyotrophy

Polyradiculopathy-diabetic amyotrophy is a mixture of pain and loss of muscle strength in the muscles of the upper leg so that the patient cannot straighten the knee. Pain extends down from the hip to the thigh. This nerve condition is second in occurrence after distal polyneuropathy in the diabetic population. Polyradiculopathy-diabetic amyotrophy generally has a short course but may continue for years and doesn't particularly improve with better diabetic control. Patients often improve only after the passage of time.

Radiculopathy nerve-root involvement

Sometimes a severe pain in a particular distribution suggests that the root of the nerve, as it leaves the spinal column, is damaged. The clinical picture is pain distributed in a horizontal line around one side of the chest or abdomen. The pain can be so severe that it is mistaken for an internal abdominal emergency. Fortunately, the pain goes away after a variable period of time — anywhere from 6 to 24 months. In the meantime, good glucose control and pain management are helpful.

Disorders of movement (mononeuropathy)

Neuropathy can affect nerves to various muscles. Disorders of movement occur when you lose motor nerves that carry the impulses to muscles to make those muscles move. When you lose those nerves, you lose the ability to move or use those muscles. These disorders are believed to originate as a result of the sudden closing of a blood vessel supplying the nerve. The clinical picture depends on which nerve or nerves are affected. If one of the nerves to the eyeball is damaged, the patient can't turn his eye to the side that nerve is on. If the nerve to the face is affected, the eyelid may droop or the smile on one side of the face may be flat. The patient can have trouble with vision or problems with hearing. Focusing the eye may not be possible. No treatment really exists, but fortunately the disorder goes away on its own after several months.

Disorders of automatic (autonomic) nerves

Even as you're reading this page, many movements of muscles are going on inside your body, but you're unaware of them. Your heart muscle is squeezing down and relaxing. Your diaphragm is rising up to empty the lungs of air and relaxing to draw air in. Your esophagus is carrying food from the mouth to the stomach and, in turn, the stomach pushes it into the small intestine, which pushes it into the large intestine. All these muscle functions are under the control of nerves from the brain, and diabetic neuropathy can affect all of them. These automatic functions are handled by the *autonomic nerves*. Sensitive tests determine that as many as 40 percent of people with diabetes have some form of autonomic neuropathy.

The clinical presentation of this type of neuropathy depends on the involved nerve. Following are some of the possibilities:

- ✔ **Bladder abnormalities, starting with a loss of the sensation of bladder fullness:** The urine is not eliminated, and urinary-tract infections result. After a while, loss of bladder contraction occurs, and the patient has to strain to urinate or loses urine by dribbling. The doctor can easily diagnose this abnormality by finding out how much urine is left in the bladder after urinating. The treatment is to remember to urinate every four hours or take a drug that increases the force of bladder contraction.

- ✔ **Sexual dysfunction, which occurs in 50 percent of males with diabetes and 30 percent of females with diabetes:** Males cannot sustain an erection, and females have trouble lubricating the vagina for intercourse. (See Chapter 6 for more information on these problems.)

- ✔ **Intestinal abnormalities of various kinds:** The most common abnormality is constipation. In one quarter of all patients with diabetes, nerves to the stomach are involved, so the stomach doesn't empty on time. This condition is called *gastroparesis*. It can lead to what's called *brittle diabetes*, where the insulin is active when there is no food. Fortunately, the drug metocloprimide helps to empty the stomach. A treatment that has worked well is the implantation of a device that stimulates the stomach electrically. It greatly diminishes the symptoms. This treatment was described in a report in *Diabetes Care* from the University of Kansas Medical Center in May 2004.

- **Involvement of the gallbladder, which leads to gallstones:** Normally, the gallbladder empties each time you eat, especially if you eat a fatty meal, because the substances in the bile (within the gallbladder) help to break down fat. If disease of the nerve to the gallbladder prevents it from emptying, these same substances form stones.

- **Involvement of the large intestine that can result in diabetic diarrhea with as many as ten or more bowel movements in a day:** Accidental loss of bowel contents can occur, and bacteria can grow abnormally in the intestine. This problem responds to antibiotic treatment. Diarrhea is treated with one of several drugs that quiet the large intestine.

- **Heart abnormalities:** If loss of nerves to the heart occurs, the heart may not respond to exercise by speeding up as it should. The force of the heart may not increase when the patient stands, and the patient then becomes lightheaded. A fast fixed heart rate also may occur, and the rhythm of the heart may not be normal. Such patients are at risk for sudden death.

- **Sweating problems, especially in the feet:** The body may try to compensate for the lack of sweating in the feet by sweating excessively on the face or trunk. Heavy sweating can occur when certain foods, such as cheese, are eaten.

- **Abnormalities of the pupil:** The pupil determines the amount of light let in by the eye. As a result of the neuropathy, the pupil is small and does not open up in a dark room.

Entrapment neuropathies

Entrapment neuropathies result from squeezing of individual nerves as they pass through bony or ligamentous areas. Those areas don't allow expansion, so the nerve is trapped if swelling takes place for any reason. The entrapment neuropathies can produce symptoms similar to the mononeuropathies described above, but they differ in several ways:

- Onset of mononeuropathies is sudden, whereas entrapment neuropathies have a gradual onset.

- Mononeuropathies are self-limited, usually resolving over six weeks, whereas entrapment neuropathies persist unless the nerve is released by surgery.

- Mononeuropathies are painful from the start, but entrapment neuropathies gradually get more and more painful.

Entrapment neuropathies are very common in people with diabetes, occurring in one in every three patients.

Following are the entrapment neuropathies:

- **Carpal tunnel syndrome:** Produces reduced sensation in the fingers and weakness touching the thumb to the fifth finger. The median nerve is trapped at the wrist.

- **Ulnar entrapment:** Produces reduced sensation in part of the fourth finger and the entire fifth finger as well as the hand between the fifth finger and the wrist. The ulnar nerve is trapped at the elbow.

- **Radial nerve entrapment:** Produces loss of sensation in the back of the hand and "wrist drop" from weakness of the muscles that straighten up the wrist. The radial nerve is trapped at the elbow.

- **Common peroneal entrapment:** Produces loss of sensation in the side of the leg and top of the foot and "drop foot" from weakness of the muscles that pull up the foot. The common peroneal nerve is trapped as it passes the head of the fibula, one of the two bones that begin at the knee joint and end at the ankle.

- **Tarsal tunnel syndrome:** Produces loss of sensation on both sides of the foot and wasting of the muscles of the foot, resulting in decreased toe movement. It's like carpal tunnel syndrome in the foot and results from trapping of the tibial nerve between two of the small foot bones.

- **Lateral femoral cutaneous nerve entrapment:** Produces loss of sensation on the outside of the thigh but no muscle weakness. It results from trapping of that nerve at the groin.

The entrapment neuropathies respond to rest, splints, drugs that promote water loss, injections of steroids, and surgery if necessary. The important thing is not to confuse them with mononeuropathies.

You can see that you can run into all kinds of problems if you develop diabetic neuropathy. None of them need ever bother you, though, if you follow the recommendations in Part III — the closest you will ever get to a nerve problem will be when you try to get a date with that cute neighbor.

Heart Disease

In the last three decades, the number of deaths due to heart disease has fallen dramatically, thanks to all kinds of new treatments as well as improved diets. However, the tremendous increase in the number of type 2 diabetes patients predicted for the next few decades may reverse this trend. In this section, you find out about the special problems that diabetes brings to the heart.

In the past, diabetic heart disease has been considered disease of the large blood vessels *(macroangiopathy)*. This sets it apart from eye, kidney, and nerve disease, which are considered diseases of the small blood vessels *(microangiopathy)*. This idea was strengthened by the fact that microangiopathy responds to good blood glucose control but macroangiopathy does not. More recently, doctors and researchers believe that both kinds of complications have much in common. The large blood vessels in the heart, brain, arms, and legs are affected by the same metabolic abnormalities (see the sidebar "How high glucose leads to complications," earlier in this chapter) and structural abnormalities that affect the small blood vessels.

Controlling the blood glucose, the blood fats, and the blood pressure early in the disease help to lessen or prevent coronary artery disease. Good evidence suggests that intensive control is not nearly as effective after an event such as a heart attack, stroke, or loss of blood flow to the leg has already occurred.

Risks of heart disease to diabetic patients

Coronary artery disease (CAD) is the term for the progressive closure of the arteries, which supply blood to the heart muscle. When one or more of your arteries closes completely, the result is a heart attack (or *myocardial infarction*). In diabetes, the incidence of CAD is increased even in the young type 1 patient. The duration of time with diabetes promotes CAD in type 1 patients. CAD affects males and females with type 1 diabetes in the same way.

Type 2 diabetes is different. CAD is the most common reason for death in type 2 patients. Women with type 2 are at increased risk for CAD compared to men. The following risk factors promote CAD in type 2 patients:

- ✔ **Increased production of insulin,** caused by insulin resistance.
- ✔ **Obesity.**
- ✔ **Central adiposity,** which refers to the distribution of fat, particularly in the waist area.
- ✔ **Hypertension** (high blood pressure).
- ✔ **Abnormal blood fats,** especially elevated LDL (bad) cholesterol. Decreased HDL (good cholesterol) appears to correlate with coronary heart disease as well, but the goal is to lower LDL. The abnormal fats may persist even when the patient's glucose is controlled. People without diabetes but with impaired glucose tolerance may show the same abnormalities.
- ✔ **Sitting time,** especially long stretches of inactivity, such as watching television for a long time.

People with diabetes have more CAD than people without diabetes. When X-ray studies of the heart blood vessels are compared, people with diabetes have more arteries involved than people without diabetes.

If a heart attack occurs, the risk of death is much greater for the person with diabetes. More than half of all people with diabetes die of heart attacks. If people without diabetes have heart attacks, they die 15 percent of the time, but people with diabetes die 40 percent of the time. The death rate is worse for people with diabetes who poorly controlled their glucose before the heart attack. The same poorly controlled people have more complications, such as shock and heart failure, from heart attacks than people without diabetes. After a heart attack occurs, the outlook is much worse for diabetic people. A second heart attack occurs in 50 percent of people with diabetes (as opposed to 25 percent of people without diabetes), and the death rate in five years is 80 percent (versus 25 percent for people without diabetes).

The picture is not a pretty one. The treatment options are the same for people with and without diabetes. Therapy to dissolve the clot of blood that is obstructing the coronary artery can be used, but people with diabetes don't do as well with *angioplasty,* the technique by which a tube is placed into the artery to clean it out and open it up. New techniques using certain chemicals in the tube are making this better therapy. People with diabetes do as well with surgery to bypass the obstruction (called *bypass surgery*) as people without diabetes, but the long-term prognosis for keeping the graft open is not as good.

It has been believed that red wine (but not white wine) is good for your heart. Recent studies suggest that white wine has substances that are heart healthy as well, and both have alcohol, which is healthy in moderate amounts (two drinks daily for men and one for women).

Although low-dose aspirin (81 milligrams) has been effective in protecting the heart of people without diabetes without preexisting heart disease, it has not been proven successful in preventing heart attack in people with diabetes. A higher dose may be needed.

Studies indicate that body-mass index is not a good predictor of heart attacks and death in obese diabetic patients. The waist in inches divided by the height in inches is the best predictor (a waist-to-height ratio under 0.5 is considered healthy), followed by the waist circumference (less than or equal to 40 inches in men and 35 inches in women is lower risk), followed by the waist-to-hip ratio (under 0.9 in men and 0.8 in women is healthy).

Metabolic syndrome

The earliest abnormality in type 2 diabetes is insulin resistance, which is found in people even before diabetes can be diagnosed. People with impaired glucose tolerance, and even 25 percent of the population with normal glucose tolerance, have evidence of insulin resistance. The condition, formerly known as the *insulin-resistance syndrome,* is now called the *metabolic syndrome.* It is particularly worrisome because it is being found in obese children and adolescents, resulting in greater danger of diabetes and an early heart attack in these children. The next 20 years will reveal how these risks play out.

Linking metabolic syndrome and insulin resistance

Several features accompany insulin resistance, which is associated with three times the incidence of coronary artery disease compared to people with normal insulin sensitivity:

- ✔ **Hypertension:** High blood pressure may be a consequence of the increased insulin required to keep the glucose normal when a patient is insulin resistant. When people are given insulin to control the glucose, a rise in blood pressure often occurs.

- ✔ **Abnormalities of blood fats:** The level of triglycerides is elevated, as is the amount of small, dense LDL (a particle in the blood that carries bad cholesterol). At the same time, you see a decline in the amount of HDL, the good cholesterol particle that helps to clean out the arteries.

- ✔ **Microalbuminuria:** The presence of microalbuminuria strongly correlates with the development of coronary artery disease. (See the section "Early indications of kidney disease," earlier in the chapter.)

- ✔ **C-reactive protein:** This marker for inflammation in the body (easily obtained by a blood test) rises as the severity of the metabolic syndrome increases. It indicates that inflammation plays an important role in coronary artery disease. The important role of inflammation is confirmed by the presence of inflammatory factors in the blood that come from fat tissue and that increase production of fats while they block glucose metabolism, as well as the presence of inflammatory cells that promote atherosclerosis in the arteries.

- ✔ **Increased plasminogen activator inhibitor-1:** This chemical, which blocks the activity of plasminogen activator, prevents the breakdown of blood clots that form in the arteries of the heart and other areas.

- ✔ **Increased abdominal visceral fat:** You can lose a lot of this fat, which is found at the waistline, by dieting and losing 5 to 10 percent of your body weight.

- ✔ **Obesity:** Many people with the metabolic syndrome are obese, but not all. Likewise, many people who are obese do not have the metabolic syndrome.

- ✔ **Sedentary lifestyle:** This feature is also often found, but an active lifestyle does not preclude the metabolic syndrome.

The preceding features, plus others, are found in people who have an increased tendency to have coronary artery disease and heart attacks. Keep in mind that the metabolic syndrome may be present even when diabetes is not. The metabolic syndrome is probably a primary abnormality and not a consequence of an elevated blood glucose over time.

When insulin resistance is present in diabetes, lowering the blood glucose may decrease the complications of a heart attack, which are related to high blood glucose. But lowering blood glucose does not impact the increased tendency to have a heart attack in the first place, which is not dependent on high blood glucose.

Finding out who's at risk

Metabolic syndrome is believed to be present in one-third of all Americans. Overweight males (with a BMI of 25 or greater) are six times as likely to have metabolic syndrome, and obese males (BMI of 30 or greater) were 32 times as likely.

The metabolic syndrome is present when three or more of the following conditions are present:

- Waist circumference in men greater than 102 cm and in women greater than 88 cm
- Fasting triglyceride greater than or equal to 150 mg/dl
- Blood pressure greater than or equal to 130/85
- HDL cholesterol less than or equal to 40 in men and 50 in women
- Fasting glucose greater than or equal to 110 mg/dl
- Abnormal glucose tolerance (glucose level of 140–199 two hours after 75 gm of glucose)

People who are at the top of the normal weight curve and slightly overweight have also been found to have the metabolic syndrome. You don't have to be obese.

Unexpectedly, people who consume diet sodas daily have been found to have an increased risk of metabolic syndrome and type 2 diabetes. The explanation is not known.

Although alcohol consumption up to the daily guideline of one drink for women and two drinks for men may be protective against heart disease, drinking more than that or binge drinking one or more days per week is associated with an increased risk of metabolic syndrome and its complication of heart disease.

Treating metabolic syndrome

A number of treatments are available for the metabolic syndrome. If you are obese and have a sedentary lifestyle, you should correct these problems. Even a small amount of weight loss or exercise can make a major contribution toward decreasing the risk of a heart attack. An exercise training program has reversed metabolic syndrome in 30 percent of patients.

Many features of the metabolic syndrome are dependent on an abnormal blood glucose. Restriction of carbohydrates reverses these features, including elevated triglyceride, elevated blood pressure, reduced HDL cholesterol, fasting glucose, and glucose tolerance.

You can treat elevated triglyceride and reduced HDL with drugs such as the class called *fibric-acid derivatives* as well as niacin.

Use of the DASH (Dietary Approach to Stop Hypertension) diet, which was developed to control high blood pressure, can also be helpful in reversing the features of the metabolic syndrome. It consists of mostly fruits and vegetables and can be found extensively discussed in my book *High Blood Pressure For Dummies* (Wiley).

Studies have found that there is variability in the prevalence of metabolic syndrome by occupation. Food preparation and food service workers have the highest risk. About 30 percent of them have been found to have the metabolic syndrome. The groups of writers, artists, entertainers, athletes, engineers, architects, and scientists have the lowest risk, at about 9 percent.

Cardiac autonomic neuropathy

I discuss cardiac autonomic neuropathy briefly in the section on neuropathy earlier in this chapter. Basically, the heart is under the control of nerves, and high glucose levels can damage these nerves. Your doctor can test for this condition in a number of ways:

- **Measure the resting heart rate:** It may be abnormally high (greater than 100).

- **Measure the standing blood pressure:** It may fall abnormally low (a decrease of 20 mm sustained for 3 minutes) compared to the sitting blood pressure.

- **Measure the variation in heart rate when the patient breathes in compared to breathing out:** The variation may be abnormally low (under 10).

The presence of cardiac autonomic neuropathy results in a diminished survival even among patients who don't have coronary artery disease.

Cardiomyopathy

Cardiomyopathy refers to an enlarged heart and scarring of the heart muscle in the absence of coronary artery disease. As a result, the heart does not pump enough blood with each stroke. The patient may be able to compensate by a more rapid heart rate, but if hypertension is present, a stable condition can deteriorate.

The key treatment in this condition is control of the blood pressure as well as control of the blood glucose. Studies in animals in which diabetic cardiomyopathy has been induced have shown healing by controlling the blood glucose.

Diabetic Blood Vessel Disease Away from the Heart

The same processes that affect the coronary arteries can affect the arteries to the brain, producing cerebrovascular disease, and the arteries to the rest of the body, producing peripheral vascular disease. I explain each condition in the following sections.

Peripheral vascular disease

Peripheral vascular disease (PVD) occurs much earlier in people with diabetes and proceeds more rapidly. This clogging of the arteries to parts of your body other than the heart and brain results in the loss of pulses in the feet; after ten years of diabetes, a third of men and women no longer feel a pulse in their feet. The most common symptom of PVD is intermittent pain in the calves, thighs, or buttocks that begins after some walking and subsides with rest. People with PVD have a reduction in life expectancy. When PVD occurs, just as when CAD occurs, it is much worse in people with diabetes because more of their arteries are involved.

The major screening test for peripheral vascular disease is the ankle-brachial index (ABI). The systolic blood pressure in the ankle is divided by the systolic blood pressure in the arm. A result of 0.95 or greater is normal. A result of less than 0.75 suggests serious peripheral vascular disease. Some people with diabetes have a lot of calcium in their arteries and get a higher blood pressure in the ankle than the arm. If the ABI is more than 1 and the systolic blood pressure in the ankle is more than 300 mm mercury or 75 greater than the arm, this condition also suggests PVD.

An ABI in a person with diabetes that is less than 0.9 is associated with a much higher risk of death from a heart attack according to a study published in *Diabetes Care* in March 2006.

In addition to diabetes, certain risk factors increase the severity of PVD. The following risk factors are unavoidable:

- **Genetic factors:** PVD is more common in some families and certain ethnic groups, especially African Americans.

- **Age:** The risk of PVD increases as you age.

WARNING!

Smoking and diabetes

As we all know, smoking has a number of ill effects on people without diabetes, but the effects are even worse in people with diabetes. Among other things, smoking has the following consequences:

✔ Reducing blood flow in arteries and blocking increased flow when it is needed

✔ Increasing pain in the legs in people with peripheral vascular disease and in the heart in people with coronary artery disease

✔ Increasing *atheromatous plaques,* the changes in arteries in the heart and other areas (like the brain and the legs) that precede closing of the blood vessels

✔ Increasing clustering of *platelets,* the blood elements that form a plug or clot that blocks the artery

✔ Increasing blood pressure, which also worsens atheromatous plaques

These problems don't even take into account the effects of smoking on the lungs, the bladder, and the rest of the body.

The following risk factors are within your control:

✔ Smoking, which promotes early foot amputation

✔ Hypercholesterolemia (high cholesterol)

✔ High glucose

✔ Hypertension

✔ Obesity

In addition to controlling the preceding factors as much as possible, you may need to take drugs that help prevent closure of the arteries and loss of blood supply. Aspirin, which inhibits clotting, is among the most useful. Pentoxifylline (Trental) improves the circulation of cells in the blood. In addition, exercise improves blood flow and promotes the development of blood vessels around an obstruction. If none of these measures reverses the symptoms, some form of surgery that opens or bypasses the blocked arteries may be necessary.

Cerebrovascular disease

Cerebrovascular disease (CVD) is a disease of the arteries that supply the brain with oxygen and nutrients. What I say about peripheral vascular disease in the preceding section also covers cerebrovascular disease, with some exceptions. The risk factors and the approach to treatment are similar.

However, the symptoms are very different because the clogged arteries in CVD supply the brain.

If a temporary reduction in blood supply to the brain occurs, the person suffers from a *transient ischemic attack,* or TIA. This temporary loss of brain function may present itself as slurring of speech, weakness on one side of the body, or numbness. TIA may disappear after a few minutes, but it comes back again some hours to days later. If a major artery to the brain completely closes, the person suffers a stroke. Fortunately, stroke victims who are seen soon enough after the stroke can take advantage of clot-dissolving materials.

People with diabetes are at increased risk for CVD just as they are for PVD. Their disease tends to be worse than the disease in a person without diabetes, and they can have blockage in many small blood vessels in the brain that leads to the loss of intellectual function, a symptom similar to Alzheimer's disease.

The treatable risk factors for CVD are the same as those for PVD (see the preceding section). You should make attempts to improve them, particularly high blood pressure.

Diabetic Foot Disease

If I ever have an opportunity to save people from the consequences of diabetes, it's in this section of the book. About 70,000 amputations occur in the United States each year, and more than half of them are done on people with diabetes. Despite the wonderful surgery to bring more blood into the feet, the number of amputations is actually rising.

Good medical care can prevent amputations. Your doctor should look at your feet as routinely as he or she measures your weight.

In the section on neuropathy, earlier in this chapter, I point out that a filament that requires a pressure of 10 grams to be felt can differentiate a patient who will not suffer damage to the feet under normal walking conditions from a patient who will. All doctors who have patients with diabetes should have this filament to test the feet at least annually. Even better, you should have your own filament and test yourself any time you feel like it. If you can't feel the filament, you had better start looking at your feet every day. See Chapter 7 for where to obtain a filament.

If your feet are dry, you may have loss of sweating. Loss of sweating is usually accompanied by the loss of touch sensation and the development of ulcers. You need to moisturize your feet, first by soaking them in water (which you test with your hand for its temperature), and then by drying them with a towel and applying a moisturizer. Soaking should always be accompanied by drying and moisturizing.

Ulcers of the foot can develop in a number of ways:

- ✔ Constant pressure
- ✔ Sudden higher pressure
- ✔ Constantly repeated moderate pressure

It takes very little pressure, if constantly applied, to damage the skin. If you have diminished sensation, some of the following tips may save your feet:

- ✔ Change your shoes about every five hours.
- ✔ If you have new shoes, change them every two hours at first. Your shoes should not be too tight or too loose.
- ✔ Never walk barefoot.
- ✔ Shake out your shoes before you put them on.
- ✔ Inspect your feet daily, with a mirror if necessary.
- ✔ Do not use a heating pad on your feet.
- ✔ Stop smoking. If you smoke, you are asking for an amputation.

If you do develop an ulcer, the treatment is to take pressure off the site by resting the foot and elevating it. When the infection is localized in a foot with adequate blood supply, a plaster cast is applied to overcome the natural tendency to want to stand or walk. The cast protects the ulcer from slight trauma that could prevent healing.

A product called becaplermin (trade name Regranex Gel) has been shown to speed the healing of deep diabetic foot ulcers when it is combined with good wound care. (Good wound care means carefully removing dead tissue and keeping your weight off the ulcer, along with treating any infection and controlling your blood glucose.) The product is applied to a clean wound bed once daily. You should see significant reduction in the size of the ulcer within 10 weeks and complete healing by 20 weeks. The long duration for healing is a problem, because Regranex Gel is very expensive. However, a typical deep diabetic ulcer is very expensive to treat in any case, and if this product can speed up your healing, it may be worthwhile.

I must reiterate that ulcers of the foot, which can lead to amputation in people with diabetes, are entirely preventable. If your feet lack sensation, your doctor must examine them at every visit, and you must examine them daily. At the first sign of a problem, take appropriate action.

Skin Disease in Diabetes

Many conditions involving the skin are unique to diabetic people because of the treatment and complications of the disease. Following are the most common and important skin complications:

- Bruises occur due to the cutting of blood vessels by the insulin needle.

- *Vitiligo* (loss of skin pigmentation) is part of the autoimmune aspect of type 1 diabetes and cannot be prevented.

- *Necrobiosis lipoidica,* which also affects people without diabetes, creates patches of reddish-brown skin on the shins or ankles, and the skin becomes thin and can ulcerate. Females tend to have this condition more often than males. Steroid injections are used to treat this condition, and the areas eventually become depressed and brown.

- *Xanthelasma,* which are small yellow flat areas called *plaques* on the eyelids, occur even when cholesterol is not elevated.

- *Alopecia,* or loss of hair, occurs in type 1 diabetes, but the cause is unknown.

- *Insulin hypertrophy* is the accumulation of fatty tissue where insulin is injected. This condition is prevented by moving the injection site around.

- *Insulin lipoatrophy* is the loss of fat where the insulin is injected. Although the cause is unknown, this condition is rarely seen now that human insulin has replaced beef and pork insulin (see Chapter 10).

- Dry skin is a consequence of diabetic neuropathy, which leads to a lack of sweating.

- Fungal infections occur under the nails or between the toes. Fungus likes moisture and elevated glucose. Lowering your glucose and keeping your toes dry prevent these infections. Medications may cure this problem, but it recurs if glucose and moisture are not managed.

- *Acanthosis nigricans,* a velvety-feeling increase in pigmentation on the back of the neck and the armpits, causes no problems and needs no treatment. This condition is usually found when insulin resistance exists. It is seen in adults and children with type 2 diabetes.

- Diabetic thick skin, which is thicker than normal skin, occurs in people who have had diabetes for more than ten years.

Gum Disease in Diabetes

The major problem that people with diabetes may have in their mouths is gum disease. This problem develops because the higher concentration of glucose in the mouth promotes the growth of germs, which mix with food and saliva to form plaque on your gums. If you don't brush your teeth twice a day and floss your teeth once a day, the plaque may harden into tarter, which is very hard for you to remove. The gums may develop gingivitis, becoming brittle and bleeding easily. You may experience pain and bad breath, and eventually the gums may become so weakened that they cannot support your teeth.

Controlling your blood glucose is a key step in preventing gum disease. Visiting your dentist for routine cleanings of your teeth twice a year is another important way to keep your gums healthy. Interestingly, people with diabetes do not seem to develop cavities more often than people who do not have the disease.

Sleep Apnea

Sleep apnea is another complication of obesity, and it can lead to metabolic syndrome and type 2 diabetes. Sleep apnea is characterized by recurrent episodes, lasting 10 to 30 second each, of failure to breathe while asleep. These episodes are due to obstruction of the airway or nerve disturbances. As many as 60 to 90 episodes may occur per hour, during which the oxygen saturation of the blood drops to as low as 50 percent (normal is greater than 95 percent).

In a study of over 300 patients with type 2 diabetes and obesity, over 86 percent of the patients had obstructive sleep apnea. Waist circumference was a key indicator of obstructive sleep apnea.

Sleep apnea makes the patient very sleepy the next day, which results in slow reactions, poor memory and concentration, and irritability. Sleep apnea also causes increased blood pressure and increased insulin resistance by unclear mechanisms. Sleep apnea increases the risk of heart disease. The reduction in oxygen in the blood may also increase damage to the kidneys, leading to nephropathy. Finally, the severity of the sleep apnea correlates with the severity of poor glucose control.

When obstructive sleep apnea is due to upper airway obstruction, it can be improved or even cured by treating an underlying condition such as low thyroid function or a tumor of the pituitary gland producing excessive growth hormone (acromegaly) if this is present. Maintaining weight loss may improve the obstructive sleep apnea. If not, then a positive pressure device worn on the face, a CPAP machine, should greatly improve the condition; unfortunately, many patients find it uncomfortable.

Chapter 6

Diabetes, Sexual Function, and Pregnancy

In This Chapter

▶ Treating impotence caused by diabetes

▶ Dealing with female sexual problems

▶ Coping with diabetes in pregnancy

▶ Recognizing polycystic ovarian syndrome

*N*othing is quite so pleasant as walking into the hospital room of a mother with diabetes holding her healthy newborn. Pregnancy associated with diabetes used to be a disaster for both the baby and the mother. No longer. With the proper precautions, diabetic pregnancies can proceed like pregnancies without diabetes. This chapter describes everything you need to know from start to finish, including overcoming obstacles to intercourse, enjoying a healthy pregnancy, and delivering a healthy baby.

Men with diabetes have sexual problems as well. Fortunately, they are manageable, so I get started here with their issues.

Examining Erection Problems

If carefully questioned, up to 50 percent of all males with diabetes admit to having difficulty with sexual function. This difficulty usually takes the form of *erectile dysfunction (ED),* the inability to have or sustain an erection sufficient for intercourse. It develops 10 to 15 years earlier in men with diabetes than in men without diabetes. After the age of 70, more than 95 percent of men with diabetes have erectile dysfunction. Many factors besides diabetes can cause the same problem, and you should rule them out before blaming diabetes.

After you eliminate the following possibilities for erectile dysfunction, you can feel confident that diabetes is the source of the problem:

✔ Trauma to the penis

✔ Medications, such as certain antihypertensives and antidepressants

✔ Hormonal abnormalities, such as insufficient production of the male hormone testosterone or overproduction of a hormone from the brain called *prolactin*

✔ Poor blood supply to the penis due to blockage of the artery by peripheral vascular disease (see Chapter 5), which can be treated very effectively by microvascular surgery

✔ *Psychogenic impotence,* an inability to have an erection for psychological rather than physical reasons (this problem should be managed by a therapist)

In order to understand how diabetes affects an erection, you need to first understand how an erection is normally produced.

Reviewing the erection process

As a result of some form of stimulation — such as touch, sight, or sound — the brain activates nerves in the *parasympathetic nervous system,* which is part of the autonomic nervous system. These nerves cause muscles to relax so that blood flow into the penis greatly increases. As blood flow increases, the veins through which blood leaves the penis compress, and the penis becomes erect. An erect penis contains about 11 times as much blood as a flaccid penis. With sufficient stimulation, muscles contract, propelling semen through the *urethra* (the tube in the penis that normally carries urine from the bladder) to the outside of the body. The pleasant sensation that occurs along with the muscle contractions *(ejaculation)* is called *orgasm.*

Orgasm and ejaculation are the result of stimulation by the other side of the autonomic nervous system, the sympathetic nervous system. As the stimulation causes contraction of the muscles, it closes the muscle over the bladder so that urine does not normally accompany expulsion of semen and the semen does not go back into the bladder.

Diabetes can damage the parasympathetic nervous system so that the male can't get an erection sufficient for sexual intercourse. The sympathetic nervous system is spared, so ejaculation and orgasm can occur, but intercourse may be unpleasant for both partners because of the psychological consequence of not being able to sustain a firm erection.

For diabetes patients, ED is affected by the following factors:

- **Degree of control of the blood glucose:** Better control is associated with fewer problems.
- **Duration of the diabetes:** The longer you have diabetes, the more likely you are to be unable to have an erection.
- **Interaction with your partner:** A positive relationship is important.
- **Use of drugs, tobacco, or alcohol:** Each may prevent erections.
- **State of mind:** A positive frame of mind is associated with successful erections.

Discussing ED with your doctor

Although sexual intercourse tends to be an embarrassing topic for many men and women, if you have diabetes and have a problem in this key area of life, you need to discuss it with your doctor. Some doctors find this topic just as embarrassing as some patients. Any doctor who treats patients with diabetes should bring the topic up (no pun intended) in the first meeting and annually thereafter. If he or she does not, you should broach the subject yourself.

Erectile dysfunction has been shown to predict coronary artery disease in men with type 2 diabetes. Diabetics with ED who had heart attacks were older and had higher blood pressure, higher total cholesterol, lower HDL cholesterol, and longer duration of diabetes. This fact makes it especially important to discuss the problem with your doctor. In men with erectile dysfunction, the occurrence of heart attacks has been reduced with the use of statins and sildenafil, vardenafil, or tadalafil (see the later section "Viagra and similar medications").

Treating for erectile dysfunction

Fortunately for men with diabetes with erectile dysfunction, numerous approaches to treatment exist, beginning with drugs, continuing with external devices to create an erection, and ending with implantable devices that provide a very satisfactory erection. Treatment is successful in 90 percent or more of men, but only 5 percent ever discuss the problem with their doctors. The following sections discuss these treatment options.

Viagra and similar medications

Sildenafil (Viagra) has been specifically studied in males with diabetes and is successful in 70 percent of patients.

Sildenafil doesn't seem to affect diabetic control, but it isn't free of side effects. Some men experience headaches, facial flushing, or indigestion, which generally decline with continued use of the drug. It has also been found to cause a temporary color tinge to a man's vision as well as increased sensitivity to light and blurred vision. These side effects also decline with continued use of the drug.

Sildenafil is taken no more than once a day, about an hour before sexual activity. While the starting dose is 50 milligrams for men, when diabetes is present, 100 mg is often required. The drug itself doesn't cause erections; an erection occurs only as a result of some kind of sexual stimulation. But it does prevent an erection from subsiding, so it lasts longer. The effects of sildenafil can last for four to six hours after taking it.

Pfizer, which makes Viagra, could not expect to have the playing field to itself for very long, given that the game is something most men want to play. Bayer Pharmaceuticals and GlaxoSmithKline have now brought vardenafil (Levitra) to the marketplace. Its characteristics are very similar to Viagra but the starting dosage is 10 mg, which probably means 20 mg for men with diabetes. Vardenafil is also marketed as Staxyn.

Eli Lilly and ICOS Corporation market tadalafil (Cialis), which works like sildenafil and vardenafil but stays active for 36 hours. In addition, its onset of action is 20 minutes, half the time of the competing drugs. Cialis has been nicknamed the "weekender pill" because it permits spontaneous sexual activity from Friday to Sunday. The starting dose for Cialis is 10 mg, but, again, men with diabetes may need to start at twice that amount. Some patients take 2.5 to 5.0 mg daily without regard to sexual activity.

Some men must not take any of these three drugs. Men who have chest pain often take nitrate drugs, the most common of which is nitroglycerine. The combination of sildenafil and nitrates may cause a significant and possibly fatal drop in blood pressure. Great care must be taken if the patient is on one of the blood pressure drugs called *alpha blockers* for the same reason. Common alpha blockers are doxazosin (Cardura), prazosin (Minipress), and tamsulosin (Flomax).

A very small number of cases have been reported of one-sided hearing loss in men who took any of the above drugs.

Injection into the penis

The patient himself can use an injection to create an erection. It is called alprostadil (Caverject or Edex), a chemical that relaxes the blood vessels in the penis to allow more flow. Alprostadil does not require sexual stimulation in order to work.

The drug is injected about 30 minutes before intercourse and no more than once in 24 hours and three times per week. An injection gives a full erection lasting about an hour in 85 to 95 percent of men, except for those who have the most severe loss of blood flow to the penis.

Complications of injections are rare but include bruising, pain, and the formation of nodules at the injection site. A very rare complication is *priapism,* where the penis maintains its erection for many hours. If the erection lasts more than four hours, the patient must see his doctor to get an injection of a *vasoconstrictor,* a drug that squeezes down the arteries into the penis so that blood flow is interrupted.

Suppository in the penis

Alprostadil — the chemical that can be injected into the penis — also comes in a suppository form. The patient inserts a tube containing this small pill into the opening of the penis after urination. When the tube is fully in the opening, the man squeezes the top so that the pill exits the tube. This preparation, called Muse, comes in several different strengths so that patients can use a higher dose if the lower dose does not result in a satisfactory erection. It may safely be used twice in 24 hours. A few men experience pain with this procedure. Sexual stimulation is unnecessary to achieve an erection.

Vacuum-constriction devices

Vacuum-constriction tubes, which fit over the penis, create a closed space when pressed against the patient's body. A pump draws out the air in the tube, and blood rushes into the penis to replace the air. When the penis is erect, a rubber band is placed around the base of the penis to keep the blood inside it. Sometimes pain and numbness of the penis occur. Because a rubber band is constricting the penis, semen does not get through, so conception can't take place. The rubber band may be kept on for up to 30 minutes.

Implanted penile prostheses

If the patient doesn't like the idea of injecting himself in his penis or using a vacuum device, and if pills don't work for him, a *prosthesis* (an artificial substitute) can be implanted in the penis to give an erection. Prostheses come in several varieties. A semi-rigid type produces a permanent erection, but some men do not like the inconvenience of a permanent erection. An inflatable prosthesis involves a pump in the scrotal sac that contains fluid. The pump can be squeezed to transfer the fluid into balloons in the penis to stiffen it. When not pumped up, the penis appears normally soft. In the past few years, the surgery to insert these prostheses has become very satisfactory.

Facing Female Sexual Problems

Sexual dysfunction in women is not as visually obvious as it is in men. But as many as half of women with diabetes have problems with sexual function, and the problems can be just as difficult to handle as they are for men. The following problems are associated with diabetes:

- Dry mouth and dry vagina because of the high blood glucose
- Irregular menstrual function when the diabetes is out of control
- Yeast infections of the vagina that make intercourse unpleasant
- A feeling of being fat and unattractive because type 2 diabetes is usually associated with obesity
- Discomfort about discussing the problem with a partner or physician
- Loss of bladder control due to a neurogenic bladder (see Chapter 5)
- A reduction in estrogen secretion and associated vaginal thinning and dryness due to increasing age made worse by the diabetes

Menopause can cause several of the same difficulties as diabetes-related sexual dysfunction, particularly the dry vagina and irregular menstrual function. You must rule out menopause before assuming that diabetes is the source of the problem.

A female with long-standing diabetes may have several other problems that are specific to her sexual organs. These problems include

- **Reduced lubrication because of parasympathetic nerve involvement:** Lubrication serves to permit easier entry of the penis, but it also increases the sensitivity of the vagina to touch, thus increasing pleasant sensations.
- **Reduced blood flow because of diabetic blood vessel disease:** Some of the lubrication comes from fluid within the blood vessels.
- **Loss of skin sensation around the vaginal area:** This loss reduces pleasure.

Most women who have problems with lubrication, whether due to diabetes or menopause, medicate themselves with over-the-counter preparations. These preparations fall into three categories:

- Water-based lubricants, like K-Y jelly and In Pursuit of Passion, which are probably the easiest to use and clean up
- Oil-based lubricants, like vegetable oils
- Petroleum-based lubricants, which are not recommended because of the possibility of bacterial infection

Estrogen, which can be taken by mouth or placed in the dry vagina in suppository form, also may be useful for menopausal women.

When psychological or interpersonal issues exist, a discussion with a therapist, the use of antidepressant medications (some of which can dry the vagina, by the way), and sex therapy with your partner are important steps to take to improve sexual pleasure.

Striving for a Healthy Pregnancy

About 0.4 percent of pregnancies occur in women with preexisting diabetes, called *pregestational diabetes,* and an additional 2 to 4 percent occur in women who develop diabetes sometime in the second half of the pregnancy, called *gestational diabetes.* Four million births occur in the United States annually, and diabetes affects 100,000 or more pregnancies each year.

If you have diabetes and want to become pregnant, you need to talk with an expert in pregnancy and diabetes before you conceive. In the following sections, I explain potential complications you may experience and some steps you should take to ensure the healthiest pregnancy possible.

Realizing the body's reaction to pregnancy

During pregnancy, hormones block insulin action. In a nondiabetic pregnancy, the woman's body makes enough insulin to overcome this effect, and her blood glucose stays normal. But a woman with type 1 diabetes can't make more insulin, and during pregnancy she needs two or three times her usual dose to counteract the effect of her hormones (although in the early first trimester, her insulin needs may decrease). This increased need for insulin in a woman with type 1 diabetes usually begins in the second trimester and stabilizes in the last several weeks of the pregnancy; by the last one or two weeks, the mother-to-be may actually begin to have hypoglycemia. After the baby and the placenta are delivered, her insulin needs plummet immediately.

A woman with type 1 or type 2 diabetes may have some retinopathy (see Chapter 5) before she becomes pregnant. If the condition is severe, her eyes may deteriorate during the pregnancy. The deterioration probably results from rapid improvement of blood glucose control in a woman who has been poorly controlled previously. If glucose control is improved or if laser photocoagulation (see Chapter 5) is carried out before the pregnancy, this deterioration does not take place. After the baby is delivered, her eyes will return to their previous state.

To find out much more about pregnancy in the woman with type 1 diabetes, check out my book *Type 1 Diabetes For Dummies* (Wiley).

If you're thinking about becoming pregnant and you have diabetes-related eye disease, that condition must be stabilized before you try to conceive.

Kidney disease, or *nephropathy* (see Chapter 5), increases the danger of complications of pregnancy for both the mother and baby. Severe, permanent worsening of the nephropathy is unusual as a result of pregnancy, but a temporary decline in kidney function in the mother may occur. The baby may have to be delivered early and may suffer some growth retardation.

Being proactive before and during pregnancy

You can take a number of steps both before and during the pregnancy to ensure a healthy baby and an uncomplicated pregnancy.

Getting your health in order

You must take action in advance to avoid potential problems by controlling your glucose before conception. (See Part III for more on how to manage your diabetes.) In addition, you need to monitor your diet after you become pregnant.

Following are some other key steps you should take to improve your chances of a problem-free pregnancy:

- ✔ **Lose weight.** Obesity, which is prevalent in type 2 patients, puts a mom-to-be at greater risk for hypertension during pregnancy.

- ✔ **Quit smoking.** Children of mothers who smoke during pregnancy are at much greater risk of developing obesity and diabetes later in life, not to mention numerous other health problems.

- ✔ **Use insulin for glucose control.** If you have type 2 diabetes and are taking oral agents to lower your glucose, you need to switch to insulin to control your glucose during pregnancy.

- ✔ **Control your blood pressure.** Elevated blood pressure before and during early pregnancy is associated with increased risk of gestational diabetes mellitus.

For more detailed information about what to do during pregnancy, see the section "Treating diabetes during pregnancy," later in the chapter.

Most diabetic pregnancies can be allowed to go to term at 39 weeks. However, if the mother-to-be has hypertension or a previous history of delivery problems, her doctor may advocate earlier delivery.

Taking special precautions if you've had bariatric surgery

Many more adolescents and young women are having bariatric surgery (see Chapter 8) to treat diabetes. They become pregnant at twice the rate of the general population after the surgery. These young women need to take the following precautions:

✔ Wait a year or two after surgery to conceive so that the growing fetus is not exposed to rapid weight loss in the mother.

✔ Be closely monitored for nutritional status and the fetus's growth (especially at the beginning of the pregnancy) if conception occurs earlier than a year or two after surgery.

✔ Consult with a nutritionist.

✔ If contraception is desired, use a method other than oral drugs because of malabsorption.

✔ Be tested for gestational diabetes. The surgery usually reduces the risk for high blood pressure, which makes any pregnancy more complicated, and the blood glucose often returns to normal. The usual tests can't be done in the patient with bariatric surgery because of the abnormal absorption. Monitoring the blood glucose at different times of day may be helpful (see Chapter 7).

Diagnosing gestational diabetes

The current consensus is to screen all women because a small but significant number of patients with gestational diabetes will be missed if all women are not screened.

Everyone agrees that if your glucose tolerance is normal in weeks 27 to 31 of the pregnancy, you don't need to do more screening. If you experienced gestational diabetes during a previous pregnancy, the screening test is done much earlier — as early as the 13th week. Other reasons for earlier screening are

✔ Previous delivery of a large baby

✔ Obesity

✔ Glucose in the urine

✔ Close family members with diabetes

The screening test is done between weeks 24 and 28 of the pregnancy. No preparation is necessary. You consume 50 grams of glucose, and a blood glucose level is obtained from a vein one hour later. If the glucose level is less than 140, it's considered normal. If it's greater than 140, a further test is done before making a diagnosis of gestational diabetes, because many women who have a value greater than 140 do not necessarily have diabetes. The definitive test is a glucose tolerance test (see Chapter 2). A diagnosis of gestational diabetes is made if two or more of the samples exceed these levels:

- ✔ **Before consuming glucose:** 95 mg/dl (5.3 mmol/L)
- ✔ **One hour after consuming glucose:** 180mg/dl (10.0 mmol/L)
- ✔ **Two hours after:** 155 mg/dl (8.6 mmol/L)
- ✔ **Three hours after:** 140 mg/dl (7.8 mmol/L)

Recognizing risks to mother and baby

Whether you have diabetes before pregnancy or develop gestational diabetes, you face many considerations regarding your own health and the health of your baby.

Persistently high blood glucose left untreated has major consequences for both mother and fetus. If high glucose is present early in the pregnancy, the result may be miscarriage or *congenital malformations* (physical abnormalities that may be life threatening) in the fetus. In the third trimester, the growing fetus may exhibit *macrosomia* (abnormal largeness) that can lead to an early delivery or damage to the baby or mother during delivery. Neonatal hypoglycemia and stillbirth are also risks of high glucose.

Babies develop normally if their fathers have diabetes but their mothers don't. The environment in which the fetus is developing is responsible for the potential abnormalities. Elevated blood glucose, abnormalities of proteins and fats that result from the elevated glucose, and the loss of sensitivity to insulin explain the problems.

Measuring the risks

The hemoglobin A1c (see Chapter 7) is an excellent measurement of overall glucose control and provides a good indicator for the risk of miscarriage. If a pregnant woman's hemoglobin A1c is high, it indicates that she was in poor glucose control at conception, and the likelihood of a miscarriage is greater. If overall glucose control is normal, the baby of the woman with diabetes is no more likely to be miscarried than that of a woman without diabetes.

The situation for congenital malformations is a little more complicated. The occurrence of these malformations rises with increasing glucose, but the level of *ketones* (the breakdown product of fats) also impacts their occurrence. However, measuring the ketones doesn't tell you if malformations will definitely occur.

Why macrosomia occurs

Macrosomia, or abnormal largeness in a fetus, has to do with the elevated glucose, fat, and amino acid levels in the second half of pregnancy for a mother with diabetes. If these levels aren't lowered, the fetus is exposed to high levels. The high levels, especially of glucose, stimulate the fetal pancreas to begin to make insulin earlier and to store these extra nutrients. The fetus becomes large wherever fat is stored, such as in the shoulders, chest, abdomen, arms, and legs. Because they are large, macrosomic babies are delivered early in order to make the delivery easier and avoid birth trauma. However, though they are large, they are not fully mature.

Early pregnancy problems

Miscarriages and congenital malformations can result from poor glucose control at conception and shortly thereafter. Both high blood glucose and low blood glucose can induce malformations. (For more on managing diabetes, see Part III.)

However, a woman in poor control of her diabetes has more trouble conceiving a baby than a woman with good glucose control, which may be the major reason that more babies aren't born with congenital malformations.

Unlike diabetes that occurs before pregnancy, gestational diabetes mellitus does not cause congenital malformations. In gestational diabetes, blood glucose doesn't start to rise until halfway through the pregnancy, long after the baby's important body structures are formed.

Late pregnancy problems

A baby is considered large if it weighs more than 4 kilograms or 8.8 pounds at birth. Keep in mind that most large babies are the healthy offspring of mothers without diabetes. Their growth is proportional throughout the pregnancy, so their shoulders aren't out of proportion to their heads and delivery isn't complicated.

However, women with pregestational diabetes or gestational diabetes need to be concerned about having a baby whose largeness is not proportional. The areas that are most responsive to insulin, where fat is stored in the baby, are the ones that enlarge the most. (See the sidebar "Why macrosomia occurs" for more information.)

Treating diabetes during pregnancy

You need to achieve a stricter level of glucose control during pregnancy than when you aren't pregnant. Your fetus is removing glucose from you at a rapid rate, so your blood glucose level is lower than usual. In addition, your body turns to fat for fuel much sooner, so you produce ketones earlier. Too many ketones can damage the fetus as well. The fact that you break down fat so early is termed *accelerated starvation.*

Monitoring your glucose and ketones

In order to maintain your blood glucose at the proper level, you must measure it more frequently. You should measure it before meals, at bedtime, and occasionally one hour after eating. Your goal is to achieve the following levels of blood glucose:

- ✔ **Fasting and premeal:** Less than 90 mg/dl (5 mmol/L)
- ✔ **One hour after eating:** Less than 120 mg/dl (6.7 mmol/L)
- ✔ **Two hours after eating:** Less than 120 mg/dl (6.7 mmol/L)

Recent studies have shown that the glucose level one hour after eating may be the most important for pregnant women with diabetes to keep under control.

You also need to check for ketones in the urine before breakfast and before supper. You can do so by placing a test strip in the stream of urine. The strip indicates whether ketones are present. If the test strip is positive, it means that you are not eating enough carbohydrates and your body is going into accelerated starvation. Too much of this condition is not good for the growing fetus.

Eating well

Your appropriate amount of weight gain depends on your weight and body mass index at the time you become pregnant. (See Chapter 3 if you're not sure how to calculate your BMI). If your BMI is normal, you should gain 20 to 25 pounds during the pregnancy. However, if you're overweight, you need to gain less weight through the pregnancy, 15 to 20 pounds. If you're obese, you should gain no more than 17 or 18 pounds. And if you're underweight, you should gain 25 to 30 pounds.

Chapter 8 tells you what you need to know about diet and diabetes, but as a pregnant woman with diabetes, you have some special requirements:

- ✔ **Your daily food intake should be 35 to 38 kilocalories per kilogram of ideal body weight.** (In this book, I use the term *kilocalories* rather than *calories,* which is typically used incorrectly.) You can use your height to determine your ideal body weight (IBW). As a woman, you should weigh 100 pounds if you are 5 feet tall, plus 5 pounds for every inch over 5 feet. For example, a 5-foot 4-inch woman should weigh 120 pounds, ideally (and *approximately,* because these numbers represent a range, not a single weight). You can change that figure to kilograms by dividing the pounds by 2.2. Then multiply that number by 35 to get the low end of the daily calorie intake and by 38 to get the high end. So if you weigh 120 pounds, you weigh 54.6 kilograms and your daily food intake should be between 1,900 and 2,100 kilocalories.

✔ **Your protein intake should be about 20 percent of your daily kilocalories, or 1.5 to 2 grams per kilogram of IBW.** A woman with the IBW of 54.6 should eat about 100 grams of protein daily. Because each gram of protein contains four kilocalories, protein takes up about 400 of the 2,000 daily kilocalories.

✔ **Your carbohydrate intake should be 50 to 55 percent of your daily kilocalories.** If you need approximately 2,000 daily kilocalories, about 1,000 kilocalories should be carbohydrate. Because each gram of carbohydrate has 4 kilocalories, just like protein, this amounts to 250 grams of carbohydrate.

✔ **Your fat intake should be less than 30 percent of the total daily kilocalories.** Using 2,000 kilocalories as our target, that amounts to 630 kilocalories of fat. Because fat contains 9 kilocalories per gram, this equals 70 grams of fat a day.

Translating grams of food into amounts of specific foods would require another whole book. Because an excellent one on the subject has already been written, I refer you to *Nutrition For Dummies,* by Carol Ann Rinzler (Wiley) to get this information.

✔ **You need to eat three meals a day plus a bedtime snack.** Frequently eating helps prevent the accelerated starvation that results from the prolonged fast between supper and breakfast.

✔ **You must maintain fasting and premeal glucose levels below 90 mg/dl.** Your glucose should be less than 120 mg/dl one hour after meals.

Ask your doctor to send you to a dietician to develop a meal plan.

In addition, you can use a good multivitamin and mineral preparation. A moderate amount of exercise is also very helpful in controlling the blood glucose and keeping you in top shape during pregnancy.

Testing for fetal defects

A blood test called a *serum alpha-fetoprotein* can be done 15 weeks into the pregnancy to determine whether the fetus has neural tube defects (openings in the brain or spinal cord more common when conception occurs in a poorly controlled diabetic). At 18 weeks, an ultrasound can show any malformations of the growing fetus. An ultrasound, by directing a sound at the fetus and catching it as it bounces back to the machine, produces a picture of the fetus that shows the presence of any abnormalities. This harmless test is not painful for the mother or the fetus.

Another useful study during the diabetic pregnancy is the nonstress test. A device is placed on your abdomen that listens to the fetus's heartbeat. When the fetus moves, its heart rate normally speeds up by 15 to 20 beats per minute. This increase in heart rate should normally occur at least three times in a 20-minute period of listening.

Handling issues of gestational diabetes

If you have gestational diabetes, you don't need to worry about congenital malformations in your baby, but you need to avoid macrosomia. You need to follow the same dietary prescription as the woman with pregestational diabetes, and you need to use insulin if a careful diet does not keep your fasting blood glucose below 90, your glucose one hour after eating below 120, or your glucose two hours after eating below 120. If you can't bring yourself to use insulin shots, glyburide (see Chapter 10) has been shown to be safe for the baby because it does not pass through the placenta, although it is not approved by the FDA for this use. Your insulin regimen will probably be simpler than that of women with pregestational diabetes because your pancreas can make its own insulin. If you are taking insulin, you will stop doing so at the time of delivery.

Early ultrasound is not necessary for women with gestational diabetes unless the doctor suspects that diabetes was actually present much earlier. An ultrasound at week 38 can show whether fetal macrosomia exists. If macrosomia is present, your doctor will probably perform a cesarean section, removing the baby through an incision made in the abdominal wall and then in the uterus.

Delivering the baby

Delivering a baby at the end of 39 weeks is best because full-term pregnancy gives the baby time to mature completely. The same is true if the mother has diabetes. If the mother doesn't go into labor spontaneously, the physician usually induces labor. The uterine contractions of pregnant women with diabetes aren't as strong as those of pregnant women without diabetes. This difference may explain the increase in rates of C-sections for these women.

If you have been taking insulin during pregnancy, nurses will monitor your blood glucose every four hours after you deliver. Your blood glucose will be maintained at 70 to 120 mg/dl with insulin, if necessary. The insulin is given in short-acting form as needed and not in large doses of long-acting insulin, which would be around in the circulation when you no longer need it.

Maintaining your health after pregnancy

If you are breastfeeding, which is always a good idea, you need to consume about 300 kilocalories *above* your usual needs. You cannot take oral agents for diabetes because they pass through the milk into the baby. For more information about breastfeeding, see *Breastfeeding For Dummies,* by Sharon Perkins and Carol Vannais (Wiley).

Gestational diabetes usually disappears when the pregnancy is over. However, a woman who develops gestational diabetes during pregnancy is at a much higher risk for developing diabetes later in life. If your fasting blood glucose is greater than 130 during pregnancy, the risk of developing diabetes again is as much as 75 to 90 percent in the next 10 to 15 years. Even modestly elevated blood glucose levels during a pregnancy that do not rise to the criteria for gestational diabetes are associated with a higher risk for future type 2 diabetes. You are also at much higher risk of heart disease, mainly due to the development of diabetes.

Women who don't breastfeed have a 50 percent increased risk of type 2 diabetes compared to women who never give birth. Women with gestational diabetes who breastfeed lower their risk of later diabetes.

If you had gestational diabetes, you need to have a test for glucose tolerance between 6 and 12 weeks after the pregnancy and annually after that if diabetes is not found.

Several factors predispose women with gestational diabetes to develop diabetes later on. Following are some factors that can't be changed:

- ✓ **Ethnic origin:** Certain ethnic groups, such as Mexican Americans, Native Americans, Asian Americans, and African Americans, are at a higher risk.
- ✓ **Prepregnancy weight:** Women with a higher prepregnancy weight are at a higher risk.
- ✓ **Number of pregnancies:** The more pregnancies you have, the higher your risk.
- ✓ **Family history of diabetes:** If a family history is present, you are at a higher risk.
- ✓ **Severity of blood glucose during pregnancy:** Higher blood glucose levels mean a higher risk.

On the other hand, you can reduce several risk factors:

- ✓ **Future weight gain:** Gain less weight in future pregnancies.
- ✓ **Future pregnancies:** Have fewer children.
- ✓ **Physical activity:** Increase your exercise.
- ✓ **Dietary fat:** Limit the fat in your diet.
- ✓ **Smoking and certain drugs:** Stop smoking and using drugs.

Using the drug metformin (see Chapter 10) can also help prevent future diabetes.

Women who have had gestational diabetes can use oral contraceptives with low levels of estrogen and progesterone to prevent conception. These drugs, along with hormonal replacement therapy after menopause, do not increase your risk of later diabetes. They may, in fact, decrease the risk and decrease blood glucose levels in those who have diabetes already. Women with type 1 and type 2 diabetes can use the same preparations.

The story is similar for postmenopausal women. A study in *Diabetes Care* in October 2003 showed that the use of estrogens (with or without progestins) by women with diabetes resulted in a decrease in coronary artery disease. Because women with diabetes are at very high risk for coronary artery disease, this finding is an important one.

Focusing on your baby's health

Increased understanding of diabetes's impact during pregnancy has resulted in a great reduction in malformations in these babies as well as the macrosomia that leads to complications at delivery. Unfortunately, many women with diabetes do not have tight glucose control at conception, so some malformations still occur. If an obvious malformation is present at birth, it is important to search for other malformations.

Also, keep in mind that the fetus was producing a lot of insulin to handle all the maternal glucose entering through the placenta. Suddenly, maternal glucose is cut off at delivery, but the high level of fetal insulin continues for a while. The danger of hypoglycemia exists in the first four to six hours after delivery. The baby may be sweaty and appear nervous or even have a seizure. It is necessary to do blood glucose tests on the baby hourly until he or she is stable and to continue testing at intervals for the first 24 hours.

Besides hypoglycemia, the baby may have several other complications right after birth:

- **Respiratory distress syndrome:** This breathing problem occurs when the baby is delivered early, but it responds to treatment. This condition is rare with good prenatal care.

- **Low calcium, with jitteriness and possible seizures:** Calcium needs to be given to the baby until its own body can take over. This condition is usually a result of prematurity.

- **Low magnesium:** This complication presents itself like low calcium and is also a result of prematurity.

- **Polycythemia:** This condition, where too many red blood cells exist, occurs for unknown reasons. Treatment requires removing blood from the baby. The amount is determined by how much extra blood is present.

✔ **Hyperbilirubinemia:** This condition is the product of too much break-down of red blood cells. It is treated with light.

✔ **Lazy left colon:** Occurring for unknown reasons, this condition presents itself like an obstruction of the bowel but clears up on its own.

If the baby was exposed to high glucose and ketones during the pregnancy, it may show diminished intelligence. This effect is not obvious at birth but is discovered later when the baby is expected to learn something.

Large babies of poorly controlled mothers with diabetes usually lose their fat by age 1. Starting at ages 6 to 8, however, these children have a greater tendency to be obese. Controlling the blood glucose in the mother may prevent later obesity and even diabetes in her offspring.

Dealing with Polycystic Ovarian Syndrome

Polycystic ovarian syndrome (PCOS) is responsible for abnormal menstrual function in 5 to 8 percent or more of women during their reproductive years. It tends to run in families. Women with this condition often have trouble conceiving a child, and they have increased hair on their faces, arms, legs, and areas of the body that are not usually hairy in women. In addition, they often experience acne and obesity. They also have more abnormal blood fats associated with coronary artery disease.

The surprise finding in PCOS is that these women are also resistant to insulin and have increased blood levels of insulin. The greater the degree of obesity, however, the more likely the metabolic syndrome (see Chapter 5). In fact, women with PCOS who do get pregnant have a prevalence of gestational diabetes that is two to three times that of those women without PCOS. They also have higher rates of other complications of pregnancy including high blood pressure, preeclampsia, preterm delivery, and small babies.

Women with PCOS who are normal in weight do not have insulin resistance or a greater tendency to develop type 2 diabetes.

Brothers of women with PCOS who have insulin resistance also have insulin resistance, suggesting that a strong component of inheritance is present.

Another feature that women with PCOS have in common with metabolic syndrome is obstructive sleep apnea. This sleep apnea results in daytime sleepiness and high blood pressure. PCOS patients with obstructive sleep apnea tend to have insulin resistance and type 2 diabetes more often than those without.

The name of the syndrome derives from the fact that early cases of PCOS were associated with multiple ovarian cysts. More recently, the presence of ovarian cysts has not been a prominent feature of the condition, but the name has stuck.

Women with PCOS have increased levels of male-associated hormones called *androgens*. Studies have shown that androgens cause decreased insulin sensitivity when they are given to women who don't have PCOS.

The major health risks for someone with PCOS, besides infertility, are the occurrence of impaired glucose tolerance and type 2 diabetes, as well as gestational diabetes. In addition, just like patients with the metabolic syndrome (see Chapter 5), these women are at greater risk for high blood pressure, abnormal blood fats, and cardiovascular disease. A group of women who had PCOS and were followed for 18 years were found to have twice the risk of diabetes compared to those without PCOS.

The most effective treatment for PCOS is lifestyle change. Weight loss and exercise often reverse the condition and prevent the development of diabetes. In very obese women with PCOS, weight-loss surgery can reverse PCOS. Oral contraceptives have been used in the past when more treatment is needed, but they don't restore fertility, which is often the main purpose of treatment. They can still be used to control the other symptoms, such as acne, irregular menses, and increased hair. Insulin sensitizing drugs, including metformin, have been very effective for treating all features of the syndrome. In a study reported in *The Journal of Clinical Endocrinology and Metabolism* in April 2005, six months of metformin was much more effective than a drug called clomiphene, a well-known inducer of ovulation, in restoring fertility. Later studies have not confirmed this.

More recently (2011), simvastatin, a cholesterol-lowering drug, has been found to be more effective than metformin in reversing PCOS and preventing complications. It must not be used if pregnancy is desired because of danger to the fetus.

Other than oral contraceptives, any treatment that is successful for reducing the acne, hairiness, and decreased insulin sensitivity in PCOS also makes the woman much more likely to get pregnant. If she doesn't want to become pregnant, she and her partner need to take the necessary precautions.

For more information on polycystic ovarian syndrome, check out *PCOS For Dummies,* by Gaynor Bussell and Sharon Perkins (Wiley).

Part III
Managing Diabetes: The "Thriving with Diabetes" Lifestyle Plan

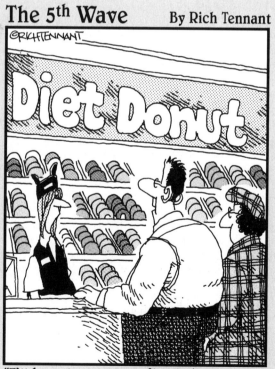

The 5th Wave   By Rich Tennant

"I'll have two lettuce filled, three carrot glazed, five celery frosted,..."

In this part . . .

Could you be healthier with diabetes than your friends who do not have diabetes are? This part shows that the answer to that question is yes. While others continue their bad habits leading to illness and perhaps premature death, you can find out exactly what you have to do not just to live with diabetes but to thrive with diabetes. The steps you need to take are simple and basic and involve changes in lifestyle, like what and how much you eat as well as your physical fitness. You will probably ask yourself as you're reading, "Why didn't I think of that?"

In this part, you find out how to choose from the vast number of products like glucose meters that help you to manage your disease. You will discover that you can have diabetes and enjoy delicious food. I introduce you to the concept of taking at least 10K (10,000) steps a day. New medications are appearing regularly, and I help you understand how to use them properly. Another function of this part is to show you that lots of people — some of whom you may not have thought of — are out there to provide the information that you need to know.

Chapter 7

Glucose Monitoring and Other Tests

*Y*ou may wonder what you have to do to prevent the complications of diabetes that I describe in Chapters 4 through 6, and the answer is a fair amount, which I discuss in this chapter. But when you weigh the benefits that add up to a longer, better-quality life against the loss of time and money from preventive care, the benefits of preventive care win by a landslide.

With preventive care, you can take advantage of an explosion of new tests and treatments that have only been available for the last 30 years, beginning with self-testing of blood glucose in 1980 right up to new tests for overall diabetic control and multiple new hardware and software tools made possible by the latest advances in computer and Internet technology.

As Woody Allen points out, "I don't want to achieve immortality through my work; I want to achieve it through not dying." On the other hand, he says, "On the plus side, death is one of the few things that can be done just as easily lying down." Well, I don't want you to take your diabetes lying down. I want to give you the benefit of every important advance. You may not achieve immortality, but you can enjoy every day that you live.

This chapter gives you all the tools you need to detect complications in their earliest stages. And if, by chance, you are reading this section for the first time and complications have already developed, this chapter also shows you how to measure the progression or, hopefully, regression of your complications.

Testing, Testing: Tests You Need to Stay Healthy

A number of tests and measurements should be done on a regular basis. To best make sure that you get your tests done regularly, you can use the chart in Figure 7-1. This form lists the tests and you can list the results underneath. Simply copy the one in Figure 7-1 and keep it up to date. Don't expect your doctor to keep this chart updated for you. He has too much on his mind and too many patients to get it exactly right for each one.

Date	Hemoglobin A1c	GlycoMark	Eye Exam	Filament	TSH	Ualb	Chol	LDL	HDL	TG

Figure 7-1:
A sample testing chart that you can copy to track your testing results.

Illustration by Wiley, Composition Services Graphics

Certain procedures, explained in this chapter, should be done by your doctor (and you, if feasible) according to the following schedule:

✔ **Blood glucose:** At each visit, evaluate the blood glucose measurements you've been taking. (See the section "Monitoring Blood Glucose: It's a Must," later in this chapter.)

✔ **Hemoglobin A1c:** Obtain hemoglobin A1c four times a year if you take insulin and twice a year if you don't. (See the section "Tracking Your Glucose over Time: Hemoglobin A1c," later in this chapter.)

✔ **GlycoMark:** The GlycoMark test may be performed every two weeks if control is poor; otherwise less often.

✔ **Eye exam:** Have a dilated eye examination by an ophthalmologist or optometrist once a year. (See the section "Checking for Eye Problems," later in this chapter.)

✔ **Filament:** Examine your bare feet at each visit and have your doctor perform a filament test. (See the section "Examining Your Feet," later in this chapter.)

In addition to looking at the feet, you should also have an ankle-brachial index performed at least every five years.

✔ **TSH:** Your doctor should check your thyroid-stimulating hormone level when your diabetes is diagnosed and every five years thereafter if it is normal.

✔ **Ualb:** Check for microalbuminuria once a year. (See the section "Testing for Kidney Damage: Microalbuminuria," later in this chapter.)

✔ **Chol/LDL/HDL/TG:** Obtain a lipid panel once a year to monitor your total cholesterol, LDL (bad cholesterol), HDL (good cholesterol), and triglycerides. (See the section "Tracking Cholesterol and Other Fats," later in this chapter.)

In addition to the preceding tests, you should also have your doctor take your blood pressure and measure your weight at each visit. (See the sections "Measuring Blood Pressure" and "Checking Your Weight and BMI," later in this chapter.)

These tests are the *minimum* standards for proper care of diabetes. If an abnormality is found, the frequency of testing increases to check on the response to treatment.

Are we doing the best job of managing diabetes? Government statistics on Preventive Care Practices from the Centers for Disease Control and Prevention (CDC) suggest that we are not. Doctors and patients are getting a little better as diabetes becomes a major health problem in the United States. The latest statistics compare the annual rates of testing for various abnormalities associated with diabetes between 1994 and 2009. They indicate some improvement, but as a whole we should be doing a whole lot better.

As diabetes knowledge has grown, the guidelines for how high various tests should be in people with diabetes have changed. Unfortunately, they seem to have no effect on the results of clinical practice:

✔ The Joint National Committee on Prevention, Detection, Evaluation and Treatment of High Blood Pressure lowered its guidelines for blood pressure in people with diabetes in 1997 and again in 2003, but as of 2008 there was no better control, according to the CDC.

✔ The American Diabetes Association lowered its goal for LDL cholesterol (see below) to less than 100 mg/dl in 1998. As late as 2009, there was no indication that patients were meeting the new goal more often than they had in 1994.

Much can be done. And that's what this chapter is all about.

Monitoring Blood Glucose: It's a Must

Insulin was extracted and used for the first time more than 80 years ago. Since that time, nothing has improved the life of the person with diabetes as much as the ability to measure his or her own blood glucose with a drop of blood.

Prior to blood glucose self-monitoring, testing the urine for glucose was the only way to determine whether your blood glucose was high, but urine testing could not tell at all whether the glucose was low. The urine test for glucose is worthless for controlling blood glucose — it actually provides misinformation. All the thousands of research papers in the medical literature before 1980, which used urine testing for glucose, are of no value and should be burned. (However, testing urine for other things, such as ketones and protein, can be of value.)

Basically, two kinds of test strips are used today. Both require that glucose in a drop of your blood reacts with an enzyme. In one strip, the reaction produces a color. A meter then reads the amount of color to give a glucose reading. In the other strip, the reaction produces electrons, and a meter converts the amount of electrons into a glucose reading.

One of the first things that was learned when frequent testing of blood glucose became feasible is that a person with diabetes, even a person who works hard to control his glucose, can experience tremendous variation in glucose levels in a relatively short time, as little as 30 minutes. This variation is especially true in association with food, but it can occur even in the fasting state before breakfast. For this reason, multiple tests are needed.

How often should you test?

How often you test is determined by the kind of diabetes you have, the kind of treatment you're using, and the level of stability of your blood glucose.

✔ **If you have type 1 or type 2 diabetes and you're taking before-meal insulin, you need to test before each meal and at bedtime.** The reason for this frequent testing is that you're constantly using this information to make adjustments in your insulin dose. No matter how good you think your control is, you cannot feel the level of the blood glucose without testing unless you're hypoglycemic. In fact, on numerous occasions I have had my patients try to guess their level before I test it. They are close less than 50 percent of the time. That degree of accuracy is not sufficient for good glucose control.

People with type 1 diabetes should occasionally test one or two hours after a meal and in the middle of the night to see just how high their glucose goes after eating and whether it drops too low in the middle of the night. These results guide you and your physician to make the changes you need.

Numerous studies have shown that increased daily frequency of blood glucose testing is significantly associated with lower levels of hemo-globin A1c and fewer complications of diabetes in patients who take insulin. There is a 0.2 percent lowering of A1c for each extra test up to a maximum of five tests.

✔ **If you have type 2 diabetes and you're on pills or just diet and exercise, testing twice a day (before breakfast and dinner) gives you the informa-tion needed to measure the effect of the treatment.** With this advice, I'm assuming that you're fairly stable as shown by mostly good blood glucose tests (in the range of 80 to 120 mg/dl) and by the hemoglobin A1c (which I discuss later in this chapter). I even have some of my most stable patients testing only once a day, alternating a pre-breakfast test with a pre-supper test on consecutive days. Any less testing than this minimal amount is not enough to keep you aware of the state of your control.

✔ **If you're pregnant, see the testing guidelines I outline in Chapter 6.** I would guess that you're probably willing to test numerous times in a day to keep your developing fetus as healthy as possible.

The blood glucose test can be useful many other times of day:

✔ If you eat something off your diet and want to test its effect on your glu-cose, do a test.

✔ If you're about to exercise, a blood glucose test can tell you if you need to eat before starting the exercise or if you can use the exercise to bring your glucose down.

✔ If your diabetes is temporarily unstable and you're about to drive, you may want to test before getting into the car to make sure that you're not on the verge of hypoglycemia. Even if your diabetes is stable, testing at the beginning and after every couple of hours of a long drive can prevent serious hypoglycemia.

You're not being graded on your glucose test results. The human body has too much variation in it to expect that each time you take the same medication, do the same exercise, eat the same way, and feel the same emotionally, you will get the same test result. If the person who reviews your results with you sees your abnormal results as bad, he or she does not understand this point. You may want to consider finding someone who does.

Keep in mind that the occasional blood glucose test done in your doctor's office is of little or no value in understanding the big picture of your glucose control. It is like trying to visualize an entire painting by Seurat (who painted using dots of color) by looking at one dot on the canvas.

How do you use a lancet?

To get the drop of blood you need to perform a glucose test, you have to use a spring-loaded device that contains a sharp lancet. You push the button of the device, and the lancet springs out and pokes your finger. Devices that allow different depths of penetration are useful for small children.

One product that seems less painful than the others is the Accu-Chek Softclix Lancet Device. It allows you to select one of 11 depth settings so that you can penetrate your finger no deeper than necessary. Many glucose meters allow testing at other sites besides your finger, which require different depths of penetration to reach blood, so these settings can be very useful. However, the Softclix uses its own type of lancet that is a little more expensive than others on the market.

Accu-Chek also offers the Multiclix device, which holds a drum of six pre-loaded lancets. Its great advantage is that there is no handling of lancets. In most devices, you have to push the lancet into the device and pull it out to discard it. In this one, as you use one lancet it re-enters the drum and the next clean lancet drops into place. When you have used all six, you throw away the drum and put a new one in the device. It too offers 11 penetration depths. The downside is that each lancet can be used only once.

Becton Dickinson (BD) makes another lancet, called BDGenie Lancet, that works like a lancet and lancing device all in one. It is less painful and a little less expensive than other devices on the market. Becton Dickinson also makes the thinnest lancets currently available, called the BD Ultra-Fine 33 Lancets.

Although you do not have to use alcohol on your fingers, they should be reasonably clean. (My patients have done millions of finger sticks, and I've never known one of them to have an infection result.) Use the side of your finger to avoid the more sensitive tips that you don't want to hurt, especially if you use a keyboard frequently. Change fingers often so that no finger becomes very sensitive.

Remember never to use a used lancet on someone else. Each lancet lasts for a few pokes and should then be discarded in a special sharps container so it can't poke someone else accidentally. Sharps containers are available in drugstores, or you can use an empty plastic laundry detergent bottle. Check with your refuse service to make sure it is okay to leave the sealed bottle in the garbage.

Make sure you wash and dry your hands if you peel fruit just before testing yourself. Glucose in the peel can significantly modify the result.

How do you perform the test?

If you don't already own a blood glucose meter, be sure to check out the next section. All meters require a drop of blood, usually from the finger. (See the previous section, "Using a lancet.") You place the blood on a specific part of a test strip and allow enough time, usually between five seconds and one minute, for a reaction to occur. Some strips allow you to add more blood within 30 seconds if the quantity is insufficient. The need for a second stick of your finger is rare if you use a test strip that requires less blood. In less than a minute, the meter reads the product of that reaction, which is determined by the amount of glucose in the blood sample. A sample that is 3.0 microliters of blood is 6 millimeters across. A sample that is 1.5 microliters is 3 millimeters across. A sample that is 0.5 microliters is 1 millimeter across.

Keep the following tips in mind when you're testing your glucose:

- **If you have trouble getting blood, you can wrap a rubber band around the point where your finger joins your hand.** You will be amazed at the flow of blood. Take off the rubber band before a major hemorrhage occurs (just joking).

- **Testing blood from sites other than your fingers is generally reliable, except for an hour after eating, immediately after exercise, or if your blood glucose is low.**

- **Some meters use whole blood, and some use the liquid part of the blood, called the _plasma_.** A lab glucose tests the plasma. The whole blood value is about 12 percent less than the plasma value, so you need to know which you're measuring. The various recommendations for appropriate levels of glucose are plasma values unless specifically stated otherwise. Most of the newer meters are calibrated to give a plasma reading, but check yours to be sure.

- **Studies have shown that the quality of test strips, which are loose in a vial, deteriorate rapidly if the vial is left open.** Be sure to cap the vial. Two hours of exposure to air may ruin the strips. Strips that are individually foil-wrapped do not have this problem.

✔ **Check the expiration date of the strips.**

✔ **Do not let other people use your meter.** Their test results will be mixed in with your tests when they are downloaded into a computer. In addition, a meter invariably gets a little blood on it and can be a source of infection.

Choosing a Blood Glucose Meter

The meter business must be a profitable one because many new meters are on the market each time I update this book. But the cost of the meter should play little part in your decision about which one to get. Most manufacturers are happy to practically give you the meter so that you're forced to buy their test strips. Each manufacturer makes a different test strip, and they're not interchangeable in other machines. Some companies even make a different strip for each different machine that they make.

Because the meters are so cheap and the science is changing so rapidly, you should get a new meter every year or two to make sure that you have state-of-the-art equipment. The cost of test strips is generally about the same from meter to meter, so the cost of strips does not have to play a big role in your meter decision, either.

Another nonconsideration is the accuracy of the various machines. All are accurate to a degree acceptable for managing your diabetes. Keep in mind, though, that they do not have the accuracy of a laboratory. Meters are probably about plus or minus 10 percent compared to the lab.

Factors that may influence your purchase

Your doctor may have a meter that he or she prefers to work with because a computer program can download the test results from the meter and display them in a certain way. This analysis can be enormously helpful in deciding how to alter your therapy for the best control of your glucose.

Any meter you buy should have a memory that records the time and date so you can read that information along with the glucose result. The memory should hold at least 100 glucose values if you test four times a day, giving you 25 days' worth of readings.

Don't buy a meter without the capability to download the results to a data-management system in a computer. Bring your meter with you to your appointments so that your doctor or an assistant can download your glucose test results and evaluate them with the aid of a data-management system. Evaluating pages of glucose readings in a log book is virtually impossible.

Your insurance company also may mandate a certain meter, in which case you may have no choice.

Ask yourself the following questions when choosing a meter:

- If a small child is to use it, can the child easily use the meter and strips?
- Are the batteries common ones, or are they hard to get and expensive?
- Does the meter have a memory that I and my doctor can check?
- Is the meter downloadable to a computer program that can manipulate the data?
- Do I have to calibrate the meter every time I change to a new box of strips (an inconvenient step)?

Studies reported in the *British Medical Journal* in 2008 showed that self-monitoring of blood glucose did not improve the blood glucose control in newly diagnosed type 2 patients and was associated with higher costs and lower quality of life in patients with non-insulin-treated type 2 diabetes. The authors concluded that self-monitoring of blood glucose in type 2 diabetics not using insulin was not cost effective. If you have type 2 diabetes and are not using insulin, you must decide for yourself whether testing your blood glucose really makes a difference.

Profiles of different meters

More than a dozen companies vie for your meter purchase. Among them, they produce more than 50 machines. Like everything in business, mergers and acquisitions have occurred and will continue to happen so that the field narrows. In the following sections, I give an overview of a number of the most common options.

Abbott Laboratories

Abbott Laboratories purchased the MediSense Company, which first made and sold blood glucose meters. This company, which has one of the longest warranties on its meters (four years), is speedy about taking care of problems that arise. The batteries are good for 4,000 tests. They can generally be replaced by you unless otherwise noted. One clue that Abbott is really interested in customer service is that you can find the owner's guides for all their meters on the Internet.

- **FreeStyle Freedom Lite:** The FreeStyle Freedom Lite requires a tiny sample of blood, and you can add more up to a minute from the first application if you don't have enough on the strip. The Freedom Lite works with a data-management program called CoPilot Health Management System. It holds up to 400 tests, eliminating the oldest as new ones are added beyond 400, just like all the other meters described in this section. You can see a 7-, 14-, and 30-day average on the screen. No calibration is required. The meter has four programmable alarms to remind you to test. It uses CR2032 coin cell batteries available at drugstores and grocery stores. You can test away from your finger with this meter.

- **FreeStyle Lite:** This meter is identical to the Freedom Lite but is smaller, with a smaller screen and smaller buttons.

- **Precision Xtra:** This meter allows measurement of blood ketones as well as glucose. It uses its own test strips that require calibration of the meter with each new vial. The vial contains a calibration strip that is inserted into the meter before using the test strips in that vial. If you want to do a blood ketone test, you use the calibration strip that comes in that vial before inserting the ketone strip. The meter remembers the last 450 tests that you do and you can view 7-, 14-, and 30-day averages on the screen. It uses its own test strips. It has its own data-management system called Precision Xtra Advanced Diabetes Management System.

AgaMatrix

AgaMatrix was the first company to manufacture a meter that attaches to the iPhone and uses the iPhone screen to provide information. AgaMatrix also manufactures three other meters that use a CR2032 lithium coin-cell battery. They also use the Zero-Click software for data management. And they all need only a 5-microliter drop of blood.

- **Wave Sense Jazz:** The Jazz requires no calibration. It can remember 1,865 tests. It has seven user-settable alarms.

- **Wave Sense KeyNote:** The KeyNote is one of the smallest meters on the market. It remembers 300 tests. It can provide 14-, 30-, and 90-day averages on the screen. It has six alarms you can set, and it alerts you if the glucose is too low or too high. You have to calibrate the KeyNote.

- **Wave Sense Presto:** The Presto also remembers 300 tests and provides the same averages as the KeyNote. It also has the same alarms. You don't have to calibrate this meter.

- **IBGStar:** With Sanofi-Aventis, AgroMatrix developed IBGStar, the tiny meter that attaches to your iPhone, turning its screen into a meter screen. It is available for sale in Europe, and it has been approved by the FDA in the U.S. but is not yet available for sale there.

Bayer HealthCare LLC

Bayer HealthCare LLC sells five meters in the United States. The meters are accurate and carry the longest warranty in the industry (five years). You can replace the batteries at home. The meters are descendants of some of the first meters available. They allow testing away from your fingers, and no coding of the meters is required. One of them, the Contour USB, is particularly interesting.

- ✔ **Breeze 2:** The Breeze 2 uses a ten-test cartridge that calibrates the meter. It remembers 420 tests. It can provide 1-, 7-, 14-, and 30-day averages. The meter uses WinGlucofacts software for data management.

- ✔ **Contour:** This meter uses individual test strips that require no coding. It remembers up to 480 tests that can be downloaded and viewed with the same data-management system as the Breeze 2. It can provide a 14-day average on the screen. It uses 3-volt lithium batteries. Contour meters use individual Contour test strips.

- ✔ **Contour USB:** The Contour USB is a small meter that plugs directly into the USB port of your computer and opens the Glucofacts Deluxe software, which analyzes your tests and shows you patterns, allowing you to make changes for better control, while charging your battery at the same time. The meter remembers 2,000 tests.

- ✔ **Didget:** Didget is a meter that plugs into the Nintendo DS and DS Lite gaming systems, rewarding your child for frequent testing, although it can be used alone. Kids who test get reward points that unlock new levels of the Nintendo games and buy in-game items. It provides 7-, 14-, and 30-day averages. It, too, uses the Contour test strips. It remembers 480 tests.

Diagnostic Devices

Diagnostic Devices makes three meters for the United States, which they call Prodigy meters. The Prodigy Pocket is a small, very portable meter that comes in five colors and remembers 120 tests. The other two meters are more interesting. None of the meters require calibration.

- ✔ **Prodigy Voice:** This meter is meant for the blind. It has raised buttons. When a strip is inserted, it turns on and verbally takes the user through the setup steps and provides the reading verbally as well. It remembers 450 tests.

- ✔ **Prodigy AutoCode:** Prodigy AutoCode talks the user through the steps of testing and speaks the result. It speaks in English, Spanish, French, and Arabic. It remembers 120 tests.

LifeScan

Johnson & Johnson purchased LifeScan, one of the older meter companies. They have a number of meters in competition with one another. The company is very reliable, taking care of problems within 24 hours. You can replace the batteries in LifeScan meters at home. This company also posts its owner's manuals online in case you need to refer to them. All of their meters require user calibration, an inconvenient step.

- ✔ **OneTouch UltraMini:** This meter is small and portable. It uses a tiny blood sample. Each new vial of UltraMini test strips must be coded in the meter. It remembers 500 tests. It uses a 3-volt CR 2032 coin-cell battery. However, it has no way to download test results to a computer and no data-management system. Therefore, I don't recommend it.

- ✔ **OneTouch Ultra2:** This system allows testing away from the fingers. It uses a tiny sample and, therefore, can work with LifeScan's ultrafine lancets. The result is displayed in five seconds, and the blood is drawn up by capillary action. The meter has a 500-test memory that allows averaging on the screen and connects to a data port using OneTouch Diabetes Management software. You can see 7-, 14-, and 30-day averages. It uses Ultra test strips. You use buttons on the meter to set the code on the meter to the code on the bottle of test strips. You can add flags to each blood glucose test to specify whether the glucose was taken before or after a meal and whether food or exercise was involved. It uses two 3-volt CR 2032 coin-cell batteries, one for the meter and one for the backlight. The test is measured from whole blood but expressed in plasma-referenced units.

- ✔ **OneTouch UltraSmart:** This meter has all the features of the OneTouch Ultra2 with the addition of other features. Using "smart buttons," you can enter information about your exercise, health, medication, and food. You are prompted to comment on out-of-range results. You can view charts and graphs that help to analyze your blood glucose on the meter's screen. The UltraSmart uses two AAA batteries. You can see averages for 7, 14, 30, 60, and 90 days, and it can store over 3,000 test results. You can also enter test results for hemoglobin A1c, microalbumin, cholesterol, blood pressure, eye exams, foot exams, weight, height, and dates of doctor's visits. You can even enter the diabetes pills you take and insulin if you use that. Furthermore, it includes a food log in which you can enter the meal and the calories of fat, carbohydrate, and protein. The meter can give you outputs of average insulin used at different times, average carbohydrates at different meals, and other data.

Nipro Diagnostics

Nipro Diagnostics makes five meters that are sold in the U.S. Three of them, the TRUEtrack, TRUEbalance, and TRUEread, have no features that differ from previous meters, but the following two are unusual:

- ✔ **TRUE2go:** The TRUE2go is claimed to be the world's smallest meter. It twists on the top of a new vial of strips. It uses a 3-volt CR 2032 coin-cell battery. The memory holds just 99 results. It does not work with a data-management system, so I don't recommend it.

✔ **Sidekick:** This meter is similar to TRUE2go in being a small meter on top of a bottle of strips, but in this case you throw away the entire meter and bottle when you use up the strips, so battery replacement is not necessary. It has a 50-test memory and no data-management system. I don't recommend it.

Roche Diagnostics

Roche Diagnostics merged with Boehringer Mannheim and now sells its meters. The batteries in these meters are replaceable at home. The meters may be used at alternate sites besides the fingers.

✔ **Accu-Chek Aviva:** This meter works with diabetes-management software (DMS). It has a very large memory, storing up to 500 blood glucose values, with 7-, 14-, and 30- day averages onscreen. It requires a tiny sample of blood. It comes with Spanish-language instructions and a phone number for a Spanish-speaking representative. It has a code key with each new bottle of test strips that are made just for this meter. You can set test reminders for up to four times a day with the built-in alarm. It uses a coin-cell 2032 battery.

✔ **Accu-Chek Compact Plus:** This meter uses a 17-test drum that requires no test-strip handling or calibration. The results are displayed in five seconds, and it has a 300-test memory that is downloadable to a DMS. You can see onscreen 7-, 24-, and 30-day averages. It uses two AAA batteries.

Roche also makes a software program for people with diabetes called Accu-Chek Compass. It helps patients to better manage their diabetes by providing reports and summaries of the glucose tests.

Four noninvasive meters: Continuous glucose monitoring

Individual blood glucose measurements represent only a moment in time and blood glucose levels can change in minutes. Potentially more useful devices that can measure blood glucose almost continuously, store the measurements, and download them to a computer are being developed. They may replace the meters in the preceding sections after they improve, but for now they often lag behind finger-stick measurements, especially after a meal or exercise. Each device still requires that you take blood glucose measurements using a finger-stick meter to calibrate these continuous meters. Many patients reject the idea of wearing the devices on their body.

Continuous monitors are most useful when the finger-stick results do not correlate well with the hemoglobin A1c measurements, which is especially the case in people with diabetes who take insulin, both type 1 and type 2. The doctor, knowing the direction of the blood glucose throughout 24 hours, can adjust the rapid-acting and long-acting insulin more accurately without causing hypoglycemia.

Several reports in *Diabetes Care* since 2006 have shown that continuous glucose monitoring is effective in lowering the hemoglobin A1c in poorly controlled patients on insulin who have type 1 diabetes and even in well-controlled type 1 patients. It is also effective in type 2 patients on multiple insulin injections. It lowers hemoglobin A1c without increased low blood glucose and has a positive effect on quality of life. A report in January 2012 in that journal showed that even type 2 patients on pills benefited from continuous monitoring. They did significantly better during the 12 weeks they were on continuous monitoring and maintained this improvement for 40 more weeks after the continuous monitoring was stopped compared to patients who continued to use finger-stick monitoring.

These studies almost always depend on the manufacturer of the device to provide the device and to fund the study. I leave it to you to decide the effect of such support on the results of the study.

Check with your insurance company before you purchase a continuous monitor. Your company may cover only a specific brand or not cover the device for type 2 diabetes.

Dexcom Seven Plus Continuous Blood Glucose Monitor

The Seven Plus monitor by Dexcom uses a sensor (changed after seven days) under the skin that wirelessly transmits glucose readings from the fluid under the skin, called the interstitial fluid, to a monitor. The monitor collects the information every five minutes and displays it onscreen. The screen can show one-, three-, and nine-hour trends as well as alert you when the blood glucose goes above or below a set level. An alarm also sounds when the glucose is below 55 mg/dl. Software called Data Manager 3 helps to display the data on a computer for further understanding of trends. The device is calibrated with a finger-stick glucose reading every 12 hours. It can store up to 30 days of data.

Freestyle Navigator

The Freestyle Navigator, sold by Abbott Diabetes Care, is a combination continuous glucose monitor and blood glucose meter. It is similar to the Dexcom monitor described in the preceding section. However, Abbott has run into a supply interruption in the United States and has discontinued the Navigator system in the U.S.

Medtronic Guardian Real-Time

The Medtronic Guardian Real-Time is a continuous glucose meter that uses a sensor that lasts three days and then must be changed. You have to calibrate the meter two hours and six hours after inserting the sensor and every 12 hours after that. The sensor transmits the blood glucose to a receiver. You set upper and lower limits, and an alarm alerts you 30 minutes before those limits are reached. It comes in a pediatric model for children and teens. Another nice feature is that the sensor and receiver can be worn under water up to 8 feet deep for up to 30 minutes.

This monitor works with data-management software to show you trends that help you to improve your glucose control. All the results can be viewed with the CareLink Personal Therapy Software. Both the transmitter and the receiver use one AAA battery.

MiniMed Paradigm Real-Time Revel

The MiniMed Paradigm Real-Time Revel is another continuous glucose meter. Medtronic, which makes this meter and the preceding one, has a long history of working in the field of insulin pumps (see Chapter 10). This meter (the transmitter) is combined with an insulin pump (the receiver) in this device to accomplish the longstanding goal of creating a "closed loop" system that has been shown to be effective in controlling the blood glucose in children, adolescents, and adults with type 1 diabetes. It is only available for research at this time.

How I use my patients' test results

I encourage my patients to keep their own records of their glucose levels so that they can see for themselves how they are doing. I maintain several years of records and can compare and contrast results for each patient. I use software to generate pictures of a patient's diabetic control. The figures in this sidebar show you graphics that depict test results for a typical patient before starting therapy and after insulin treatment had time to work. You can easily see how helpful the graphic information can be.

The first figure shows the patient's blood glucose levels in three different formats. The top, the Trendgraph, shows the blood glucoses each day, in this case, between 6/11 and 7/1. The shaded area represents the blood glucoses from 80 to 180 mg/dl. The line below the shaded area is the 50 mg/dl line. Each X represents a distinct blood glucose test. You can see that the glucose is often high, going up to 300, and sometimes low, going down to 50 with large excursions. This graph also shows that the mean of the tests is 159 and that 5 percent of the time, the patient is less than 80; 63.4 percent of the time, she is between 80 and 180; and 31.7 percent of the time, she is above 180.

The next figure, the Standard Day, puts all those glucose levels in a 24-hour day so that tests taken between certain hours, regardless of the day, appear close to one another. This grouping allows me to see whether the patient has a tendency to be high or low at a given time each day. The software averages out the blood glucose at different times, providing a number to compare to other time periods. This information permits me to adjust her insulin to correct for that particular time.

(continued)

(continued)

The bottom figure, the Pie Chart, clearly shows how much of the time this patient is high, how much of the time she is within the target of 80 to 180, and how much of the time she is below 80.

These three figures provide an excellent picture of the patient's diabetic control and permit me to easily compare it to the result of treatment.

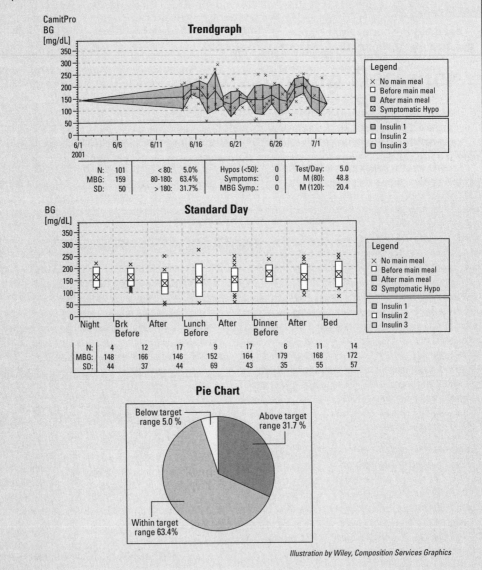

CamitPro
BG
[mg/dL]

Trendgraph

N:	101	< 80:	5.0%	Hypos (<50):	0	Test/Day:	5.0
MBG:	159	80-180:	63.4%	Symptoms:	0	M (80):	48.8
SD:	50	> 180:	31.7%	MBG Symp.:	0	M (120):	20.4

BG
[mg/dL]

Standard Day

N:	4	12	17	9	17	6	11	14
MBG:	148	166	146	152	164	179	168	172
SD:	44	37	44	69	43	35	55	57

Pie Chart

Below target range 5.0 %

Above target range 31.7 %

Within target range 63.4%

Illustration by Wiley, Composition Services Graphics

The next set of figures represents tests taken after treatment with a new form of insulin, insulin glargine (Lantus), for one week. The results are dramatic. Now almost all the glucoses are in the shaded area, and there is little excursion of the tests. A few Xs fall above 180, and a few fall below 80. The Standard Day now shows fairly low averages throughout, except perhaps after lunch. The Pie Chart shows much more in the target range and far fewer above the target range. Comparing the two graphs, the *above target range* area has dropped from 31.7 percent to 6.5 percent.

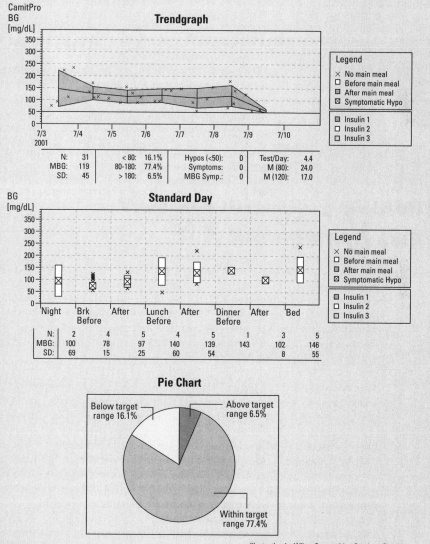

Illustration by Wiley, Composition Services Graphics

I can print all these graphs and charts. In later visits, I can compare the current control with the way the patient was doing before. When patients can see so clearly how they're improving from time to time, it keeps them motivated to take their medicine and follow their diet and exercise plan.

A report in *Diabetes Care* (December 2011) confirms the potential of the closed-loop system. In this case, the system was used in 6 of 12 pregnant women with type 1 diabetes who were well controlled (with hemoglobin A1c 6.4 percent). The other six women used conventional continuous insulin infusion without connecting to the meter. Both groups remained well controlled during their pregnancy, but the closed-loop group had less severe hypoglycemia and spent less time with low blood glucose levels.

This monitor uses the same CareLink Personal software as the Guardian Real-Time, and its features are similar.

In January 2012, the FDA approved a remote continuous diabetes monitor called MySentry Remote Glucose Monitor that works with the Revel system. Now a parent sleeping in another room can monitor the glucose of her small child, as the device alerts her with an alarm if the glucose is too low or too high. If the parents of small children with diabetes can afford to shell out about $3,000 for the device, it should provide great peace of mind.

Tracking Your Glucose over Time: Hemoglobin A1c

In order to follow your improvement with treatment, you need a test that gives you the big picture, the average blood glucose over time. As I explain in Chapter 2, the hemoglobin A1c is that test. Figure 7-2 shows you the correlation between the hemoglobin A1c and the estimated average blood glucose. By correlating the A1c with the estimated average blood glucose, you can think of the A1c in the same units as the blood glucose that you measure several times a day.

As you can see in the figure, a normal hemoglobin A1c of less than 6 percent corresponds to an estimated average blood glucose of less than 126, while a fair hemoglobin A1c of 7 percent reflects an average blood glucose of 155.

Large-scale studies have shown that the average hemoglobin A1c in the United States for type 2 diabetes is around 9.4 percent, which means the average blood glucose is 223. The American Diabetes Association recommends taking action to control the blood glucose if the hemoglobin A1c is 8 percent or greater, with the goal being less than 7 percent.

The American Association of Clinical Endocrinologists suggests a goal of 6.5 percent or less. Although I wish all of my patients would achieve a level of 6.5 percent, I try to get them as low as possible but still consistent with a decent quality of life, which means few to no severe hypoglycemic episodes.

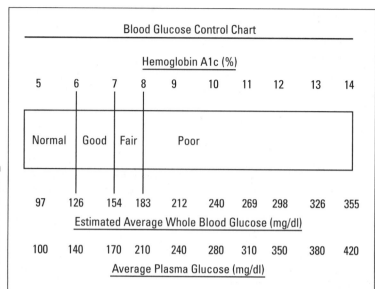

Blood Glucose Control Chart

Hemoglobin A1c (%)

| 5 | 6 | 7 | 8 | 9 | 10 | 11 | 12 | 13 | 14 |

| Normal | Good | Fair | Poor |

| 97 | 126 | 154 | 183 | 212 | 240 | 269 | 298 | 326 | 355 |

Estimated Average Whole Blood Glucose (mg/dl)

| 100 | 140 | 170 | 210 | 240 | 280 | 310 | 350 | 380 | 420 |

Average Plasma Glucose (mg/dl)

Figure 7-2: Comparison between hemoglobin A1c and blood glucose.

Illustration by Wiley, Composition Services Graphics

Your physician should test for hemoglobin A1c as follows:

✔ Four times a year if you have type 1 or type 2 diabetes and are on insulin

✔ Two times a year if you have type 2 diabetes and are not on insulin

In my own practice, I test all patients every three months. A good hemoglobin A1c is highly motivating to keep up good self-care, whereas a poor result gives immediate feedback as to the need for tighter control.

The National Glycohemoglobin Standardization Program, created by the American Association for Clinical Chemistry, has standardized the hemoglobin A1c test so that a 6 percent result means the same thing for every patient.

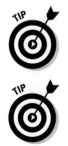

A study published in *Diabetes Care* in January 2011 showed that the hemoglobin A1c changes much more frequently in gestational diabetes. The authors recommend weekly testing of the A1c to guide treatment. If you have gestational diabetes, discuss this issue with your doctor.

Bayer sells a clever home version of the hemoglobin A1c called *A1c Now*. You do a finger stick to produce a large drop of blood. The blood is mixed with a solution that is provided, and a sample of that mixture is placed in the testing device. Five minutes later, the hemoglobin A1c result appears in the device window. The device is then discarded. The device appears to be highly accurate and may save the trouble of going to a lab for this test. Because it's so quick, your doctor can have the test results while you're at his office and can act on them immediately, instead of waiting for a lab to return the test results at a later time. The test kit is available at pharmacies without a prescription, for about $30 a test. It is annually certified by the National Glycohemoglobin Standardization Program.

Another option is to collect your own blood specimen and send it to a company that runs the test and gives you and your doctor a result. Following are some companies currently doing this test:

✔ **AccuBase A1c Glycohemoglobin:** Each test costs $29.59 and includes lab analysis and reporting. It can be ordered on the Internet at Amazon. com or American Diabetes Wholesale.

> Phone 888-872-2443

> Website www.diabetestechnologies.com

✔ **A1c at Home:** This testing service costs $24.95 each including lab analysis and reporting.

> Phone 772-221-8893 or 877-212-8378

Another test similar to the hemoglobin A1c is the *fructosamine*. This test, which measures the glucose combined with protein in the blood, reflects the level of blood glucose for the past three weeks. Fructosamine is a relatively new test that has not seen a lot of use, so its place in diabetes care has not been established. However, the test should prove very useful for the pregnant woman with diabetes, for example, where you need to know the effect of a treatment change very rapidly. As doctors become more familiar with its use, more fructosamine tests may be ordered.

The Food and Drug Administration has approved a home-testing device called the Duet Glucose Control Monitoring System, which can measure both the blood glucose and the fructosamine. The machine costs around $300, and a set of eight test strips is $64. How useful it will be is yet to be determined.

Testing Average Glucose Another Way: The GlycoMark Test

This test is another marker for glucose control, but it differs from the hemoglobin A1c test in two important ways:

✔ Results take two weeks rather than three months to change.

✔ Better control is marked by a higher rather than a lower number for the GlycoMark test.

The test is based on the normal presence of 1.5 anhydroglucitol (1,5 AG) in the blood. As blood glucose rises and more of it gets into the kidneys, it blocks the return of 1,5 AG to the bloodstream and the measured blood level of 1,5 AG falls.

Table 7-1 shows the values for GlycoMark in people without diabetes and at different levels of glucose control.

Table 7-1	GlycoMark Test Results	
GlycoMark (ug/ml)	*Control*	*Glucose (mg/dl)*
14 or higher	Normal	Under 180
10.0–13.9	Well controlled	185
6.0–9.9	Moderately controlled	190
2.0–5.9	Poorly controlled	200
1.9 or lower	Very poorly controlled	225

The GlycoMark test has been shown to be an excellent indicator of the blood glucose levels, especially after meals, even when the hemoglobin A1c test was similar in these patients. It gives the doctor and the patient a much earlier indication of whether therapy is working than does the slow-changing hemoglobin A1c. It is especially useful as an indicator of the blood glucose two hours after eating for the past two weeks. Drugs that treat the blood glucose after meals can be monitored with this test.

GlycoMark is not useful in patients with kidney disease, pregnancy, or advanced liver disease.

The test is available at major clinical laboratories, including Esoterix, LabCorp, Quest, and Specialty Laboratories.

Testing for Kidney Damage: Microalbuminuria

The finding of very small but abnormal amounts of protein in the urine, called *microalbuminuria,* is the earliest sign that high glucose may be damaging your kidneys (see Chapter 5). When microalbuminuria is found, you still have time to reverse any damage.

As soon as you are diagnosed with type 2 diabetes, and within five years of being diagnosed with type 1, your doctor must order a urine test for microalbuminuria (a Ualb test). If the test is negative, it must be repeated annually. If the test is positive, it should be done a second time to verify the result. If the second test is positive, your doctor should do the following:

- **Put you on a drug called an ACE inhibitor:** After you have been on this drug for some months, the test for microalbuminuria can be repeated to see whether it has turned negative. The ACE inhibitor can be stopped and restarted later if microalbuminuria appears again. If ACE inhibitors aren't tolerated, then ARBs, another class of antihypertensives, may be used. Both classes have been shown to reverse microalbuminuria and the ongoing kidney damage it reflects.

- **Bring your blood glucose under the tightest control possible.** Bringing it under control helps to reverse the damaging process as well.

- **Normalize your body fats so that your cholesterol and triglycerides are made normal.** Elevated cholesterol and triglycerides have been found to damage the kidneys. (See the section "Tracking Cholesterol and Other Fats," later in this chapter.)

- **Bring your blood pressure under control.** Lowering your blood pressure will help to minimize the damage to your kidneys that occurs when they are exposed to elevated blood pressure.

Doing this simple little test can protect your kidneys from damage. Ask your doctor about it if you think you've never had it done. Show him or her this page if the doctor is unclear as to why it is performed.

Up to 25 percent of patients with diabetes can have ongoing kidney damage without showing an elevated microalbumin. For this reason, the idea that all patients with diabetes should receive an ACE inhibitor may not be far-fetched.

Women who have gestational diabetes and show microalbuminuria have been found to have heart disease and kidney disease later, even if they don't develop diabetes. Persistent microalbuminuria predicts later heart disease even in the absence of gestational diabetes.

Checking for Eye Problems

All people with diabetes need to have a dilated eye exam done annually by an ophthalmologist or optometrist. No other physician, including the endocrinologist (yours truly excepted, of course), can do the exam properly.

For this exam, the doctor instills drops into your eyes and uses various instruments to examine the pressure, the appearance of your lens, and, most importantly, the retina of your eye.

All kinds of treatments can be done if abnormalities are found, but they must be discovered first. (See Chapter 5 for more information on eye problems.)

This test is something you must demand. Your doctor must refer you to an ophthalmologist or optometrist every year. Better yet, set up the appointment yourself with the eye doctor's nurse at the end of your first visit so that you are reminded about it each year. People who have mild type 2 diabetes and no retinopathy may be tested at three-year intervals rather than annually.

Examining Your Feet

Failing to take care of your feet leads to problems that often end in amputation. An amputation is really evidence of inadequate care. (For more on foot problems, see Chapter 5.) The doctor is not necessarily at fault here. The doctor sees you once in a while; you're with yourself much more often.

If you have any problem sensing touch with your feet, you need to take the following precautions:

✔ You must use your eyes to examine your feet every day.

✔ You must use your hand to test hot water before you step into it so that you do not get burned.

✔ You must shake out your shoes before you step into them to make sure no stone or other object is inside them.

✔ You must not go barefoot.

✔ You must keep the skin of your feet moist by soaking them in water, drying them a towel, and applying a moisturizing lotion. (Soaking should always be accompanied by drying and moisturizing.)

Your doctor can test your ability to feel an injury by using a 10-gram filament, but, again, that is done only when you have an appointment. You can obtain one of these filaments for yourself. A couple of the places where you can get them include

✔ Lower Extremity Amputation Prevention (LEAP) Program: `www.hrsa.gov/hansensdisease/leap`

✔ Medical Monofilament Manufacturing, LLC: www.medicalmono
filament.com, or call 508-746-7877

✔ Sensory Testing Systems: 225-923-1297

If you have any suggestion of a loss of sensation, at each visit to the doctor who takes care of your diabetes, you should take off your shoes and socks and have your feet inspected.

The other part of a foot examination involves checking the circulation of blood to your feet. To check the circulation, your doctor does a measurement called an *ankle-brachial index* at least once every five years. The systolic blood pressure is measured in the ankle and the arm. (See the sidebar "The meaning of your blood pressure," later in this chapter, for an explanation of systolic blood pressure.) The value for the ankle is divided by the value for the arm. An index of greater than 0.9 is considered normal. A value between 0.4 and 0.9 indicates peripheral vascular disease (see Chapter 5), and a value less than 0.4 indicates severe disease.

The ankle-brachial index should be done for any person with diabetes over age 50. Patients under 50 require the study if risk factors such as smoking, high cholesterol, and high blood pressure are present.

Tracking Cholesterol and Other Fats

Most people these days know the level of their total cholesterol, but other tests that show levels of various types of fats in the blood are needed as well.

Cholesterol is a type of fat that circulates in the blood in small packages called *lipoproteins*. These tiny round particles contain fat (*lipo*, as in liposuction) and protein. Because cholesterol does not dissolve in water, it would separate from the blood if it were not surrounded by the protein, just like oil separates from water in salad dressing. (That's why you have to shake the salad dressing each time you use it.)

A second kind of fat found in the lipoproteins is *triglyceride*. Triglyceride actually represents the form of most of the fat you eat each day. Although you may eat only a gram or less of cholesterol (an egg yolk has one-third of a gram of cholesterol), you eat up to 100 grams of triglyceride a day. (For more on the place of fats in your diet, see Chapter 8.) The fat in animal meats is mostly triglycerides.

Four types of lipoproteins exist:

✔ **Chylomicrons:** The largest of the fat particles, these lipoproteins contain the fat that is absorbed from the intestine after a meal. They are usually cleared from the blood rapidly. Ordinarily, chylomicrons are not a concern with respect to causing *arteriosclerosis* (hardening of the arteries).

✔ **Very-low-density lipoprotein (VLDL):** These particles contain mostly triglyceride as the fat. They're smaller than chylomicrons.

✔ **High-density lipoprotein (HDL):** Known as "good" cholesterol, this lipoprotein is the next smallest in size. This particle functions to clean the arteries, helping to prevent coronary artery disease, peripheral vascular disease, and strokes.

✔ **Low-density lipoprotein (LDL):** Known as "bad" cholesterol, this smallest particle is the particle that seems to carry cholesterol to the arteries, where it's deposited and causes hardening.

As you may imagine, doctors need to know which particle your cholesterol comes from in order to understand whether you have too much bad cholesterol (LDL) or a satisfactory level of good cholesterol (HDL).

You don't have to fast to test for total cholesterol and HDL cholesterol. However, you do need to fast for eight hours to find out your LDL cholesterol and triglycerides, because the blood has to be cleared of chylomicrons, which rise greatly when you eat.

You should have a *fasting lipid panel* at least once each year. A fasting lipid panel gives you your total cholesterol, your LDL cholesterol, your HDL cholesterol, and your triglyceride levels. If your values indicate you are at low risk (LDL less than 100, HDL greater than 50), the fasting lipid panel may be done every two years.

Table 7-2 lists the current recommendations for the levels of these fats in terms of the risk for coronary artery disease.

Table 7-2	Levels of Fat and Risk for Coronary Artery Disease		
Risk	*LDL Cholesterol*	*HDL Cholesterol*	*Triglycerides*
Higher	Greater than 130	Less than 35	Greater than 400
Borderline	100 to 130	35 to 45	150 to 400
Lower	Less than 100	Greater than 45	Less than 150

You can see in Table 7-2 that the risk goes up as the LDL cholesterol goes up and the HDL cholesterol goes down. A huge study of thousands of citizens of Framingham, Massachusetts, shows that you can get a good picture of the risk by dividing the total cholesterol by the HDL cholesterol. If this result is less than 4.5, the risk is lower. If it's greater than 4.5, you're at higher risk for coronary artery disease. The higher it is, the worse the risk.

In March 2004, the story got a little more complicated. The *New England Journal of Medicine* published results of a study of more than 4,000 men who had just had heart attacks. In the study, some patients' LDL cholesterol was reduced maximally (to a mean of 62) with a large dose of a powerful drug called *atorvastatin*. The result was a major reduction, starting in just 30 days after treatment with the drug, in subsequent heart attacks, chest pain, and strokes compared to a group whose LDL was lowered only to 95. This result calls for a major reappraisal of what LDL is considered normal. Experts agree that the lowest possible LDL level is best and that this policy applies to everyone, not only people who have just had a heart attack.

Diabetes adds its own complication because of metabolic syndrome (see Chapter 5). In the metabolic syndrome, the total cholesterol may not be very high, but the HDL cholesterol is low and the triglycerides are elevated. These patients also have a lot of a dangerous form of LDL cholesterol, so they are at higher risk for coronary artery disease. This increased risk must be taken into account in considering treatment for the fats.

In deciding whether and how to treat the fats, you have to consider other risk factors for coronary artery disease. You're at high risk if you have diabetes and fit any of the following conditions:

✔ You already have coronary artery disease, stroke, or peripheral vascular disease.

✔ You are a male over 45.

✔ You are a female over 55.

✔ You smoke cigarettes.

✔ You have high blood pressure.

✔ You have HDL cholesterol less than 35.

✔ You have a father or brother who had a heart attack before age 55.

✔ You have a mother or sister who had a heart attack before age 65.

✔ You have a body-mass index greater than 30.

You're at low risk if you have none of the preceding risk factors.

The treatment for abnormal fats then depends on your risk category and level of LDL cholesterol (see Table 7-3).

Table7-3	Your Treatment Based on Risk Category	
Risk	**Dietary Treatment if LDL Is Greater Than:**	**Diet and Drug Treatment if LDL Is Greater Than:**
Low	160	190
High	130	160
Very high	100	130

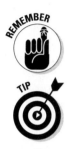

All these decisions depend on obtaining a lipid (fat) panel.

These treatment guidelines will change as the experts have a chance to evaluate the LDL study of heart-attack victims that I discuss in this section.

After LDL cholesterol is lowered, even below 70, a higher level of HDL cholesterol has been found to be associated with fewer heart attacks than a lower level.

Measuring Blood Pressure

The United States is experiencing an epidemic of high blood pressure *(hypertension)* similar to the epidemic of diabetes. The reasons are the same:

✔ Americans are getting fatter.

✔ Americans are storing fat in the center of our bodies, the so-called *abdominal visceral fat.*

✔ Americans are getting older as a population. The fastest-growing segment of the population is over 75 years of age. Of people age 50 to 55 with diabetes, 50 percent have high blood pressure. Of people older than 75 with diabetes, 75 percent have high blood pressure.

✔ Americans are more sedentary than before.

People with diabetes have high blood pressure more often than the nondiabetic population for a lot of other reasons besides the preceding ones:

✔ People with diabetes get kidney disease.

✔ People with diabetes have increased sensitivity to salt, which raises blood pressure.

✔ People with diabetes lack the nighttime fall in blood pressure that normally occurs in people without diabetes.

Doctors generally agree that a normal blood pressure is less than 140/90. For years, the *diastolic blood pressure* (the lower reading) was considered more damaging, and an elevation in that pressure was treated with greater importance than an elevation in the *systolic blood pressure* (the higher reading). More recent studies have shown that the systolic blood pressure, not the diastolic blood pressure, may be more important. (See the sidebar "The meaning of your blood pressure" for more detailed explanations of each type of blood pressure.)

All the complications of diabetes are made worse by an elevation in blood pressure, especially diabetic kidney disease but also eye disease, heart disease, nerve disease, peripheral vascular disease, and cerebral arterial disease (see Chapter 5).

Evidence of the importance of controlling blood pressure in diabetes comes from the United Kingdom Prospective Diabetes Study, published in late 1998. This study found that a lowering of blood pressure by 10 mm systolic and 5 mm diastolic resulted in a 24 percent reduction in any diabetic complication and a 32 percent reduction in death related to diabetes.

Controlling the blood pressure is absolutely essential in diabetes. The goal in diabetes is an even lower blood pressure than in the person without diabetes because studies have shown that lower normal blood pressures result in less diabetic damage than higher normal blood pressures. Your blood pressure should be no higher than 130/80.

How well are doctors doing at controlling blood pressure in people with diabetes? A study has shown that only 15 percent of people with diabetes with hypertension have a blood pressure as low as 140/90, and only 5 percent have a blood pressure down to 130/80.

Your doctor should measure blood pressure at every visit. Better yet, get a blood pressure device and measure it yourself. If you detect an elevation, bring it to the attention of your doctor.

Pregnant women with diabetes who have high blood pressure should not take ACE inhibitors or ARBs (two classes of drugs). They're known to be harmful to the growing fetus. If you have high blood pressure and plan to become pregnant, discuss your blood pressure medication with your doctor before conceiving.

For much more information on every aspect of high blood pressure, see my book *High Blood Pressure For Dummies* (Wiley).

The meaning of your blood pressure

What does the blood pressure measurement mean, and what is high blood pressure? When you get a reading, it usually looks something like 120/70 — it has an upper reading and a lower reading.

✔ The upper reading, called the *systolic pressure,* is the amount of force exerted by the heart when it contracts to push blood around the body. A cuff around your arm connects to a column of mercury. You, your doctor, or a machine listens for the first sound you hear on the side of the cuff away from your heart. That sound is the sound of blood finally able to overcome the pressure in the cuff and get through to the other side. The systolic blood pressure is the height of the column of mercury, read in millimeters, just as the blood comes through. (Sometimes the cuff is not connected to a column of mercury but to a gauge that is calibrated so the reading on the gauge is in millimeters of mercury even though no mercury is present.) In our example, the systolic blood pressure reading is 120 mm of mercury.

✔ The lower reading, called the *diastolic blood pressure,* is the pressure in the artery when the heart is at rest. A valve in the heart keeps the blood from flowing backwards so that the pressure does not fall to zero (you hope). When the sound stops, the height of the mercury column gives the diastolic blood pressure, in this case 70 mm of mercury.

Checking Your Weight and BMI

To give you a general idea of how much you ought to weigh, you can use the following formula:

✔ If you're a woman, give yourself 100 pounds for being 5 feet tall and add 5 pounds for each inch over 5 feet. For example, if you're 5 feet 3 inches, your appropriate weight should be approximately 115 pounds.

✔ If you're a man, give yourself 106 pounds for being 5 feet tall and add 6 pounds for each inch over 5 feet. A 5-foot 6-inch male should weigh around 142 pounds.

Body-mass index (BMI) is a measurement that relates weight to height. A tall person has a lower BMI than a short person of the same weight. (See Chapter 3 for more on BMI, including instructions for calculating your own BMI.) A person with a BMI under 18.5 is considered underweight. A person with a BMI from 18.5 to 24.9 is normal. A person with a BMI from 25 to 29.9 is overweight, and a person with a BMI of 30 or over is obese. By this definition, more than half the people in the United States are overweight or obese.

Non-white populations like South Asians, Chinese, and blacks develop diabetes at a lower BMI. Ethnicity must be considered in developing prevention techniques and targets for ideal body weight.

You can't get a reading of your BMI by stepping on a scale, but you can get your weight. This measurement is one of the easiest in medicine. Your doctor should measure your weight at every visit.

The National Heart, Lung, and Blood Institute makes knowing your BMI easy. Using the calculator at `www.nhlbisupport.com/bmi`, just fill in your weight in pounds and your height in feet and inches, click "Compute BMI," and get your result.

Maintaining a BMI in the normal range makes controlling your diabetes and blood pressure easier. Also, you must eliminate obesity as a risk factor for coronary artery disease.

Testing for Ketones

When your blood glucose rises above 250 mg/dl (13.9 mmol/L), or if you are pregnant with diabetes and your blood glucose is below 60 mg/dl (3.3 mmol/L), your doctor should probably check for *ketones* — products of the breakdown of fats. Finding ketones means that your body has turned to fat for energy. If you have high glucose and find ketones, you may need more insulin. If you have low glucose and find ketones during pregnancy, you may need more carbohydrates in your diet.

Testing for ketones is done by inserting a test strip into your urine and observing a purple color. The deeper the color, the greater the ketone level. If you find a large amount of ketones, you should contact your physician.

Even better, you can use a meter such as the Precision Xtra Blood Glucose and B-Ketone Monitoring System described earlier in this chapter to test your blood ketone level.

Testing the C-Reactive Protein

C-reactive protein (CRP) is a substance in the blood that is produced by the liver when infection or inflammation is present. It can be measured with a simple blood test. Diabetes is associated with several features that suggest that inflammation plays an important role in the disease. People who develop diabetes have higher C-reactive protein than those who don't. (Other substances associated with inflammation are also elevated in diabetes.)

Half the people with diabetes who have heart attacks have low or low-normal levels of LDL (bad) cholesterol. It is believed that inflammation plays a major role in many of these patients. Elevated CRP in the blood has been shown to directly contribute to blood-vessel damage and the formation of blood clots that cause heart attacks.

Drugs that improve diabetes lower the amount of C-reactive protein, which is also considered a marker for coronary artery disease.

 Have your C-reactive protein measured with other blood tests about once a year. If the level is elevated, it may serve as a predictor of future diabetes or coronary artery disease. You need to work even harder to lower your blood glucose, improve your LDL and HDL cholesterol, and lower your blood pressure. About 90 percent of healthy individuals have CRP levels less than 3, and 99 percent have levels less than 10.

Checking the TSH

A screening test called the *thyroid-stimulating hormone (TSH) level* is done at the time that diabetes is diagnosed and every five years thereafter if it is normal. This test is done because people with diabetes (type 1) have a higher incidence of thyroid disease than the general population, because thyroid disease is often confused with other conditions, and because hypothyroidism can lead to weight gain, which obviously isn't good for diabetes.

TSH is produced by the pituitary gland in the brain. When the thyroid gland makes the right amount of thyroid hormone, the pituitary produces the right amount of TSH to keep it working properly. The normal level in the blood is 0.5–2.5 microunits per milliliter (mU/ml).

When the thyroid makes inadequate amounts of thyroid hormone, the pituitary increases its production of TSH to stimulate the thyroid, and values of 10 or more mU/ml are not uncommon. When the thyroid makes too much thyroid hormone, it causes the pituitary to turn down its production of TSH, and values less than 0.5 mU/ml are found.

Too much thyroid hormone leads to insulin resistance, making diabetes worse than before. Too little thyroid hormone increases insulin sensitivity, so people with low thyroid function have reduced levels of blood glucose.

 Low levels of thyroid hormone cause an elevation in the hemoglobin A1c in patients who don't have diabetes as well as those who do. Replacing the thyroid hormone lowers the A1c to normal if diabetes is not present.

Much more about thyroid disease and its treatment can be found in my book *Thyroid For Dummies* (Wiley).

Evaluating Testosterone in Men with Type 2 Diabetes

About one third of men in the United States over the age of 65 have low levels of testosterone, and a similar percentage of those men have diabetes. Low testosterone is associated with changes in body composition that promote diabetes like increased fat and decreased muscle. According to tests done so far, giving testosterone to these men has not resulted in persistent improvement in glucose metabolism.

Older men who have significant reduction in muscle mass and increase in fat should have their testosterone measured. If very low, treatment with testosterone may be considered by you and your doctor. Such patients should at least make a major effort to increase exercise and decrease caloric intake, which often results in a rise in testosterone.

Checking Vitamin D

Recent studies suggest a relationship between low levels of vitamin D and the development of both type 1 and type 2 diabetes. Communities that live furthest from the equator, getting less sun to make vitamin D, have the highest incidence of type 1 diabetes. Vitamin D protects the body from autoimmunity (where the body attacks itself), and type 1 diabetes is an autoimmune disease. High levels of vitamin D are associated with a lower risk of developing type 2 diabetes. In a study, people who were prediabetic were given vitamin D over three months showed a significant improvement in glucose metabolism and reduction in hemoglobin A1c. Severe vitamin D deficiency has been shown to predict death and heart attacks in both type 1 and type 2 diabetes.

A study in the *Journal of Clinical Endocrinology and Metabolism* in September 2010 showed that blood vitamin D levels were low in obese women. The greater the degree of obesity, the lower the vitamin D. When weight was lost, the vitamin D level rose and the insulin resistance declined.

Have your vitamin D level measured with a blood test if you have prediabetes or diabetes. Take supplemental vitamin D if the level is low.

Chapter 8

Diabetes Diet Plan

*B*oy, are we big and getting bigger! The Centers for Disease Control tells us that more than six in ten Americans are overweight or obese. Most adults are 25 pounds heavier than people in the 1960s. And yet more than half of these overweight people think they are at a healthy weight.

The good news, according to a study in the *Journal of the American Medical Association* in January 2012, is that the prevalence of obesity and high body-mass index in the United States was the same — that is, no worse — in 2009 and 2010 as it was from 2003 to 2008. The bad news is that it is not improving.

Language specialists claim that the five sweetest phrases in the English language are

✔ I love you.

✔ Dinner is served.

✔ All is forgiven.

✔ Sleep until noon.

✔ Keep the change.

To that, most people would certainly add, "You've lost weight."

For the diabetic population, most of whom are overweight, appropriate nutrition and weight loss are not an option but a necessity. The Diabetes Control and Complications Trial clearly demonstrated that a person with diabetes who follows a careful nutrition program can reduce his or her hemoglobin A1c (see Chapter 7) by as much as 1 percent compared to the person with diabetes who is careless about diet.

In this chapter, you find out all you need to know to make your diet work for you, not only to improve your diabetes and control your blood glucose but also to feel generally that you have an improved quality of life.

Considering Total Calories First

Wanda B. Thinner, age 46, was a new type 2 diabetic patient who came to me because of high blood glucose levels, some blurring of her vision, and some numbness in her toes. She was 5 feet 5 inches tall and weighed 165 pounds. She was taking pills for the diabetes, but they were not helping. Her doctor had told her she needed to lose weight but gave no further instructions. I started her on a diet based on the principles in this chapter. She was willing to follow the diet and lost 20 pounds, which she has kept off. Her blood glucose is now in the range of 110 most of the time. She no longer suffers from blurred vision, and her toes are beginning to improve. She is not taking the diabetes medication and feels much better.

No matter how you slice it, your weight is determined by the number of calories you take in minus the number of calories you use up by exercise or loss of calories in the urine or bowel movements. If you have an excess of calories coming in and have insulin with which to store them, you gain weight. If you have fewer calories in than out, you lose weight. (See Chapter 7 if you're not sure how much you should weigh.) If you are overweight, you will benefit from even a small weight loss for the following reasons:

- ✔ Weight loss markedly reduces the risk of developing type 2 diabetes.

- ✔ Weight loss prevents the progression of prediabetes (see Chapter 2) into type 2 diabetes.

- ✔ Weight loss can reverse the failure to respond to drugs for diabetes that develops after responding at first (see Chapter 10).

- ✔ Weight loss reduces the risk of death from diabetes.

- ✔ Weight loss increases life expectancy in patients with type 2 diabetes.

- ✔ Weight loss has beneficial effects on high blood pressure and abnormal fats (see Chapter 7).

In an article in the *International Journal of Obesity* in June 2006, the authors from the University of Alabama and the University of Wisconsin offered ten reasons that may play a role in the obesity epidemic besides taking in excess calories:

✔ **Reduced length of nightly sleep:** An inverse relationship exists between weight and hours of sleep. People are sleeping less than they did before.

✔ **Hormones and other substances in food:** Substances like estrogens, which are put in animal feed to fatten the animals, have the same fattening effect on the humans who eat those animals.

✔ **Decreased exposure to high and low temperatures:** High temperatures cause sweating, and low temperatures cause shivering, both of which contribute to weight loss. Modern heat and air conditioning diminish our exposure to extremes of temperature, which is actually good for us.

✔ **Decreased smoking:** This phenomenon has a good side and a bad side. Cigarette smoking is the greatest public health menace that exists, but smokers do tend to be leaner than nonsmokers.

✔ **Use of drugs that cause weight gain:** Many of the drugs used for mental states like depression and high blood pressure cause marked weight gain and even diabetes.

✔ **Increases in age and ethnic groups that tend to be more overweight or obese:** Hispanic Americans, who are increasing in the population, have a much higher obesity prevalence than Caucasians. At the same time, the general population is older.

✔ **Increasing age of new mothers:** Older mothers tend to produce more obese children.

✔ **Effects in the uterus:** Maternal obesity may cause changes in the growing fetus that promote obesity.

✔ **Heavier women have more offspring:** These offspring, in turn, tend to be heavier.

✔ **Humans tend to choose heavier mates:** Heavier mates have reproductive advantages. And if your mate is heavier, you tend to become heavier.

Portion sizes have increased significantly both in restaurants and at home. Here are correct portion sizes for several foods:

✔ Three ounces of meat is the size of a deck of playing cards.

✔ A medium apple or peach is the size of a tennis ball.

✔ One ounce of cheese is the size of four dice.

✔ One-half cup of ice cream is the size of a tennis ball.

✔ A cup of mashed potatoes is the size of your fist.

✔ A teaspoon of butter or peanut butter is the size of the tip of your thumb.

✔ One-half cup of nuts is the size of a golf ball.

To have an approximate idea of how many *kcalories* (kilocalories) you need each day (not *calories,* which are much smaller, and which are incorrectly used as the common unit of food energy), you need to figure your desirable weight. Using the method described in Chapter 7, a 5-foot 6-inch male with a moderate frame should weigh around 142 pounds. Follow these steps to find the number of kcalories needed:

1. **Multiply your weight times 10.** In our example, this gives a value of about 1,400 kcalories.

2. **Add kcalories for your level of exercise:**

   - A sedentary male adds 10 percent of the basal kcalories.

   - A moderately active male adds 20 percent.

   - A very active male adds 40 percent or more, depending on the length and the degree of exercise.

If the male in our example is moderately active, he needs 1,400 kcalories plus 1,400 times 20 percent (or about 300) more for a total of about 1,700 kcalories.

These formulas are true for women as well, but women usually require fewer calories to maintain the same weight as men. Be aware that this calculation is an approximation that differs not only for different people but even for the same person on different days.

Caloric needs are different for people of different ages and different levels of activity. A woman who is pregnant or breastfeeding obviously needs more kcalories (as I discuss in Chapter 6). If a person is trying to lose weight, reducing the total kcalories per day can help accomplish this goal. I say a lot more about this topic in the section on weight reduction later in this chapter.

After you determine the total kcalories you need, the question becomes how to divide the calories among various foods. Basically, three types of foods contain calories: carbohydrates, proteins, and fats. Within these foods, you have many variables, which I explain in this section.

Consuming the right amount of carbohydrates

No area in nutrition is more controversial for the diabetic person than carbohydrates. For years, the American Diabetes Association (ADA) told people with diabetes that they should eat 55 to 60 percent of their calories as carbohydrate. Other experts said that amount was too much or too little. The ADA has now modified its recommendation so that it says in the Clinical Practice

Recommendations for 2012, "The recommended daily allowance for carbo-hydrate is 130 grams per day and is based on providing adequate glucose as the required fuel for the central nervous system without reliance on glucose production from ingested protein or fat."

Carbohydrates are the sources of energy that start with *glucose,* the sugar in your bloodstream that is one sugar molecule, and include substances containing many sugar molecules called *complex carbohydrates, starches, cellulose,* and *gums.* Some of the common sources of carbohydrate are bread, potatoes, grains, cereals, and rice.

Physicians know a lot of information about carbohydrate in the body:

- Carbohydrate is the primary source of energy for muscles.
- Glucose is the carbohydrate that causes the pancreas to release insulin.
- Carbohydrate causes the triglyceride (fat) level to rise in the blood.
- When insulin is not present or is ineffective, more carbohydrate raises the blood glucose higher.
- If simple sugars are in the diet in increased amounts, they are not harmful as long as the total calorie count is satisfactory. (The major reason to reduce simple sugars in the diet is the harmful effect on dental cavities. Cavities are no more severe or common in people with diabetes than in people without diabetes.)

Although the fat intake of the U.S. population has declined because of the fear of coronary artery disease caused by cholesterol, Americans are getting fatter. In fact, 68 percent of Americans are considered overweight or obese according to the U.S. Department of Health and Human Resources. Because Americans are not eating more protein, the culprit is most likely excess carbohydrate, such as that found in concentrated sweets, such as pastry and candy, as well as the more complex carbohydrate found in bread. Within the body, carbohydrate can be turned into fat and stored. This function was great when everyone lived in caves and got little food for prolonged periods of time, but it doesn't fit today's lifestyle, consisting as it does of abundant food (and minimal foraging for it in the supermarket).

Because carbohydrate is the food that raises the blood glucose, which is responsible for the complications of diabetes, it seems right to recommend a diet that is lower in carbohydrate than previously suggested. Furthermore, a major source of coronary artery disease in diabetes is the metabolic syndrome (see Chapter 5). Because increased carbohydrate triggers increased triglyceride, which is the beginning of a number of abnormalities that lead to increased coronary artery disease, recommending less carbohydrate on this basis as well seems prudent.

My experience has been that a diet of between 40 and 50 percent carbohydrate makes controlling my patients' blood glucose much easier. It also leads to weight loss because you don't tend to substitute protein or fat for the reduced amount of carbohydrate in the diet. My patients on lower-carbohydrate diets are able to reduce the amounts of drugs they take, such as insulin, which can cause weight gain and complicate controlling their diabetes. They also have a better fat profile.

Thinking back to the example earlier in this chapter, a man on a diet of 1,700 kcalories should eat about 850 kcalories as carbohydrate. Because each gram of carbohydrate is 4 kcalories, he eats about 210 grams of carbohydrate a day. This amount, which I recommend in this case based on my experience, is higher than the recommendation by the ADA. Translating this amount into the foods you know and love, it's the same as two slices of whole-wheat bread, 1 cup of brown rice, five fruits, and a cup of baked beans a day.

Glycemic index

All carbohydrates are not alike in the degree to which they raise the blood glucose. This fact was recognized some years ago, and a measurement called the *glycemic index* was created to quantify it. The *glycemic index* (GI) uses white bread as the indicator food and assigns it a value of 100. Another carbohydrate of equal calories is compared to white bread in its ability to raise the blood glucose and is assigned a value in comparison to white bread. A food that raises glucose half as much as white bread has a GI of 50, whereas a food that raises glucose 1½ times as much has a GI of 150.

A recent study reported in the *Archives of Internal Medicine* in November 2007 showed that a group of Chinese women who tended to eat a lot of high-glycemic index rice had a significant increase in the risk of developing type 2 diabetes. Another study in the same issue showed that increasing the level of low glycemic cereal in the diet reduced the risk of type 2 diabetes in a group of black women, a group that is getting type 2 diabetes in epidemic numbers.

The point is to select carbohydrates with low GI levels to try to keep the glucose response as low as possible. A glycemic index of 70 or more is high, 56 to 69 is medium, and 55 or less is low.

Good clinical studies have shown that knowledge of the glycemic index of food sources can be very valuable. Evaluation of the diet of people who develop diabetes compared with those who don't shows that, all other things being equal, the people with the highest GI diet most often develop diabetes. After diabetes is present, patients who eat the lowest GI carbohydrates have the lowest levels of blood glucose. Patients in these studies have not had great difficulty changing to a low GI diet. The other thing that happens when low GI food is incorporated into a diet is that the levels of triglycerides and LDL (or "bad" cholesterol) fall in both type 1 and type 2 diabetes.

I believe that switching to low GI carbohydrates can be very beneficial for controlling the glucose. You can easily make some simple substitutions in your diet, as shown in Table 8-1.

Table 8-1	Simple Diet Substitutions
High-GI Food	*Low-GI Food*
White bread	Whole-grain bread
Processed breakfast cereal	Unrefined cereals like oats and processed low-GI cereals
Plain cookies and crackers	Cookies made with dried fruits or whole grains like oats
Cakes and muffins	Cakes and muffins made with fruit or whole grains like oats
Tropical fruits like bananas	Temperate-climate fruits like apples and plums
Potatoes	Pasta and legumes
White rice	Basmati and other low-GI rice

Because bread and breakfast cereals are major daily sources of carbohydrates, these simple changes can make a major difference in lowering your glycemic index. Foods that are excellent sources of carbohydrate but have a low GI include legumes such as peas or beans, pasta, grains like barley, parboiled rice (rice that is partially boiled in the husk, making it nutritionally similar to brown rice), bulgar, and whole-grain breads.

Even though a food has a low GI, it may not be appropriate because it is too high in fat. You need to evaluate each food's fat content before assuming that all low GI foods are good for a person with diabetes.

The position of the American Diabetes Association, stated in its position paper in 2011, is that "the use of the glycemic index may provide a modest additional benefit over that observed when total carbohydrate is considered alone."

And though a food has a high GI, it may still be acceptable in your diet if it contains very little total carbohydrate. For example, cantaloupe has a GI of about 70, but the amount of total carbohydrate is so low that it doesn't raise your blood glucose significantly when you eat a normal portion. This concept is called the *glycemic load* (GL), a number that takes both glycemic index and total carbohydrates into account. A GL of 20 is high, 11 to 19 is medium, and 10 or less is low.

If you want to go into this subject in deeper detail, you can find a listing of many foods by category of food and by level of GI, portion size, and GL on the web at www.glycemicindex.com.

Fiber

Fiber is the part of the carbohydrate that is not digestible and, therefore, adds no calories. Fiber is found in most fruits, grains, and vegetables. Fiber comes in two forms:

- ✔ **Soluble fiber:** This form of fiber can dissolve in water and has a lowering effect on blood glucose and fat levels, particularly cholesterol.

- ✔ **Insoluble fiber:** This form of fiber cannot dissolve in water and remains in the intestine. It absorbs water and stimulates movement in the intestine. Insoluble fiber also helps prevent constipation and possibly colon cancer. This fiber is called *bulk* or *roughage*.

Before the current trend to refine foods, people ate many sources of carbohydrate that were high in fiber. These sources were all plant foods such as fruits, vegetables, and grains. Animal foods contain no fiber.

Because too much fiber causes diarrhea and gas, you need to increase the fiber level in your diet fairly slowly. The recommendation for daily fiber is 20 to 30 grams. Most Americans eat only about 15 grams daily.

Many of the foods listed in the previous section as having a low glycemic index contain a lot of fiber, which helps to reduce the blood glucose.

The way to eat the right amount of carbohydrate without increasing your blood glucose or triglycerides is to make it a low-glycemic, high-fiber carbohydrate. Such a diet has been shown to reduce the need for insulin in women with gestational diabetes without any negative effect on the fetus or mother. Increased dietary fiber intake has been shown to reduce the risk of death, not only from heart and blood vessel disease but also from infectious respiratory diseases.

Portioning proteins

Excluding vegetable sources of protein like soybeans, legumes, nuts, and seeds, protein in your diet is usually the muscle of other animals, such as chicken, turkey, beef, or lamb. For this reason, people used to believe that you could build your own muscle by eating lots of another animal's muscle. (The truth is that you can build up your muscle only by exercising or weight-lifting.) You need little protein to maintain your current level of muscle (or to increase it, for that matter).

Your choice of protein is very important because some is very high in fat and some is practically fat-free. The following lists can give you an idea of the fat content of various sources of protein. (In the next section, I explain how to integrate fat into your diet.)

- ✔ **Very lean:** One ounce of very lean meat, fish, or substitutes has about 7 grams of protein and 1 gram of fat. Examples include

  - Skinless white-meat chicken or turkey

  - Flounder, halibut, or tuna canned in water

  - Lobster, shrimp, or clams

  - Fat-free cheese

- ✔ **Lean:** An ounce of lean meat, fish, or substitutes has about 7 grams of protein and 3 grams of fat. Examples include

  - Lean beef, lean pork, lean lamb, or lean veal

  - Dark-meat chicken without skin or white-meat chicken with skin

  - Sardines, salmon, or tuna canned in oil

  - Other meats or cheeses with 3 grams of fat per ounce

- ✔ **Medium-fat:** An ounce of medium-fat meat, fish, or substitutes has about 7 grams of protein and 5 grams of fat. Examples include

  - Most beef products

  - Regular pork, lamb, or veal

  - Dark-meat chicken with skin or fried chicken

  - Fried fish

  - Cheeses with 5 grams of fat per ounce, such as feta and mozzarella

- ✔ **High fat:** High-fat meat, fish, or substitutes contain about 8 grams of fat and 7 grams of protein per ounce. Examples include

  - Pork spareribs or pork sausage

  - Bacon

  - Processed sandwich meats

  - Regular cheeses like cheddar or Monterey Jack

Based on the fat, you can guess that low-fat and high-fat proteins have a huge difference in kcalories. An ounce of skinless white-meat chicken contains about 40 kcalories, whereas an ounce of pork spareribs has 100 kcalories. Because most people eat a minimum of four ounces of meat at a meal, they're eating from 160 to 400 kcalories depending on the source.

My recommendation is that 20 percent of your kcalories come from protein. This would be about 350 kcalories for the gentleman who weighs 142 pounds and needs 1,700 kcalories each day. Because a gram of protein is 4 kcalories, he can eat about 90 grams of protein. Translating that into ounces of meat, because each ounce has 7 grams of protein, he can eat about 13 ounces of meat daily. For example, he can eat 6 ounces of flounder at one meal and 5 ounces of dark-meat chicken at another, with 2 cups of milk providing the rest of his protein.

Many authorities suggest less protein in the diet because protein has a damaging effect on the kidneys. Several studies have shown this to be the case, but a very large study in the *Annals of Internal Medicine* in March 2003 came to a different conclusion. It showed that high-protein diets caused increasing damage in kidneys that already had some damage but not in normal kidneys. The jury remains out on this question of lower versus higher protein diets.

Filling the fat requirement

People with type 2 diabetes have to be very aware of the fats in their diet. Fortunately, the amount of fat you need is a lot less controversial than the carbohydrate and protein in your diet. Everyone agrees that you should eat no more than 30 percent of your diet as fats. (Currently, the U.S. population eats 36 percent of its diet as fats.)

Keep in mind that some fats are more dangerous in their tendency to promote coronary artery disease than others. These fats should make up less of the dietary fat than the safer fats.

Cholesterol is the fat everyone knows. It has been shown to be the culprit in the development of coronary artery disease, as well as peripheral vascular disease and cerebrovascular disease (see Chapter 5). The recommendation is that no more than 300 milligrams a day of fat come from cholesterol. One egg can take care of that prescription. Most other foods that you eat regularly do not contain a lot of cholesterol, but whole milk and hard cheeses like Jack and cheddar contain saturated fat, which raises the cholesterol in the body.

You also must pay attention to foods that increase triglycerides, which lead to the production of small, dense LDL particles that are connected to coronary artery disease. Abnormal fats are one component of the metabolic syndrome. Triglycerides comes in several forms:

✔ **Saturated fat** is the kind of fat that usually comes from animal sources. The streaks of fat in a steak are saturated fat. Butter is made up of saturated fat. Bacon, cream, and cream cheese are other examples. Vegetable sources of saturated fat include coconut, palm, and palm-kernel oils. Eating a lot of saturated fat increases your blood cholesterol level.

- **Trans fatty acid** is produced when polyunsaturated fat (which I describe in the next bullet) is heated and hydrogen is bubbled through it. Fully hydrogenated, it becomes solid fat; partially hydrogenated, it has a consistency like butter and can be used in butter's place.

Trans fatty acids may contribute more to the development of heart disease than saturated fats. Keep them out of your diet! Some examples of foods high in trans fats are some cake mixes and dried soup mixes, many fast foods and frozen foods, baked goods like donuts and cookies, potato chips, crackers, breakfast cereals (even some with seemingly health-conscious names), candies, and whipped toppings. The government now requires food labels to list trans fats, so read those labels! Fortunately, food manufacturers are increasingly removing trans fats from their products.

- **Unsaturated fat** comes from vegetable sources. It comes in several forms:

  - **Monounsaturated fat** does not raise cholesterol. Avocado, olive oil, and canola oil are examples. The oil in nuts like almonds and peanuts is monounsaturated.

  - **Polyunsaturated fat** also does not raise cholesterol but causes a reduction in the good or HDL cholesterol. Examples of polyunsaturated fats are soft fats and oils such as corn oil and mayonnaise.

Eskimos eat a lot of fat (more than is recommended), and yet they have a low incidence of coronary artery disease. It has been shown that their protection comes from *essential fatty acids*. These acids are found in fish oils, which Eskimos consume to a great extent. Essential fatty acids reduce triglycerides, reduce blood pressure, and increase the time that it takes for blood to clot, which protects against a blood clot in the heart. You can have the benefits of fish oil by substituting fish for meat two or three times a week in your diet. Pills containing fish oil have not been shown to provide the same benefit. If you don't like fish (which means you have probably never tasted salmon cooked on a barbecue), you can't get this benefit.

Keeping in mind that 30 percent of your total daily calories should come from fat, less than a third of that amount should come from saturated fats. You should also keep your dietary cholesterol under 300 milligrams per day.

For the gentleman who weighs 142 pounds and needs 1,700 kcalories, who is slowly starving waiting for us to figure out how much to feed him, his final 500 kcalories can come from fat. Fat has 9 kcalories per gram, so he can eat about 56 grams of fat daily.

Remember that he has already taken in 40 grams of fat with his flounder and chicken, so he is left with only 16 grams, 8 of which come with his milk. That leaves about a teaspoon of butter from the fat sources.

Getting Enough Vitamins, Minerals, and Water

Your diet must contain sufficient vitamins and minerals, but the amount you need may be less than you think. If you eat a balanced diet that comes from the various food groups, you generally get enough vitamins for your daily needs. Table 8-2 lists the vitamins and their food sources.

Table 8-2	Vitamins You Need	
Vitamin	*Function*	*Food Source*
Vitamin A	Needed for healthy skin, bones, and eyes	Milk and green vegetables
Vitamin B₁ (thiamin)	Converts carbohydrates into energy	Meat and whole-grain cereals
Vitamin B₂ (riboflavin)	Needed to use food properly	Milk, cheese, fish, and green vegetables
Vitamin B₆ (pyridoxine), pantothenic acid, and biotin	All needed for growth	Liver, yeast, and many other foods
Vitamin B₁₂	Keeps the red blood cells and the nervous system healthy	Animal foods (for example, meat)
Folic acid	Keeps the red blood cells and the nervous system healthy	Green vegetables
Niacin	Helps release energy	Lean meat, fish, nuts, and legumes
Vitamin C	Helps maintain supportive tissues	Fruit and potatoes
Vitamin D	Helps with absorption of calcium	Fortified dairy products, and made in the skin when exposed to sunlight
Vitamin E	Helps maintain cells	Vegetable oils and whole-grain cereals
Vitamin K	Needed for proper clotting of the blood	Leafy vegetables, and made by bacteria in your intestine

As you look through the vitamins in Table 8-2, you can see that most of them are easily available in the foods you eat every day. In certain situations, such as if you are pregnant, you need to be sure that you are getting enough every day, so you take a vitamin supplement. Some evidence also suggests that extra vitamin C protects against colds.

As far as the other vitamins go, the proof just does not exist that large amounts of the vitamins are beneficial, and in some cases, they may be harmful. I do not recommend that you take megadoses of these vitamins.

Minerals are also key ingredients of a healthy diet. Most are needed in tiny amounts, which are easily consumed from a balanced diet. Keep the following in mind:

- ✔ **Calcium, phosphorus, and magnesium build bones and teeth.** Milk and other dairy products provide plenty of these minerals, but evidence suggests that people are not getting enough calcium. Adults should get 1,000 milligrams of calcium every day, and you should get 1,500 milligrams if you are growing up (adolescents) or out (pregnant women). Older people must be sure to eat 1,500 milligrams a day. Increased magnesium in the diet has a protective role in the development of type 2 diabetes.

- ✔ **Iron is essential for red blood cells and is gotten from meat and some nuts, legumes, and vegetables.** However, a menstruating woman tends to lose iron and may need a supplement.

- ✔ **Sodium regulates body water.** You need only about 220 milligrams a day, but you likely take in 20 to 40 times that much, which probably explains a lot of the high blood pressure in the United States. Because hypertension is so prevalent in both types of diabetes and it makes diabetic complications occur earlier, reduction of salt intake is an important consideration. Don't add salt to your food (it already has plenty in it), and you will enjoy the taste a lot more without it.

- ✔ **Chromium is needed in tiny amounts.** No scientific evidence shows that chromium is especially helpful to the person with diabetes in controlling the blood glucose, despite reams of articles in health food magazines to the contrary.

- ✔ **Iodine is essential for production of thyroid hormones.** It is added to salt in order to assure that people get enough of it. In many areas of the world where iodine is not found in the soil, people suffer from very large thyroid glands known as *goiters*.

- ✔ **Various other minerals, like chlorine, cobalt, tin, and zinc, are found in many foods.** These minerals are rarely lacking in the human diet.

Water is the last important nutrient I discuss in this section, but it is by no means the least important. Your body is made up of 60 percent or more water. All the nutrients in the body are dissolved in water. You can live without food for some time, but you will not last long without water. Water can help to give a feeling of fullness that reduces appetite. In general, people do not drink enough water. You need to get a minimum of 10 cups, or 2½ quarts, of water a day from all sources (that is, from all the foods and liquids you ingest).

Counting Alcohol as Part of Your Diet

Alcohol is a chemical that has calories but no particular nutritional value; although it has been shown that a moderate amount (a glass or two of wine a day) may reduce the risk of a heart attack. Notice that I call alcohol a *chemical.* That's because alcohol is often taken to excess and does major damage to the body. It wrecks the liver and can lead to bleeding and death.

This book is not the place for a discussion of the social issues that surround the use of alcohol. Suffice it to say that excess alcohol destroys lives and families. In this section, I want to explain the part that alcohol plays in the life of the person with diabetes.

Because alcohol has calories, if you drink some, you must account for those calories in your diet. The proof of the alcohol is the percentage of alcohol in an ounce of the drink multiplied by 2. Wine that is 12.5 percent alcohol is 25 proof. Beer is around 12 proof most of the time. Liquor is often 80 proof. To determine the calories, use the following formula:

Calories = 0.8 × proof of the drink × number of ounces

For example, for a 12-ounce can of beer, you use the formula 0.8 × 12 × 12 for a total of 115 kilocalories. For a couple of 6-ounce glasses of wine, you use the formula 0.8 × 25 × 12 to come up with 240 kilocalories. You can see that the alcohol calories add up pretty quickly. You may even wonder why alcoholics are not often overweight. The answer is that alcohol becomes a staple of their diet and they develop wasting diseases associated with inadequate intake of protein, carbohydrate, fat, vitamins, and minerals.

In addition to the calories, alcohol plays other roles in diabetes. If alcohol is taken without food, it can cause low blood glucose by increasing the activity of insulin without food to compensate for it. Some alcoholics, even without diabetes, go to bed with several drinks in their systems and are unconscious the next morning because of very low blood glucose. They can have brain damage unless their bodies are able to manufacture enough glucose to wake them up.

If you're having a couple glasses of wine or other alcohol, make sure that you eat some food along with it.

A study in *Diabetes Care* in 2009 confirmed previous research findings that moderate alcohol intake (two glasses of wine daily for men and one glass for women) was protective against diabetes while more than that was harmful.

Using Sugar Substitutes

Fear of the "danger" of sugar in the diet has led to a vast effort to produce a compound that can add the pleasurable sweetness without the liabilities of sugar. Interestingly enough, despite the availability of a number of excellent sweeteners, some containing no calories at all, the incidence of diabetes continues to rise. Still, if you can reduce your caloric intake or your glucose response by using a sweetener, doing so has advantages. Sweeteners are divided into those that contain calories and those that do not.

Among the calorie-containing sweeteners are the following:

- **Fructose, found in fruits and berries:** Fructose is actually sweeter than table sugar *(sucrose)*. However, it is absorbed more slowly from the intestine than glucose, so it raises the blood glucose more slowly. It is taken up by the liver and converted to glucose or triglycerides.

- **Xylitol, found in strawberries and raspberries:** Xylitol is about like fructose in terms of sweetness. It is taken up slowly from the intestine so that it causes little change in blood glucose. Xylitol does not cause cavities of the teeth as often as the other sweeteners containing calories, so it is used in chewing gum.

- **Sorbitol and mannitol, sugar alcohols occurring in plants:** Sorbitol and mannitol are half as sweet as table sugar and have little effect on blood glucose. They change to fructose in the body. (If you read Chapter 5, you may remember sorbitol. When taken as a food, sorbitol does not accumulate or damage tissues.)

The non-nutritive or artificial sweeteners are often much sweeter than table sugar. Therefore, much less of them is required to accomplish the same level of sweetness as sugar. Following are some of the current artificial sweeteners:

- **Saccharin:** This sweetener is 300 to 400 times sweeter than sucrose. It is rapidly excreted unchanged in the urine. Brand names include Sweet'N Low and Sugar Twin.

- **Aspartame:** This sweetener is more expensive than saccharin, but many people seem to prefer its taste. It's 150 to 200 times sweeter than sucrose. The brand name is Equal when used as a tabletop sweetener or NutraSweet when used in food and beverages.

- **Acesulfame:** This sweetener is 200 times sweeter than sucrose and does not leave an aftertaste. It can be used in cooking and is found in numerous foods and beverages. Its brand name is Sunett or Sweet One. It should not be used by people with a rare genetic disorder called phenylketonuria.

- ✔ **Sucralose:** This sweetener is obtained from sugar and is 600 times sweeter. It is very stable and can be used in place of sugar in any food. It leaves no unpleasant aftertaste. The brand name is Splenda.

- ✔ **Neotame:** Authorized by the FDA in July 2000, neotame has 7,000 to 13,000 times the sweetening power of sucrose. It is not in commercial products yet, but food manufacturers are working with it because it can be used cooked or uncooked with no loss of sweetening. The brand name is not yet determined.

- ✔ **Cyclamate:** Because it has been associated with cancer when given in huge doses, cyclamate is banned in the United States. It is 30 times as sweet as sucrose. The association with cancer has not been substantiated.

- ✔ **Tagatose:** Tagatose is a naturally occurring sweetener present in small amounts in fruits and dairy products. The FDA has recognized tagatose as safe. It can be purchased as most health food stores. It has about the same sweetening power as table sugar and is called Naturlose.

- ✔ **Stevia:** This sweetener is derived from the stevia plant, native to South America. It is marketed as SweetLeaf Stevia. It is 150 to 400 times sweeter than sugar and can be used in cooking and baking.

For people with diabetes, recommendations regarding using sugar have been changed so that some sugar is permitted. The point is to count the calories eaten as sugar and subtract that from your permissible intake. If you do this calculation, you'll have little use for either the nutritive or the non-nutritive sweeteners.

Eating Well for Type 1 Diabetes

A person with type 1 diabetes takes insulin (see Chapter 10) to control the blood glucose. At this time, doctors and their patients can't match the human pancreas in the way that it releases insulin just when the food is entering the bloodstream so that the glucose remains between 80 and 120 mg/dl. Therefore, diabetic patients need to make sure that their food enters as close to the expected activity of the insulin as possible. This book is most concerned with type 2 diabetes, so I refer you to my book *Type 1 Diabetes For Dummies* (Wiley) for a thorough discussion of food and insulin treatment in type 1 diabetes.

Reducing Your Weight

Because most people with type 2 diabetes are overweight, weight control and reduction should be the major consideration. The benefits of weight loss are rapidly seen, even when relatively little has been lost. The blood glucose falls rapidly. The blood pressure declines. The cholesterol falls. The triglycerides drop, and the good cholesterol (HDL) rises. As I point out in Chapter 5, even a modest reduction of 10 percent of body weight has a significant positive effect on coronary artery disease.

In addition to the many other benefits, weight loss also results in significant improvement in obstructive sleep apnea.

Weight reduction is difficult for many reasons. In my experience, most patients do very well initially but tend to return to old habits. Evidence suggests that this tendency to regain weight is built into the human brain. When fat tissue is decreased or even increased, a central control system in the brain acts to restore the fat to the previous level. If liposuction is done, for example, the remaining cells swell up to hold more fat.

Still, losing weight and keeping it off is possible. At one time, it was calculated that only 1 out of 20 people who lost weight would keep it off. Now the figure is closer to 1 out of 5. The information in the following sections can help you find a weight-loss plan that will work for you.

In the next chapter, I cover the value of exercise in a weight-loss program. At this point, you need to realize that successful maintenance of weight loss requires a willingness to make exercise a part of your daily life. A recent study showed that 92 percent of people who maintain weight loss exercise regularly, while only 34 percent of those who regain their weight continue to exercise. If, for some reason, you cannot move your legs to exercise, you can get a satisfactory workout using your upper body alone.

Types of diets

The numerous methods that are available for weight loss certainly suggest that no one method is especially better than all the rest. Some are fairly drastic in the degree to which they cut calories, and weight loss is fairly rapid. But these methods are particularly prone to result in restoration of the original weight. Among the many more drastic diets are the following:

- ✔ **Very-low-calorie diets:** These diets provide 400 to 800 kcalories daily of protein and carbohydrate with supplemental vitamins and minerals. They are safe when supervised by a physician and are used when you need rapid weight loss — for example, for a heart condition. They result in rapid initial weight loss with a fall in the need for medications. Weight restoration commonly occurs, however.

- ✔ **Animal-protein diets like the Atkins diet:** Food is limited to animal protein sources in an effort to maintain body protein, along with vitamins and minerals. Carbohydrates are strongly discouraged. Patients often complain of hair loss. Weight is rapidly regained when the diet is discontinued. This diet is not balanced, and I don't recommend it for more than a few weeks. Because the Atkins diet encourages foods that are high in fats, a variation called the *South Beach Diet* was developed that emphasizes decreased carbohydrates along with decreased fats.

✔ **LEARN diet:** The name stands for lifestyle, exercise, attitudes, relationships, and nutrition. It recommends a diet of 55 to 60 percent carbohydrate and less than 10 percent from fat.

✔ **Fasts:** A *fast* means giving up all food for a period of time and taking only water and vitamins and minerals. A fast is such a drastic change from normal eating habits that patients do not remain on the fast for very long, and weight is regained.

✔ **DASH diet:** The Dietary Approach to Stop Hypertension was designed to lower blood pressure. It consists of lean meat, poultry, and fish; whole grains; fruits and vegetables; dairy; and legumes, nuts, and seeds. High-salt foods and foods rich in saturated fats are out.

Several diets are associated with large organizations and may require that you purchase only their foods. The support given by these organizations seems to be extremely helpful in weight-loss maintenance. In addition, the slower loss of weight and the connection to more normal eating seems to result in a greater tendency to stay with the program and keep the weight off. Following are the leading contenders for this type of diet:

✔ **Jenny Craig:** This organization provides the food that you eat, which you must pay for. It offers some information on behavior modification and has special diets for people with diabetes. In 1997, the government required Jenny Craig to tell its customers that the weight-loss methods may be only temporary, because customers had no way to judge from its advertising that many people regain their weight.

✔ **Weight Watchers:** This organization emphasizes slow weight loss, exercise, and behavior modification. It charges for weekly attendance at its meetings, which are held all over the world. It does not require that you purchase any products, but Weight Watchers foods are available for purchase. Its point program for increasing fiber in your diet may be especially helpful to the person with diabetes.

U.S. News and World Report asked 22 experts in diet, nutrition, and diabetes to rank these and other diets for their ability to prevent and manage diabetes. The DASH diet beat all the rest. It is a diet you can stay on, and it works. (See my book *High Blood Pressure For Dummies* [Wiley] for much more on this diet.)

The National Weight Control Registry, which has been running since 1993, shows that people can lose a lot of weight and keep it off. The average loss is 60 pounds and is maintained for more than five years. These "losers" do it on their own half the time. They use a combination of a low-fat diet and at least 45 minutes of exercise daily, usually walking, to keep the weight off, even though the initial weight loss was accomplished in many different ways such as a liquid diet in an organized program, other types of organized programs, or on their own. Most of them (68 percent) eat breakfast every day. The longer they kept the weight off, the easier it became to continue weight maintenance.

Vegetarian diets

Time and again vegetarian diets have been shown to reduce the risk of type 2 diabetes and to improve all aspects of the disease when diabetes is already present. Increasing the daily intake of green leafy vegetables has been especially helpful.

A report in *Diabetes Care* in 2009 looked at the diets of 60,000 men and women. The mean body-mass index was lowest in vegans (no dairy), higher in lacto-ovo vegetarians (who ate dairy and eggs), still higher in vegetarians who ate fish, and highest in nonvegetarians. The prevalence of type 2 diabetes was lowest in the vegans and rose with the mean BMI so that it was highest in the nonvegetarians. The risk of metabolic syndrome was also found to be lowest in the vegans and rose with increased meat eating.

Consider shifting your diet in the direction of more vegetables and less animal protein. The benefits may be huge.

Pills for weight loss

Currently only one weight-loss drug is approved for long-term use. It's called orlistat and goes by the trade names Alli and Xenical. Many other drugs have come and gone because they haven't worked or they caused damage to the body of the patient. Orlistat works by inhibiting the absorption of fat. The result is that the patient feels bloated and has gas and diarrhea. I tried it on several patients, but they hated the side effects and didn't lose much weight. I don't recommend it.

Metabolic surgery for diabetes

Metabolic surgery has been so successful in preventing and reversing diabetes that many surgeons and diabetes specialists consider diabetes a surgical disease. This surgery leads to marked and long-lasting weight reduction.

When the effects of metabolic surgery are compared with standard (non-surgical) care, the results are unequivocal. In one study, operated patients reduced their BMI from 34.6 to 25.8 and their hemoglobin A1c from 8.2 to 6.1 percent, while no change occurred in the patients receiving standard care. In another study, BMI fell by 11.4 for the operated group while standard care again produced no long-term change.

You may want to consider surgery if you fit these descriptions:

- ✔ You have a body-mass index (see Chapter 7) that is greater than 40 or greater than 35 with a serious health problem linked to obesity.

- ✔ You have an obesity-related physical problem, such as inability to walk.

- ✔ You have a high-risk, obesity-related health problem like heart disease or sleep apnea.

The best surgical treatment for obesity is the *gastric bypass operation,* in which the upper stomach is stapled to create a small, thumb-sized pouch at the top and a larger pouch below. Because the upper pouch is small, you have a feeling of early fullness, and you tend to eat less. The upper pouch is connected to the small intestine so that the lower stomach and a length of the small intestine are bypassed. Patients are forced to eat very small portions and can't eat sugar and other carbohydrates, which cause dizziness and other symptoms. Most of the weight is lost in the first year.

The surgery is performed without opening the abdomen except for the small tubes needed to perform it laparascopically. A laparoscope shows the surgical area on a TV screen, and the surgeon operates with other tubes that have cutting devices and sewing devices at their end. The abdomen is raised above the site with CO_2 gas to allow the surgeon to work.

Following are some problems associated with the gastric bypass operation:

- ✔ Leaks where organs are sewed together

- ✔ Gastrointestinal bleeding

- ✔ Closure of the opening between organs

- ✔ Long-term malabsorption of vitamins and minerals

More recently, the *laparoscopic gastric banding* procedure has been used. A constricting band containing an inflatable balloon is placed around the upper end of the stomach to create a small upper pouch and a larger lower pouch. It can be inflated or deflated to control the size of the upper stomach. The usual weight loss is two-thirds of the excess within two years. By removing the band, the procedure can be reversed. This operation is simpler than gastric bypass and is less likely to result in a surgical complication. Some of the problems of gastric banding include the following:

- The pouch may stretch.
- The band may slip.
- The reservoir in the constricting band that permits inflation may leak.
- Weight loss may not occur (if the patient chooses to overeat).
- The patient may experience acid reflux from the stomach into the esophagus.
- The patient may experience persistent vomiting.

The results of surgery greatly favor gastric bypass over gastric banding. People in one study who had gastric bypass lost 64 percent of their excess body weight in a year compared to 36 percent for gastric banding. Complication rates were similar in both groups, and no deaths were recorded. Within one year after bypass surgery, 75 percent showed remission of diabetes while only 50 percent of the banding group showed remission. Gastric banding can be overcome relatively easily with resultant weight gain. If you are going to have surgery for diabetes and weight loss, choose gastric bypass.

You won't be cured of your diabetes after either of these surgeries. The benefit will be improved control of your blood glucose and weight loss. If you have that as your expectation, you will be much more satisfied.

The International Diabetes Federation stated in 2011 that "Bariatric surgery should now be considered earlier in the treatment of type 2 diabetes and should no longer be seen as a last resort." Some members suggested that a BMI of 30 with diabetes was enough to warrant surgery.

When you have surgery for obesity, you must be committed to lifelong medical follow-up. You must be willing to give up large meals and be determined to lose weight.

Behavior modification

From my years of working with obese patients, I've seen that weight loss requires more than a commitment to a sound diet and routine exercise; it requires changes in behavior with respect to food. To lose weight and keep it off, you must change your eating behavior to make your diet easier to follow. Following are some of the best techniques:

✔ Eat according to a schedule to avoid unplanned eating.

✔ Find a single place to eat all food. (Don't eat in front of the TV.)

✔ Slow down your eating to make the meal last.

✔ Put high-calorie foods away. Remove serving dishes and bread from the table.

✔ Don't dispense food to others to avoid exposure for yourself.

✔ Leave some food on your plate.

✔ Set realistic goals for weight loss. (A reasonable rate is ½ to 1 pound per week.)

✔ When eating out, be careful of salad dressing, alcohol, and bread. Share a meal.

✔ Get a ten-pound weight and carry it around for a while to appreciate the importance of losing even that little.

✔ At the market, buy from a list, carry only enough money for the food on that list, and avoid aisles containing loose foods like candy (loose fruits and vegetables are okay, though).

✔ Eat off a salad plate (a visual cue to cut portion sizes).

Incorporate one technique into your life each week (or even longer) until you feel you have mastered it and have added it to your eating style. Then go on and take up another technique.

As you go about this difficult task of losing weight and keeping it off, remember to seek the help of those around you. A loving partner provides great help through the roughest days.

In an effort to lose weight, some people with diabetes skip their insulin shots. If you do so, your body will turn to fat for fuel because glucose can't be used (see Chapter 2), and you will lose weight. However, the result is that you also lose muscle mass and your blood glucose rises very high. This situation is dangerous and not a healthy approach to weight loss.

Coping with Eating Disorders

You can't be too rich or too thin. How much damage has this statement done to society, especially the *thin* part? Young people, particularly girls, are preoccupied with their body weight. When this preoccupation becomes too great, it can result in an eating disorder.

The dangers of anorexia and bulimia

Young girls have eating disorders about ten times as often as young boys do. They either starve themselves and exercise excessively or eat a great deal and then induce vomiting and/or take laxatives and water pills. Someone who starves herself has *anorexia nervosa,* whereas someone who binges and purges has *bulimia nervosa.* By themselves, these conditions can result in severe illness and even death when carried to extremes. When combined with diabetes, the danger increases greatly.

Here are some of the clues that someone has one of these disorders:

- She eats by herself.
- She feels guilty or disgusted after overeating.
- She eats more rapidly than others do.
- She eats until uncomfortably full.
- She eats large amounts of food even when she is not hungry.

Anorexia is usually found in middle- and upper-class girls. They have a distorted body image and are fearful of weight gain. The prevalence may be as high as 1 in 200 in these girls. Their parents are usually very concerned with slimness. The girls may appear unusually thin and do not menstruate. Their malnutrition may be so severe that they die from it.

People with anorexia are in a constant state of starvation. When they have diabetes, their condition is just like that of people with type 1 diabetes before the availability of insulin. They have very low blood glucose levels, so little or no insulin is required (see Chapter 10). They develop problems with their hearts and have low blood pressure and low body temperature. They lose a lot of body musculature after the fat is gone.

People with severe anorexia may require intravenous feeding until they are stabilized a little bit, which sometimes leads to very high blood glucose levels, necessitating the use of insulin. After the life-threatening starvation is under control, good blood glucose control can be achieved with help from the patients themselves and from therapists who can help them understand their distorted body image. If the patient suffers from clinical depression, antidepressant medication may be necessary.

Bulimia involves eating large quantities of easily digested food and then purging it by vomiting and taking laxatives or water pills. These patients are usually not as severely thin as patients with anorexia. However, their backgrounds are often similar to those of anorexia patients: They may represent up to 40 percent of college-age female students. Because their weight is closer to normal, they usually menstruate normally.

Bulimia has a negative effect on diabetes because management of diabetes requires a certain amount of routine from day to day. There is no way to achieve such systematization when the amount of food coming into the body is so uncertain. However, food intake in bulimia is less severe than that in anorexia, so blood glucose levels do not fluctuate as much in this case.

However, people with bulimia are more likely to go on to adult obesity and are harder to treat psychologically. They actually do not do as well with therapy as those with anorexia, and they end up with more psychiatric problems later in life.

Sources of help

A major source of useful information is the National Eating Disorders Association. The association's website, www.nationaleatingdisorders.org, contains extensive information on this subject of eating disorders. You can contact the association at 165 West 46th St., New York, NY 10036, or call its help hotline at 800-931-2237.

The National Association of Anorexia Nervosa and Associated Disorders provides information online, including referrals to support groups, therapists, and treatment centers, at www.anad.org. You can also contact the association through the website or by calling 630-577-1330. The mailing address is 800 E Diehl Rd. #160, Naperville, IL 60563.`

Chapter 9

Keep It Moving: Creating Your Exercise Plan

*I*n the Standards of Medical Care in Diabetes 2012, the American Diabetes Association makes the following recommendations:

✔ People with diabetes should perform at least 150 minutes each week of moderate-intensity aerobic physical activity (50 to 70 percent of maximum heart rate), spread over at least three days per week, with no more than two consecutive days without exercise.

✔ In the absence of a medical reason not to, people with type 2 diabetes should perform resistance training at least twice per week.

If your time is limited, you don't have to set aside an hour daily to do your physical activity, although that amount would be best. Since the last edition of this book, numerous studies have suggested that many other approaches to exercise can greatly improve control of type 2 diabetes and prevent prediabetes from turning into diabetes. Here are some of the best approaches:

✔ Doing just two 20-second sprints (high intensity) on an exercise bike three times a week has been shown to prevent type 2 diabetes and to lower the blood glucose if diabetes is present.

✔ Doing one minute of high-intensity exercise followed by one minute of rest, performed for 20 minutes (for a total of 10 minutes of intense exercise), three times a week, dropped average blood glucose levels from 137 mg/dl to 119 mg/dl.

✔ Using a pedometer to ensure a minimum amount of daily walking may reduce your chance of getting diabetes by half.

In this chapter, you discover why exercise is important, how much and what kinds you need to do to make a difference, and which specific exercises are best for you.

Getting Off the Couch: Why Exercise Is Essential

More than 60 years ago, the great leaders in diabetes care declared that diabetes management has three major aspects:

✔ Proper diet

✔ Appropriate medication

✔ Sufficient exercise

When the diabetes experts wrote their recommendations for proper care, the isolation and administration of insulin had just recently begun, and they were focusing specifically on how to control type 1 diabetes. Since that time, many studies have shown that exercise doesn't normalize the blood glucose or reduce the hemoglobin A1c (see Chapter 7) in type 1 diabetes. Many other studies have shown that exercise *does* normalize blood glucose and reduce hemoglobin A1c in type 2 diabetes.

Although exercise cannot replace medication for the type 1 diabetic, its benefits are crucial for patients with both types of diabetes.

Preventing macrovascular disease

The major benefit of exercise for both types of diabetes is to prevent *macrovascular disease* (heart attack, stroke, or diminished blood flow to the legs). Macrovascular disease affects everyone, whether they have diabetes or not, but it's particularly severe in people with diabetes. Exercise prevents macrovascular disease in numerous ways:

✔ Exercise helps with weight loss, which is especially important in type 2 diabetes.

✔ Exercise lowers bad cholesterol and triglycerides, and it raises good cholesterol.

✔ Exercise lowers blood pressure.

✔ Exercise lowers stress levels.

✔ Exercise reduces the need for insulin or drugs.

✔ Exercise reduces C-reactive protein, a cause of heart and blood vessel disease in diabetes (see Chapter 7).

Providing other benefits

In addition to its major benefits in the prevention of macrovascular disease, exercise provides a number of other very important benefits:

✔ Exercise has been shown to improve pancreatic beta-cell function, the very cells that produce insulin.

✔ Exercise is medicine for the brain. It stimulates the production of nerve cells, which prevent loss of memory, improve thinking, and enhance judgment.

✔ Higher levels of physical activity at midlife are associated with exceptional health among women at age 70 or older.

✔ Increased physical activity prevents weight gain as you age and weight regain if you diet.

✔ Exercise, even without weight loss, reduces the risk of diabetes.

✔ Higher levels of physical activity before pregnancy or in early pregnancy significantly lower the risk of gestational diabetes.

Taking charge of your health

John Plant is a 46-year-old male who has had type 1 diabetes for 23 years. He takes insulin shots four times daily and measures his blood glucose multiple times a day. He follows a careful diet.

Prior to developing diabetes, he was a very active person, participating in vigorous sports and doing major hiking and mountain climbing. At the time of his diagnosis, his doctor warned him that he would have to give up many of the most strenuous activities because he would never know his blood glucose level and it might drop precipitously during heavy exercise. He ignored this advice and continued his active way of life. He found that he could do with much less insulin than his doctor prescribed and rarely became hypoglycemic. He has been able to continue these activities without limitation. His blood glucose level is generally between 75 and 140. His last hemoglobin A1c was slightly elevated at 5.7 (see Chapter 7). A recent eye examination showed no diabetic retinopathy (see Chapter 5). He has no significant microalbuminuria in his urine and no tingling in his feet (see Chapter 5).

Is John lucky? You bet he is. But like most "luck," his is based on a self-realization that the human body is made up of both a mind and a body. If humans were meant to spend their lives munching potato chips in front of a TV set, why would they have all these muscles?

When a new diabetic patient enters my office, I give him a bottle of 50 pills. I instruct him not to swallow the pills but to drop them on the floor three times daily and pick them up one at a time. The condition a person is in can be judged by which thing he or she takes two at a time: pills or stairs.

Understanding your body mechanics during exercise

The feeling of fatigue that occurs with exercise is probably due to the loss of stored muscle glucose.

With exercise, insulin levels in nondiabetics and people with type 2 diabetes decline because insulin acts to store and not release glucose and fat. Levels of glucagon, epinephrine, cortisol, and growth hormone increase to provide more glucose. Studies show that glucagon is responsible for 60 percent of the glucose, and epinephrine and cortisol are responsible for the other 40 percent. If insulin did not fall, glucagon could not stimulate the liver to make glucose.

You may wonder how insulin can open the cell to the entry of glucose when insulin levels are falling. In fact, two things are at work here. Glucose is getting into muscle cells without the need for insulin, and the rapid circulation that comes with exercise is delivering the smaller amount of insulin more frequently to the muscle. The muscle seems to be more sensitive to the insulin as well, which is exactly what the person with type 2 diabetes hopes to accomplish when insulin resistance is the major block to insulin action.

One way to preserve glucose stores is to provide calories from an external source. Any marathoner knows that additional calories can delay the feeling of exhaustion. The timing is important. If the glucose is given an hour before exercise, it will be metabolized during the exercise and increase endurance. However, if it's given 30 minutes before exercise, it may decrease stamina by stimulating insulin, which blocks liver production of glucose.

Fructose can replenish you when you're doing prolonged exercise. This sweetener can replace glucose because it is sweeter but is absorbed more slowly and does not provoke the insulin secretion that glucose provokes. Fructose is rapidly converted into glucose inside the body. (See Chapter 8 for more on fructose.)

Reaping the benefits

As your body becomes trained with regular exercise, the benefits for your diabetes are very significant. Your body starts to turn to fat for energy earlier in the course of your exercise. At the same time, the hormones that tend to raise the blood glucose during exercise are not produced at the same high rate because they aren't needed. Because you don't require as much insulin, your insulin doses can be reduced, and avoiding hypoglycemia during exercise becomes much easier.

Exercising When You Have Diabetes

If you have diabetes and have not exercised previously, you should check with a doctor prior to beginning a new exercise program, especially if you're over the age of 35 or if you've had diabetes for ten years or longer. You should also check with a doctor if you have any of the following risk factors:

- ✔ The presence of any diabetic complications like retinopathy, nephropathy, or neuropathy (see Chapter 5)
- ✔ Obesity
- ✔ A physical limitation
- ✔ A history of coronary artery disease or elevated blood pressure
- ✔ Use of medications

You need to discuss these issues with your doctor in order to choose the appropriate exercises. I say more about the choice of exercise in the section "Is Golf a Sport? Choosing Your Activity" later in this chapter.

When you begin to exercise, whether you have type 1 or type 2 diabetes, you can take many steps to make your experience safe and healthful. Following are some important steps to take:

- ✔ Wear a bracelet identifying your first and last name, type of diabetes, food or drug allergies, and emergency contact numbers for your doctor and a family member or close friend.
- ✔ Test your blood glucose very often.
- ✔ Choose proper socks and shoes.
- ✔ Drink plenty of water.
- ✔ Carry treatment for hypoglycemia.
- ✔ Exercise with a friend.

And here are some things to avoid when you exercise:

- ✔ Don't assume that you have to buy lots of special clothing to exercise. The right shoes and socks are essential, but other than that, you need special clothing only if your sport demands it (such as soft pants for cycling).

- ✔ Don't expect to lose weight in certain spots by repetitively exercising them.

- ✔ Don't exercise to the point of pain.

- ✔ Don't get too focused on using exercise gadgets, like belts or other objects, that do not require you to move.

Working out with type 1 diabetes

People with type 1 diabetes or type 2 on insulin depend on insulin injections to manage blood glucose. They don't have the luxury of a "thermostat" that automatically shuts off during exercise and turns back on when exercise is finished. After an insulin shot is taken, it is active until it's used up.

If you have type 1 diabetes, you have to avoid overdosing on insulin before exercise, which can lead to hypoglycemia, or underdosing, which can lead to hyperglycemia. If your body doesn't have enough insulin, it turns to fat for energy. Glucose rises because it is not being metabolized but its production is continuing. If exercise is particularly vigorous in a situation of not enough insulin, the blood glucose can rise extremely high.

Reducing your insulin dosage prior to exercise helps prevent hypoglycemia. One study showed that an 80 percent reduction of the dose allowed the person with diabetes to exercise for three hours, whereas a 50 percent reduction forced the person with diabetes to stop after 90 minutes due to hypoglycemia. Each person with diabetes varies, and you must determine for yourself how much to reduce insulin by measuring the blood glucose before, during, and after exercise.

Another way to prevent hypoglycemia, of course, is to eat some carbohydrate (see Chapter 8). You need to have some carbohydrate (which quickly raises blood glucose) available during exercise.

In addition, the site of the insulin injection is important because it determines how fast the insulin becomes active. If you are running and inject insulin into your leg, it will be taken up more quickly than an injection into the arm would be.

What are aerobic and anaerobic exercise?

Aerobic exercise is exercise that can be sustained for more than a few minutes, uses major groups of muscles, and gets your heart to pump faster during the exercise, thus training the heart. I give you many examples of aerobic exercise throughout this chapter.

Anaerobic exercise, on the other hand, is brief (sometimes a few seconds) and intense and usually cannot be sustained. Lifting large weights is an example of an anaerobic exercise. A 100-yard dash is another example.

You can exercise whenever you will do it faithfully. If you like to sleep late and you schedule your exercise at 5:30 a.m., you probably won't consistently do it. Your best time to exercise is probably about 60 to 90 minutes after eating because the glucose is peaking at this time, providing the calories you need; if you exercise then, you avoid the usual post-eating high in your blood glucose, and you burn up those food calories. If you take insulin and prefer early-morning exercise, check your blood glucose and eat a snack if you are below 150 mg/dl. Don't exercise just before bedtime; it may cause hypoglycemia while you are sleeping.

Working out with type 2 diabetes

Other than the insulin discussion, many of the suggestions for type 1 patients in the previous section apply to type 2 patients as well.

With sufficient exercise and diet, some people with type 2 diabetes can revert to a nondiabetic state. This state doesn't mean that they no longer have diabetes, but it certainly means that they will not develop the long-term complications that can make them so miserable later in life (see Chapter 5).

Determining How Much Exercise to Do

Unless you have a physical abnormality, you have no limitation on what kind of exercise or how much you can do. You should select one or more activities that you enjoy and will continue to perform.

Exerting enough effort

In the recent past, exercise physiologists said that you needed to make sure that you monitored your exercise intensity by periodically checking your heart rate. Your exercise heart rate was supposed to be based on your age. The usual formula to figure this out is to take the number 220, subtract your age, and multiply that number by 60 to 75 percent to get the recommended exercise heart rate for aerobic exercise. (See the sidebar "What are aerobic and anaerobic exercise?" if you're not sure what aerobic exercise is.)

Now studies have shown that people can sustain aerobic exercise at higher heart rates. Perhaps the best way to know whether you're meeting your exercise goals is to use the perceived exertion scale described in the sidebar "Checking the value of your exercise."

The younger you are, the faster your exercise heart rate may be. Like everything in this book, your exercise heart rate is an individual number. If you are a world-class athlete training for your ninth marathon, your exercise heart rate may be higher. If you have some heart disease, your exercise heart rate may be significantly lower.

Checking the value of your exercise

Measuring your pulse during exercise (or even at rest) may be hard for you. Instead, you can use the perceived exertion scale. Exercise is given a descriptive value from *extremely light* to *extremely hard* with *very light, light, somewhat hard,* and *very hard* in between. You want to exercise to a level of *somewhat hard,* and you will be at your target heart rate in most cases. As you get into shape, the amount of exertion that corresponds to *somewhat hard* will increase.

Here is a description of these various levels of exercise:

✔ **Extremely light exercise** is very easy to do and requires little or no exertion.

✔ **Very light exercise** is like walking slowly for several minutes.

✔ **Light exercise** is like walking faster but at a pace you can continue without effort.

✔ **Somewhat hard exercise** is getting a little difficult but still feels okay to continue.

✔ **Very hard exercise** is difficult to continue. You have to push yourself, and you're very tired. At this level, you have trouble talking. The very hard level of exercise is most beneficial.

✔ **Extremely hard exercise** is the most difficult exercise you've ever done.

Do not continue exercising if you have tightness in your chest, chest pain, severe shortness of breath, or dizziness.

Devoting an hour a day

When you know your maximal exercise heart rate, you can choose your activity and use the perceived exertion scale to be sure that you achieve that level during exercise. I must repeat that the best choice of exercise for you is an exercise you enjoy and will continue to perform.

The choices are really limitless. The number of kcalories you use for any exercise is determined by your weight, the strenuousness of the activity, and the time you spend actually doing it. In the past it was suggested that in order to have a positive effect on your heart, you need to do a moderate level of exercise for 20 to 45 minutes at least three times a week. In 2002, the Institute of Medicine (the medical division of the National Academies) recommended that in order to maintain health and a normal body weight, you need to do one hour of exercise a day.

An hour (not an apple) a day keeps the doctor away! Moderate aerobic exercise done for an hour every day provides enormous physical, mental, and emotional benefits.

You need to warm up and cool down for about five minutes before and after you exercise. Stretching is one possibility for both warm-up and cool-down. I am not going to discuss stretching in detail because the importance of stretching for the healthy exerciser is not clear. One study showed that a group of runners who did not stretch did better than a group who did. Most doctors agree that stretching after an injury is appropriate, but whether all the advice about stretching before exercise for an uninjured person is much ado about nothing is yet to be determined. If you do stretch, do not stretch to the point that it hurts, or you risk tearing muscle. See the excellent book *Fitness For Dummies,* by Suzanne Schlosberg and Liz Neporent (Wiley), for more about stretching.

Making moderate exercise your goal

Moderate exercise has a moving definition. If you're out of shape, moderate exercise for you may be slow walking. If you're in good shape, moderate exercise may be jogging or cross-country skiing. Moderate exercise is simply something you can do and not get out of breath. For ideas on the types of exercise you can do, see the following section.

How long can you stop exercise before you start to decondition? It takes only about two to three weeks to lose some of the fitness your exercise has provided. Then it takes up to six weeks to get back to your current level, assuming that your holiday from exercise does not go on too long.

Is Golf a Sport? Choosing Your Activity

The following factors can help you determine your choice of activity:

- ✔ Do you like to exercise alone or with company? Pick a competitive or team sport if you prefer company.

- ✔ Do you like to compete against others or just yourself? Running or walking are activities you can do alone.

- ✔ Do you prefer vigorous or less-vigorous activity? Less-vigorous activity over a longer period is just as effective as more-vigorous activity.

- ✔ Do you live where you can do activities outside year-round, or do you need to go inside a lot of the year? Find a sports club if weather prevents year-round outside activity.

- ✔ Do you need special equipment or just a pair of running shoes?

- ✔ What benefits are you looking for in your exercise: Cardiovascular, strength, endurance, flexibility, or body fat control? You should probably look for all these benefits, but you may have to combine activities to get them all in.

- ✔ Do you have any balance problems? Swimming and water aerobics are great choices for you.

Perhaps a good starting point in your activity selection is to focus on the benefits. Table 9-1 gives you some ideas.

Table 9-1	Match Your Activity to the Results You Want
If You Want to . . .	*Then Consider . . .*
Build up cardiovascular condition	Vigorous basketball, racquetball, squash, cross-country skiing, handball, swimming
Strengthen your body	Low-weight, high-repetition weight lifting; gymnastics; mountain climbing; cross-country skiing
Build up muscular endurance	Gymnastics, rowing, cross-country skiing, vigorous basketball
Increase flexibility	Gymnastics, yoga, judo, karate, soccer, surfing
Control body fat	Handball, racquetball, squash, cross-country skiing, vigorous basketball, singles tennis

You can tell from Table 9-1 that living in places with plenty of snow is helpful because cross-country skiing is on almost every list. On the other hand, so is vigorous basketball, so you don't have to give up exercise if you live in a warm climate like Florida.

The special needs of many of these sports may turn you off to exercise. The curious thing is that the best exercise that you can sustain for life is right at your feet. A brisk daily walk improves heart function, adds to muscular endurance, and helps control body fat. So many people drive their cars to the gym and try to park as close as possible so that they can get to the building with as little effort as possible. Seems a little strange, doesn't it?

Of course, the social benefits of exercise are very important. You are together with people who are concerned with health and appearance. These people usually share many of your interests. People who like to jog often like to hike and climb and camp, too. Many lifetime partnerships begin on one side of a tennis court (and some end there as well).

Cross-training, where you do several different activities throughout the week, is a good idea. Cross-training reduces the boredom that may accompany doing one thing day after day. It also permits you to exercise regardless of the weather because you can do some things indoors and some outside.

Table 9-2 lists a variety of activities, including some that don't exactly fit into the category of *exercise* but offer some interesting comparisons. Next to each activity, I include the amount of kcalories that a 125-pound person and a 175-pound person burn in 20 minutes.

Table 9-2   Calories Burned in 20 Minutes at Different Body Weights

Activity	*Kcalories Burned (125 pounds)*	*Kcalories Burned (175 pounds)*
Standing	24	32
Walking, 4 mph	104	144
Running, 7 mph	236	328
Gardening	60	84
Writing	30	42
Typing	38	54
Carpentry	64	88
House painting	58	80
Playing baseball	78	108
Dancing	70	96
Playing football	138	192
Golfing	66	96
Swimming	80	112
Skiing, downhill	160	224
Skiing, cross-country	196	276
Playing tennis	112	160

Everything you do burns calories. Even sleeping and watching television use 20 kcalories in 20 minutes if you weigh 125 pounds.

Your choice of an activity must take into account your physical condition. If you have diabetic neuropathy (see Chapter 5) and can't feel your feet, you don't want to do pounding exercises that may damage them without your awareness. You can swim, bike, row, or do armchair exercises where you move your upper body vigorously. One of my favorite machines that give you a good workout without trauma to your joints is the elliptical trainer, but you may have to join a club to get at one unless you buy one for home.

If you have diabetic retinopathy (see Chapter 5), you won't want to do exercises that raise your blood pressure (like weight lifting), cause jerky motions in your eyes (like bouncing on a trampoline), or change the pressure in your eyes significantly (like scuba diving or high mountain climbing). You also should not do exercises that place your eyes below the level of your heart, such as when you touch your toes.

Patients with nephropathy (see Chapter 5) should avoid exercises that raise the blood pressure for prolonged periods. These exercises are extremely intense activities that you do for a long time, like marathon running.

Some people have pain in the legs after they walk a certain distance. It may be due to diminished blood supply to the legs so that the needs of the muscles in the legs cannot be met. Although you need to discuss this problem with your doctor, you do not need to give up walking. Instead, determine the distance you can walk up to the point of pain. Then walk about three-quarters of that distance and stop to give the circulation a chance to catch up. After you rest, you can go about the same distance again without pain. By stringing several of these walks together, you can get a good, pain-free workout. You may even find that you are able to increase the distance after a while because this kind of training tends to create new blood vessels.

Is there a medical condition that should absolutely prevent you from doing exercise? Short of chest pain at rest, which must be addressed by your doctor, the answer is no. If you can't figure out an exercise that you're able to do, get together with an exercise therapist. You will be amazed at how many muscles you can move that you never knew you had.

Walking 10K a Day

The idea of walking 10,000 steps a day may seem like a huge, unattainable goal to you, but you may be surprised. This goal is certainly worth striving toward because, as I discuss previously in this chapter, walking is one of the most beneficial exercises you can do. All of your steps count, and 10,000 steps can be all the daily exercise you need to do in addition to resistance training (weight lifting, for example).

The first step toward reaching this goal is to buy a *pedometer,* a device that you wear on your waist that counts each step you take. Don't buy a fancy one with a lot of bells and whistles. All you need is to be able to count your steps and, if you want, to convert the steps into miles. To do this, you need to know how far you walk each time you take a step. Walk ten steps, measure the distance, and divide by ten to get your stride length. Input this number in the appropriate place in the pedometer, and it will give you the miles that correspond with the steps you walk.

Accusplit pedometers work very well. The model I like is the Accusplit Eagle, which does nothing but record your steps. You can find it at www. accusplit.com. You also can find pedometers at sporting goods stores.

Begin by doing your usual amount of exercise each day. Remember to record the steps at the end of the day and reset the button on the pedometer to zero. After seven days, add up the steps and divide by seven to get your daily count. You will probably find that you are doing between 3,000 and 5,000 steps a day.

Next, you want to build up your daily number. Use the catchy phrase *10k a day* to remind you to do extra walking to reach 10,000 steps. Here are some tips to help:

- ✔ Get a good pair of walking shoes or sneakers and replace them when they begin to wear out.
- ✔ Leave your car parked. If you can make a trip in an hour or less by foot, save your gas money and add substantially to your daily step count.
- ✔ Try to add a few hundred steps a week. Begin by identifying a baseline day in your first week when you did the most steps, and make every day like that one. Each week, add a few hundred more.
- ✔ Find an exercise buddy to walk with you. It's much more fun.
- ✔ Keep a record of the number of steps involved in various walks you take so you can easily get the steps you are missing on any given day.
- ✔ Use stairs instead of the elevator, whether you're going up or down.
- ✔ Take a walk at lunchtime daily.
- ✔ Stop if you feel pain, and check with your doctor before continuing.

If you don't have a pedometer, or if you want to count other types of exercise toward your walking goal, use the following conversions:

- ✔ 1 mile = 2,100 average steps
- ✔ 1 block = 100 average steps
- ✔ 10 minutes walking = 1,200 steps on average
- ✔ Biking or swimming = 150 steps per minute
- ✔ Weight lifting = 100 steps per minute
- ✔ Roller skating = 200 steps per minute

If you like tangible rewards for what you do (besides the reward of a lower blood glucose, a lower cholesterol, a lower blood pressure, and possibly a lower weight), join the President's Challenge at www.presidentschallenge.org. It provides a place to record your activity, and it offers all kinds of information on activities for every age. You choose what you like to do, and every time you do it you record your progress. It gives you points toward awards.

If you prefer to follow an actual trail, take a virtual walk on the American Discovery Trail, a 5,048-mile walk across America from Delaware to California. You can find it at www.discoverytrail.org. Every time you walk, convert your steps into miles and see how far they take you along that trail. The website has links to all the sights you would see.

A study in the *Archives of Internal Medicine* in June 2003 provides the best evidence for the benefits of walking. Diabetics who walked at least two hours a week had a 40 percent lower death rate than inactive diabetics.

Another study in *Diabetes Care* in June 2005 entitled "Make Your Diabetic Patients Walk" followed 179 patients with type 2 diabetes who were divided into six groups and followed for two years. The groups differed in the amount of increased exercise they did. For example, the first group did a little more exercise by the end of the study, whereas the last group did much more exercise by the end of the study. The other groups fell in between those extremes. The results were that the highest exercisers had the lowest blood pressure, greatest weight loss, greatest reduction in total cholesterol and bad cholesterol, greatest increase in good cholesterol, greatest reduction in blood glucose, and greatest reduction in money spent on drugs. Although the people who did the least exercise had no change in the cost of their annual medications, the highest exercisers had a reduction of $660 per year. What are you waiting for? Take the first steps!

Lifting Weights

Weight lifting is a form of anaerobic exercise. (See the sidebar earlier in this chapter if you're not sure what anaerobic exercise is.) It involves the movement of heavy weights, which can be moved only for brief periods of time. It results in significant muscle strengthening and increased endurance.

Doctors are looking for drugs that can increase insulin sensitivity (see Chapter 10). You need look no further. Lifting weights has been shown in several studies to accomplish this. Writing in *Diabetes Care* in September 2007, a group of investigators from the Centers for Disease Control showed that muscle-strengthening activity significantly increased insulin sensitivity, thereby lowering the blood glucose and the hemoglobin A1c in 4,500 adults between the ages of 20 and 70.

Older adults from age 50 and above who were given only eight weeks of flexibility and resistance training had substantial improvement in strength and flexibility while their glucose levels improved as well.

Because weight lifting causes a significant rise in blood pressure as it is being done, people with severe diabetic eye disease should not do it unless your blood pressure is under very good control. Check with your doctor.

Weight training, which uses lighter weights, can be a form of aerobic exercise. Because the weights are light, they can be moved for prolonged periods of time. The result is improved cardiovascular fitness along with strengthening of muscles, tendons, ligaments, and bones. Weight training is an excellent way to protect and strengthen a joint that is beginning to develop some discomfort.

I recommend that you do seven different exercises with light weights every other day, or daily if possible. Choose weights that permit you to do each exercise ten times in a row, for three sets of ten with a rest in between each set. You should need only five to ten minutes to complete all seven, and the benefits will be huge. These exercises are the bicep curl, shoulder press, lateral raise, bent-over rowing, good mornings, flys, and pullovers. You may want to do them initially with a trainer to make sure you do them correctly.

Figure 9-1 shows the bicep curl. To do this exercise:

1. **Hold the dumbbells along the sides of your body, palms facing forward.**

2. **Raise the dumbbells until your elbows are fully bent.**

3. **Slowly lower the dumbbells to the original position.**

Figure 9-2 shows the shoulder press. To do this exercise:

1. **Hold the dumbbells with your palms facing each other and your elbows bent.**

2. **Raise the dumbbells over your head, turning your palms to face forward.**

3. **Lower the dumbbells to the original position.**

Figure 9-3 shows the lateral raise. To do this exercise:

1. **Hold the dumbbells along the sides of your body, palms facing each other.**

2. **Lift the dumbbells out to the sides, palms facing the floor, until they are above your head.**

3. **Lower the dumbbells down to your sides.**

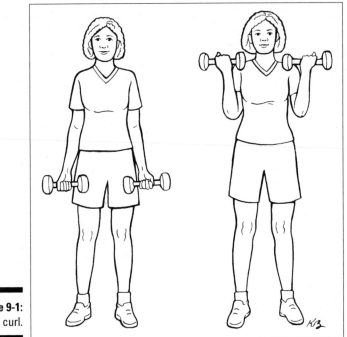

Figure 9-1:
Bicep curl.

Illustration by Kathryn Born

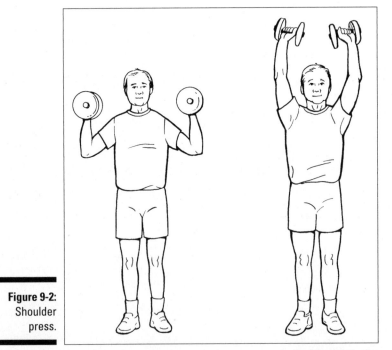

Figure 9-2:
Shoulder
press.

Illustration by Kathryn Born

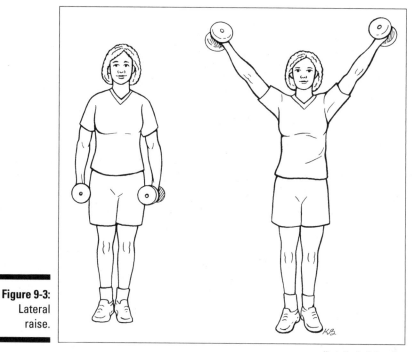

Illustration by Kathryn Born

Figure 9-3:
Lateral
raise.

Figure 9-4 shows bent-over rowing. To do this exercise:

1. **Hold a dumbbell in each hand, arms hanging down, legs straight, and back bent as necessary toward the floor.**

2. **Raise the dumbbells up to your chest with your back parallel to the floor.**

3. **Lower the dumbbells toward the floor.**

Figure 9-5 shows good mornings. To do this exercise:

1. **Hold the ends of one dumbbell above your head, arms straight.**

2. **Lower the dumbbell forward as you bend so that your back is parallel to the floor.**

3. **Raise the dumbbell to the original position.**

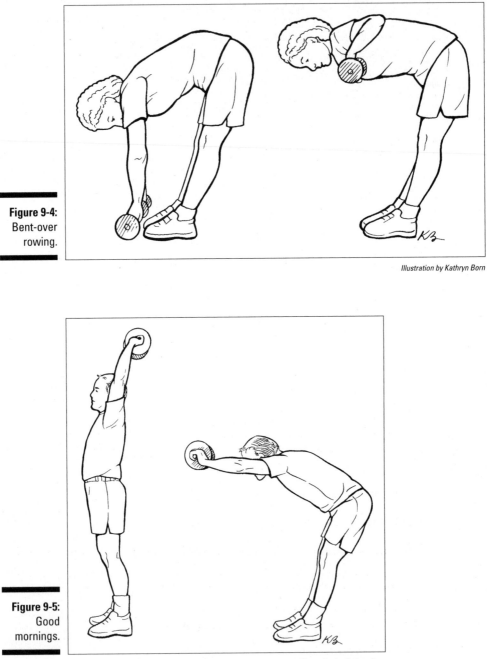

Figure 9-4:
Bent-over
rowing.

Illustration by Kathryn Born

Figure 9-5:
Good
mornings.

Illustration by Kathryn Born

Figure 9-6 shows flys. To do this exercise:

1. **Lie on your back and hold the dumbbells out to each side at the shoulder.**

2. **Lift the dumbbells together until they are above your head.**

3. **Lower them to the sides again.**

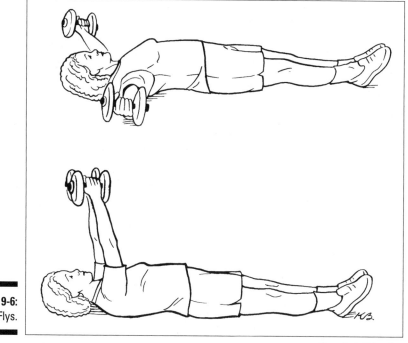

Figure 9-6: Flys.

Illustration by Kathryn Born

Figure 9-7 shows pullovers. To do this exercise:

1. **Lie on your back holding one dumbbell with both hands straight up above your head.**

2. **Lower the dumbbell with your arms straight to the floor behind your head.**

3. **Raise the dumbbell back above your head.**

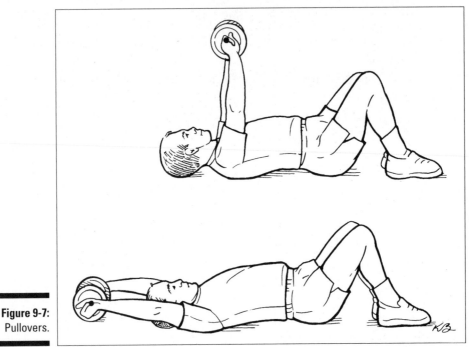

Figure 9-7:
Pullovers.

Illustration by Kathryn Born

Older people in nursing homes who are given weights of just a few pounds have shown excellent return of strength to what appeared to be atrophied muscles. The benefits for you will be that much greater.

Weight training may be good for the days that you do not do your aerobic exercise, or you can add it for a few minutes after you finish your activity. Weight training is also good for working on a particular group of muscles that you feel is weak. Very often, these muscles are in the back. Weight-training exercises can isolate and strengthen each muscle.

If you do a lot of aerobic exercise that involves the legs, you may want to use upper-body weight training only. I can tell you from personal experience that you gain both a stronger upper body and an enhanced ability to do your usual exercise.

Chapter 10

Medications: What You Should Know

. . . .

In This Chapter

▶ Taking pills to control blood glucose

▶ Using insulin injections

▶ Combining insulin and oral agents in type 2 diabetes

▶ Avoiding drug interactions

. . . .

*Y*ou don't know how lucky you are (but I'm about to tell you). You are the beneficiary of the greatest advances in diabetes medications in the history of the disease. From 1921, when insulin was isolated and used for the first time, to 1955, when a class of glucose-lowering drugs called *sulfonyl-ureas* became available, insulin was the only option for treating diabetes. For another 40 years, nothing new showed up in the United States — until 1995. Now many newer classes of drugs, each in its own way, lower blood glucose.

Since the last edition of this book, new medications have been introduced and older medications have run into trouble. You find the latest information on all those changes in this chapter.

If you have diabetes and diet and exercise aren't keeping your blood glucose under control, you need to see your doctor about taking medication. In this chapter, you find out all you need to know to use diabetes medications effectively and safely.

This chapter helps you become an educated consumer. Not only can you find out about the medication you're taking and how it works, but you also discover when to take it, how it interacts with other medications, what side effects it may cause, and how to use several medications together, if necessary, to normalize your glucose. Right now, today, you have all the tools needed to control your diabetes, and there are more to come. In the immortal words of the great entertainer Al Jolson, "You ain't seen nothin' yet."

Taking Drugs by Mouth: Oral Agents

For years, insulin shots were the only treatment available for diabetes. Most people do not care for shots. You may be an exception, but I doubt it. Fortunately, drugs that can be taken by mouth have been available for some time. One thing you should know about these pills: You can take them or leave them, but they work much better if you take them.

Sulfonylureas

Scientists discovered sulfonylureas accidentally when they noticed that soldiers who were given certain sulfur-containing antibiotics developed symptoms of low blood glucose. When scientists began to search for the most potent examples of this effect, they came up with several different versions of this drug. Sulfonylureas all have the following characteristics:

- They work by making the pancreas release more insulin.

- They are not effective in type 1 diabetes where the pancreas is not capable of releasing any insulin.

- Sometimes they don't work when first given (primary failure), but they almost always stop working within a few years after you start them (secondary failure). Sulfonylureas continue to be used because, for most people, they improve glucose control for at least those first few years.

- They are all capable of causing hypoglycemia.

- When you use any of a class of antibiotics called *sulfonamides,* the glucose-lowering action of the sulfonylureas is prolonged.

- They should not be taken by pregnant women or nursing mothers, with the exception of glyburide, which has been shown to be safe. Check with your doctor.

- They can be fairly potent when given in combination with one of the other classes of oral agents.

Following are the sulfonylureas that are currently in use:

- **Glyburide (brand names Micronase, Diabeta, and Glynase):** Among the foreign brand names for glyburide are Antibet, Azuglucon, Betanase, Gliban, Glibil, Gluben, and Orabetic. Pretty confusing, huh? Glyburide comes in 1.25, 2.5, and 5 mg. The usual starting dose is 2.5 to 5 mg with breakfast, and the maintenance dose is 1.25 to 20 mg. Glyburide leaves the body equally in the bowel movement and the urine, so patients with either liver or kidney disease are at greater risk for low blood glucose. Glyburide is carried around the bloodstream bound to proteins, so if you take other drugs that bind to proteins, such as aspirin, the activity of glyburide may increase. When these drugs are withdrawn, the activity of glyburide may decrease. Other than hypoglycemia, the incidence of negative effects is very low.

Glynase is a form of glyburide that is slightly more active because it is absorbed better, so less is required for the same effect. The starting dose is 1.5 mg, and it's available in 1.5-mg, 3-mg, or 6-mg tablets with a maximum dose of 12 mg.

You can take either form of glyburide once a day in the morning, but sometimes it works better when given twice a day.

A French study published in the *Journal of Clinical Endocrinology and Metabolism* in November 2010 showed that the death rate due to heart attacks in people taking glyburide was three times greater than those taking glipizide or glimepiride (see the following bullets). If you are on glyburide, discuss switching to one of the others with your doctor.

✔ **Glipizide (brand names Glucotrol and Glucotrol XL):** Among the foreign brand names are Digrin, Glibenase, Glican, Glyco, Glynase (which is the same name as glyburide in the United States!), Mindiab, Napizide, and Sucrazide. Glipizide is similar to glyburide but slightly less potent, so pills come in 5 and 10 mg. You take it 30 minutes before food. The starting dose is 5 mg. Up to 40 mg can be given daily in several doses. Because it's less potent, glipizide is preferred for elderly patients.

Glucotrol XL is an extended release form of glipizide that lasts for 24 hours, so it usually is given as 5 or 10 mg once a day.

✔ **Glimepiride (brand name Amaryl):** This drug also lasts a longer time and is fairly potent, so it is given once a day. It comes in 1-, 2-, and 4-mg sizes with a maximum daily dose of 8 mg.

Amaryl is combined with rosiglitazone (trade name Avandia, discussed in the later section "Rosiglitazone") to form a medication called Avandaryl. It's also combined with pioglitazone (trade name Actos, discussed in "Pioglitazone") as the drug Duetact. However, because both rosiglitazone and pioglitazone have unacceptable side effects, I do not recommend these combination drugs.

Choosing among the second-generation sulfonylureas, I generally select glimepiride because of its long duration of action. All three of the drugs are available as generic preparations

Metformin

Metformin, brand names Glucophage, Fortamet, and Glumetza, is an entirely different kind of glucose-lowering medication. Outside the United States, it's called Benoformin, Dextin, Diabex, Diaformin, Fornidd, Glucoform, Gluformin, Metforal, Metomin, and Orabet.

More than 20 years ago, the United States banned a sister medication called *phenformin* because of an association with a fatal complication. Metformin has been used in Europe for years without much trouble and was finally approved in the U.S. in 1995. Metformin is rarely, and perhaps never, associated with the fatal complication *lactic acidosis* that caused phenformin to be banned. A study reported in the *Archives of Internal Medicine* in November 2003 stated that no evidence exists to date that metformin therapy leads to lactic acidosis.

Metformin has the following characteristics:

- It lowers the blood glucose mainly by reducing the production of glucose from the liver (the *hepatic* glucose output).

- It works for both type 1 and type 2 diabetes because (unlike the sulfonylureas) it does not depend on stimulating insulin to work.

- It may increase the sensitivity of the muscle cells to insulin and slow the uptake of glucose from the intestine.

- It's available in 500-mg, 850-mg, and 1,000-mg tablets. It is also available as a liquid containing 500 mg per 5 milliliters called Riomet and as an extended release form containing 750 mg.

- The maximum dose is 2,500 mg taken in divided doses with each meal.

- A relatively inexpensive generic form is available, which is just as good as any of the brand name forms.

- Used by itself (a treatment called *monotherapy*), it does not cause hypoglycemia. However, when given in combination with the sulfonylureas, hypoglycemia can occur. If low blood glucose is persistent, the dose of sulfonylurea is reduced.

- It must be taken with food because it causes gastrointestinal irritation, but this side effect declines with time.

- It's often associated with weight loss, possibly from the gastrointestinal irritation or because of a loss of taste for food.

- It's not recommended if you have significant liver disease, kidney disease, or heart failure.

- It's usually stopped for a day or two before surgery or an X-ray study using a dye and restarted two days later.

- It's not recommended for use by alcoholics.

- It's not recommended for use in pregnancy or by nursing mothers except for women with polycystic ovarian syndrome in the first trimester and gestational diabetes.

✔ Metformin reduces the occurrence of heart and blood-vessel disease as well as cancer in diabetes and should probably be continued if insulin is added in type 2 diabetes.

✔ After gastric bypass, uptake of metformin in the intestine is increased, so a reduction in dosage may be necessary.

Metformin was previously stopped when kidney disease occurred. The drug is considered to be so useful that experts now recommend continuing to use it and perhaps lowering the dose except in very severe kidney disease, when it must be stopped. Discuss continuing it with your doctor if you have kidney disease and diabetes.

Metformin can be a very useful drug, especially when *fasting hyperglycemia* (high blood glucose upon awakening) is present. Metformin has some positive effects on the blood fats, causing a decrease in triglycerides and LDL cholesterol and an increase in HDL cholesterol. About 10 percent of patients fail to respond to it when it is first used, and the secondary failure rate is 5 to 10 percent a year. It occasionally causes a decrease in the absorption of vitamin B_{12}, a vitamin that is important for the blood and the nervous system.

Bristol-Myers Squibb, the maker of Glucophage (one of the trade names of metformin), and other drug makers have come up with new preparations of metformin, which, they believe, have some advantages over the original drug:

✔ **Glucophage XR:** The original preparation of metformin has to be taken at each meal. However, Glucophage XR lasts for 24 hours and comes in a 500-mg strength. Its longer-lasting effects help overcome the problem of patients not taking their medication the required multiple times a day as well as reducing gastrointestinal side effects. Glumetza is the same drug by Biovail Pharmaceuticals.

✔ **Glucovance:** This pill combines glyburide (a sulfonylurea described in the previous section) with metformin at a dose of 250 or 500 mg. The various combinations are 1.25 mg of glyburide with 250 mg metformin, 2.5 mg glyburide with 500 mg metformin, and 5 mg glyburide with 500 mg metformin. The advantage is the convenience of having to take only one pill instead of two. Glyburide/metformin is the generic form. But note the warning about glyburide in the previous section.

✔ **Metaglip:** Made by Bristol-Myers Squibb, this drug combines metformin 250 mg and glipizide 2.5 mg. Glipizide/metformin is the generic form that also comes in 500 mg/5 mg.

✔ **Avandamet:** This drug is a combination of 4 mg of rosiglitazone (Avandia; which I describe in the section "Rosiglitazone," later in this chapter) and 500 mg of metformin. It's a potent combination of two drugs that act differently to improve insulin sensitivity. Rosiglitazone has been associated with increased heart attacks. I do not recommend Avandamet.

- ✔ **ACTOplus Met:** This pill combines 500 or 850 mg metformin with 15 mg pioglitazone (Actos), which I discuss in the later section "Pioglitazone." It is made by Takeda. Pioglitazone has unacceptable side effects, so I don't recommend this combination.

- ✔ **Janumet:** Janumet combines 500 or 1,000 mg metformin with 50 mg sitagliptin, a member of a new class of drugs called DPP-4 inhibitors (which I address in a later section). It is made by Merck.

In my experience, the combination drugs work better than giving two drugs separately. This effect may reflect the greater compliance that results when a single pill is given compared to two separate pills. If you are already taking both of the drugs separately that are available in a combination pill, ask your doctor about getting the single pill that contains both.

Alpha-glucosidase inhibitors

Alpha-glucosidase inhibitors are drugs that block the action of an enzyme in the intestine that breaks down complex carbohydrates into simple sugars that can be absorbed. Taking alpha-glucosidase inhibitors results in a slowing of the rise in glucose after meals. The carbohydrates are eventually broken down by bacteria lower down in the intestine, producing a lot of gas, abdominal pain, and diarrhea — the main drawbacks of these drugs.

The following two alpha-glucosidase inhibitors are currently being used:

- ✔ **Acarbose (brand name Precose):** This drug seems to have much greater popularity in Europe than it does in the United States. It was the first alpha-glucosidase inhibitor on the market. Following are its main characteristics:

  - It's supplied in 25-, 50-, and 100-mg strengths.

  - The recommended starting dose is 25 mg at the beginning of each meal. This dose can be increased to 50 or 100 mg three times daily, depending on the blood glucose. The highest dose is not given unless the patient weighs more than 130 pounds.

  - It does not require insulin for its activity, so it works for both type 1 and type 2 diabetes.

  - It does not cause hypoglycemia when used alone but does in combination with sulfonylureas. If hypoglycemia is persistent, the dose of sulfonylurea is decreased.

  - It should not be used by people with intestinal disease.

- Many people do not like it because of the gastrointestinal effects.

- The lowering of glucose and hemoglobin A1c is modest at most.

✔ **Miglitol (brand name Glyset):** This medication was the second alpha-glucosidase inhibitor introduced. Its characteristics are identical to acarbose. It comes in 25, 50, and 100 mg. Curiously, Bayer is the manufacturer of both drugs.

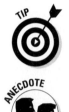

Because these drugs block the breakdown of complex carbohydrates, hypoglycemia occurring with acarbose or miglitol and sulfonylurea combinations must be treated with a preparation of glucose, not more complex carbohydrates.

In my own practice, I have not found a use for either of the drugs in this section. I tried acarbose on a number of patients, and even though they started at a low dose and gradually built up to a more effective level, they complained about the gas and abdominal pain and asked me to take them off the drug. Because I was not seeing much change in the blood glucose, I did not object. I see no reason to expect that miglitol would be any different.

Thiazolidinediones (The glitazones)

This group of drugs for diabetes is the first type of medication that directly reverses insulin resistance. Unfortunately, I can't recommend any of them.

Troglitazone

Troglitazone, brand name Rezulin (called Prelay outside the United States), was the first oral agent for type 2 diabetes that actually reversed the basic lesion in this disease, namely the insulin resistance. It does so by causing changes within the muscle and fat cells where the insulin resistance resides. These changes take several weeks to occur, and if the patient stops taking troglitazone, they take several weeks to subside.

In March 2000, because of continuing occurrences of severe liver disease sometimes leading to death in a small number of patients taking troglitazone, the FDA removed troglitazone from the market. The other glitazone drugs currently on the market have not had this problem, although the FDA requires monitoring the patient's liver function when these drugs are first used.

Rosiglitazone

Rosiglitazone was the second thiazolidinedione to be approved by the FDA. It is marketed by GlaxoSmithKline as Avandia. Rosiglitazone has been found to have unacceptable side effects and its use is limited to physicians who receive special permission. I will not discuss it further, therefore.

Pioglitazone

Pioglitazone, manufactured by Eli Lilly and Takeda in the United States, was the third thiazolidinedione to come to market. The brand name is Actos, and it has the following properties:

- The initial dose is 15 mg once a day with or without food, but most patients require 30 or even 45 mg. It comes in all three sizes.

- In addition to restoring fertility in some women who are infertile due to insulin resistance, pioglitazone reduces estrogen levels in women taking estrogen and may result in making hormone-based contraception, such as birth-control pills or Depo-Provera, less effective.

- Pioglitazone has been shown to reduce bad (LDL) cholesterol particles in people with or without diabetes (as reported in *Diabetes Care,* September 2003).

- Pioglitazone has been shown to be associated with increased osteoporosis in women.

- Pioglitazone has not been shown to be associated with a higher incidence of heart attacks.

- It is authorized for use alone, with insulin, with metformin, or with a sulfonylurea.

Pioglitazone, like rosiglitazone, has been associated with decreased bone mineral density and increased fractures in older women. After 18 months of treatment with pioglitazone, patients have a two or three times greater risk of a fracture than people who never used the drug. The fractures occur especially in the hip or wrist. Pioglitazone has also been found to cause or worsen heart failure (which is why it is contraindicated for use in patients with heart failure) and has been associated with increased bladder cancer. For these reasons, *I do not recommend it.*

Pioglitazone 30 mg has been combined with glimepiride 2 or 4 mg in a pill called Duetact made by Takeda.

Meglitinides

Each of the drugs in the meglitinides group has about the same activity, although they are chemically somewhat different. They are chemically unrelated to the sulfonylureas but work by squeezing more insulin out of the pancreas just like the sulfonylureas do. They are taken just before meals to stimulate insulin for only that meal.

Following are the two drugs in this class:

✔ **Repaglinide (brand name Prandin):** This medication was the first meglitinide. Here are the characteristics of repaglinide:

- It is available as 0.5-, 1-, and 2-mg tablets and is taken just before or up to 30 minutes before meals.

- The starting dose is 0.5 mg with a mild elevation of blood glucose or 1 or 2 mg if the initial blood glucose is higher. The dose may be doubled once a week to a maximum of 4 mg before meals.

- Because it acts through insulin, repaglinide can cause hypoglycemia.

- It's not recommended during pregnancy or for nursing mothers.

- It's not used with the sulfonylureas but can be combined with metformin.

- Repaglinide lowers the blood glucose and the hemoglobin A1c effectively when used in combination with metformin.

- It's mostly broken down in the liver and leaves the body in the bowel movement. Therefore, if liver disease is present, the dose has to be adjusted downward.

- Despite the lack of excretion through the kidneys, increases in the dose have to be made more carefully when kidney impairment is present.

Experience with repaglinide has shown that it causes no problems when given with nondiabetes medications. It's bound to protein in the blood, so medications like aspirin (which also bind to protein) may, theoretically, increase its activity. I have not seen this as a problem with my patients who are on this medication.

A combination of repaglinide and metformin is called PrandiMet, and it has two strengths, 1 mg or 2 mg of repaglinide plus 500 mg of metformin. It is taken two or three times daily, 15 to 30 minutes before meals.

✔ **Nateglinide (brand name Starlix):** This drug is very similar to repaglinide in its activity. However, it comes in 60 and 120 mg. The starting dose is usually 120 mg before each meal; if a meal is skipped, no dose is taken. If hypoglycemia occurs, the dose is lowered to 60 mg. The features of repaglinide also apply to nateglinide, other than the dosage. A report in Diabetes Care in July 2003 showed that repaglinide combined with metformin is a more potent combination than nateglinide with metformin.

Nateglinide is available as a generic, but repaglinide is not, so the less expensive choice is nateglinide.

DPP-4 inhibitors

This class of drugs has a different mechanism from any of the previous classes of oral agents. They affect a hormone called *glucagon-like peptide-1* (GLP-1), which is made in the small intestine and has a number of positive effects for people with diabetes:

- ✔ It slows the movement of food in the intestine.

- ✔ It reduces the production of glucagon from the pancreas. Glucagon raises the blood glucose.

- ✔ It increases insulin levels.

- ✔ It decreases food intake (by decreasing appetite), leading to weight loss.

- ✔ It normalizes the blood glucose in many patients.

The only problem with GLP-1 is that it's rapidly broken down by an enzyme called DPP-4. Therefore, under usual circumstances, GLP-1 is not around long enough to have these effects in a major way.

The class of drugs called DPP-4 inhibitors block the rapid breakdown of GLP-1 and prolong its actions. They cause hypoglycemia when used with sulfonylureas, so the dose of the latter drug is usually reduced. They reduce the hemoglobin A1c about the same as the sulfonylureas but less than metformin. Over the long term, they have been found to reduce atherosclerosis and inflammation, a deterrent to heart disease. They are excreted by the kidneys, so their dosage has to be reduced when kidney disease is present, with the exception of linagliptin (see below).

Currently, three DPP-4 inhibitors are on the market:

- ✔ **Sitagliptin (brand name Januvia):** Approved in 2006, this Merck drug comes in 25, 50 and 100 mg. The dose is 100 mg daily. Because it's excreted by the kidneys, people with kidney disease must take lower doses. It can cause stomach discomfort. It can be taken in combination with a sulfonylurea, metformin, or insulin

    The problem with sitagliptin is that the amount of lowering of the hemoglobin A1c is less than 1 percent. In addition, it does not result in weight loss, which, I believe, is the major advantage of GLP-1.

    Sitagliptin is available in combinations as the following drugs:

    - • Janumet, containing 50 mg of sitagliptin and 1,000 mg of metformin or 50/500

    - • Juvisync, containing 100 mg of sitagliptin and 10 mg of simvastatin or 100/20 or 100/40

✔ **Saxagliptin (brand name Onglyza):** Saxagliptin was approved in 2009. It comes as 2.5- and 5-mg tablets. The recommended dose is 2.5 or 5.0 mg once daily. It may be given with a sulfonylurea, metformin, or insulin.

Saxagliptin is available in combination with extended-release (XR) metformin as Kombiglyze XR, containing 2.5 mg saxagliptin and 1,000 mg metformin or 5 mg saxagliptin and 500 or 1,000 mg metformin.

✔ **Linagliptin (brand name Tradjenta):** This drug was approved in 2011. It comes as 5-mg tablets and the recommended dosage is 5 mg once daily. It may be used in the same combinations as the other DPP-4 inhibitors. At the end of January 2012, the FDA approved a combination of linagliptin 2.5 mg and metformin, either 500 mg or 1,000 mg, which is called Jentadueto.

Only one head-to-head trial of the DPP-4 inhibitors has been done, saxagliptin versus sitagliptin. They were found to have the same potency.

Bile acid sequestrants

Bile acid sequestrants are drugs that are used to reduce the total cholesterol and the LDL cholesterol. When they were being used for that purpose, it was noted that they also lowered the blood glucose and the hemoglobin A1c. Although the lowering of hemoglobin A1c is modest, about 0.5 percent, these drugs may have a place in prediabetes or mild type 2 diabetes. They do not cause hypoglycemia.

The FDA has authorized the use of colesevelam (brand name Welchol) for this treatment. It can be used for both type 1 and type 2 diabetes. Side effects include constipation and nausea. Colesevelam comes as 625-mg tablets as well as 1,875- and 3,750-mg powder packets. The dose is 3,750 mg once daily. It may be used alone or with other oral hypoglycemic agents and does not cause weight gain.

Bromocriptine

Bromocriptine is another drug long used for a different illness that has been found to have glucose-lowering effects. It has been used to treat Parkinson's and to treat brain tumors that produce too much growth hormone or prolactin. It was discovered to lower the blood glucose and the hemoglobin A1c to a slightly greater extent (hemoglobin A1c reduced 0.6 to 0.7 percent) than the bile acid sequestrants but by a different mechanism. It also reduces triglycerides and free fatty acids without causing hypoglycemia or weight gain.

Side effects include nausea, dizziness, and headache in less than 15 percent of patients. The dose of bromocriptine (called Cycloset) is one 0.8-mg tablet increased by one tablet per week up to a maximum of 4.8 mg. It may be used by itself or with other oral agents. The generic version of bromocriptine does not work for people with diabetes.

Combining oral agents

Taking one oral agent alone often does not control the blood glucose sufficiently to prevent complications of diabetes. (A hemoglobin A1c of less than 7 percent is the goal; see Chapter 7.) In this section, I explain how you can use two or more of these drugs together.

You should never take a drug, or a combination of drugs, as a convenient way of avoiding the basic diet and exercise that are the keys to diabetic control. (See Chapters 8 and 9 for more information on these crucial points.)

I currently start all new type 2 patients who are mildly out of control on metformin. I give this medication at least two weeks to work. Many patients need no more treatment than this in addition to their diet and exercise. I usually begin with a dose of 500 mg twice daily and raise it to 1,000 mg twice daily if the blood glucose is still elevated after two weeks.

If 2,000 mg of metformin does not control the patient's blood glucose, sitagliptin or another DPP-4 inhibitor is an excellent second drug to add at this point, usually at a dose of 3,100 mg once daily.

When a patient is taking these two drugs but still has slightly elevated blood glucose, I add a sulfonylurea. I like to use a longer-acting form, such as glimepiride, because I always prefer a drug that can be taken only once a day over drugs that require multiple dosing. I have found that 2 to 4 mg of glimepiride combined with the other drugs is all the treatment needed to achieve the goal.

A few patients still have elevated blood glucose and hemoglobin A1c levels, even with the preceding treatments. For them, repaglinide in place of the sulfonylurea usually does the trick. Starting with a dosage of 1 mg before each meal, those patients have found this medication to be very helpful.

If low blood glucose starts to be a problem, the dose of the sulfonylurea or repaglinide is lowered because the other medications are not responsible for hypoglycemia.

If there is still a little way to go to get the hemoglobin A1c down to 7 percent, colesevelam or bromocriptine may do the trick.

Many diabetes specialists believe that the pancreas gradually fails to make insulin in type 2 diabetes and that most patients need to take insulin sooner or later (see the sidebar "Combining insulin and oral agents in type 2 diabetes"). My experience is that giving insulin early on is not necessarily needed and that the modern medications, particularly metformin, can delay or eliminate the need for insulin. Certainly, numerous people with diabetes are well controlled with only a small dose of an oral medication. And I have seen many others who used insulin when nothing else was available but have since stopped taking it and do not appear as though they will ever need it again. Some people need no drugs at all. Several of my patients with long-standing, poorly controlled type 2 diabetes, who have been able to change their lifestyle and lose weight with diet and exercise, have been able to stop all medications as well.

Some patients still don't lower their hemoglobin A1c to 7 or below despite all the above medications, or do so initially but not later. These patients are given insulin or the injectable drugs described in the next section.

New injectable drugs

In the earlier discussion of DPP-4 inhibitors, I mention that these drugs work by blocking the breakdown of the natural hormone GLP-1. The effects of GLP-1, such as increasing the secretion of insulin and decreasing the uptake of glucose, have been called the *incretin effect*. Recent studies suggest that the incretin effect is lost early in type 2 diabetes. Because incretins have been shown to preserve beta-cell function, some experts believe they should be used early in the treatment of type 2 diabetes. The following sections introduce you to several forms of GLP-1 that are in use.

Exenatide

Amylin Pharmaceuticals and Eli Lilly have been able to extract a substance from the venom of a lizard called the Gila monster that acts like GLP-1 but does not break down nearly as fast. This substance is used in the medication exenatide (trade name Byetta). The pharmaceutical companies have also been able to produce a second injectable substance called *pramlintide* with many similar properties.

Exenatide is a powerful form of GLP-1 that lasts for several hours. It is taken within an hour before breakfast and supper. It may only be used in type 2 diabetes and comes in pens containing either 5 or 10 micrograms per dose. It may be used with metformin or a sulfonylurea or combinations of those drugs. It can sometimes cause substantial weight loss and eliminate the need for all of those drugs. It is associated with nausea, and in rare cases it can't be used because the nausea is so severe. Hypoglycemia is frequent when it is used with a sulfonylurea. The dosage of the sulfonylurea is then reduced. At present it may be used with long-acting insulin but not short-acting or rapid-acting insulin.

Exenatide has been found to be linked to pancreatitis (true for all GLP-agonists), an inflammation of the pancreas that causes abdominal pain, nausea, and vomiting and can be fatal. Whether and how exenatide may cause pancreatitis is not clear.

This drug has proved to be very valuable in the treatment of type 2 diabetes. It is sometimes necessary to use more than the maximum recommended dose of 20 micrograms a day.

Liraglutide

Liraglutide (brand name Victoza) is another form of GLP-1. Liraglutide can be injected once a day without relation to meals. It has been shown to lower the hemoglobin A1c to a greater extent than twice-daily exenatide. It also causes more weight loss, increased reduction in fasting plasma glucose, and more blood pressure lowering. Nausea is a minor side effect.

Liraglutide is started at a dose of 0.6 mg by injection and raised to 1.8 mg daily over two weeks.

Liraglutide has been associated with tumors of the thyroid gland in animals but not humans.

Extended-release exenatide

Once-weekly extended-release exenatide (brand name Bydureon) was approved by the FDA in January 2012. It is more effective than twice-daily exenatide but has about the same potency as daily liraglutide. The obvious advantage is one shot a week instead of 14. It had previously been rejected by the FDA twice in 2010 until the manufacturer, Amylin Pharmaceuticals, satisfied the FDA's objections. It is a new formulation, and time will tell its place in the management of type 2 diabetes.

Other extended release forms of GLP-1, including albiglutide and taspoglutide, are currently in different stages of clinical trials.

Pramlintide

Pramlintide (brand name Symlin) is an extract from the same beta cells of the pancreas that produce insulin. The hormone in its natural state in the body is called *amylin*. It has a number of valuable properties for type 1 and type 2 diabetes, including the following:

✔ It blocks the secretion of glucagon, a major hormone that tends to raise blood glucose (see Chapter 2 for details).

✔ It slows the emptying of the stomach so that glucose is absorbed more slowly.

✔ It causes loss of appetite and weight loss.

Pramlintide, therefore, has an important effect on the rate at which glucose appears in the blood after eating. These effects occur when pramlintide reaches certain centers in the brain.

Because amylin comes from the same cells that make insulin, it's absent in type 1 diabetes just as insulin is absent in type 1 diabetes. It was thought that providing amylin to a patient with T1DM might improve the blood glucose. However, naturally occurring amylin has chemical properties that make it unusable as a pill or an injection. Mainly, it couldn't be made to dissolve in any liquid. A small change in the chemical structure made it possible to dissolve the new chemical while retaining all the properties of amylin.

Pramlintide is taken before meals that contain at least 30 grams of carbohydrate or 250 kilocalories. It does not mix with insulin. Because pramlintide is so potent, the insulin dose must be reduced by half. It can cause nausea and hypoglycemia.

The starting dose of pramlintide for type 1 diabetes is 15 micrograms before meals, and it's increased by 15 micrograms every three days. The maximum daily total dose is 180 micrograms. For type 2 diabetes, the starting dose is 60 micrograms before major meals, and it can be increased to 120 mcg if necessary.

Pramlintide has not been studied in pregnancy or while breastfeeding, so it should not be used for these conditions. Children may use it.

You should probably not use pramlintide if you have hypoglycemia unawareness (see Chapter 4) or a form of diabetic neuropathy called gastroparesis (see Chapter 5), which makes the stomach empty slowly.

Taking Insulin

If you have type 1 diabetes, insulin is your savior. If you have type 2 diabetes, you may need insulin at some point in the course of your disease. Insulin is a great drug, but most people take it through a needle, and that's the rub (or the pain). Inventors have come up with many different ways to administer insulin, but using a syringe and a needle has been the standard for so long that most patients continue to do so. In this section, I tell you about the newer methods, which you should at least consider because they are easier and possibly more accurate than the old method. However, the new syringes and needles are just about painless.

Until a few years ago, insulin could be obtained only by extracting it from the pancreas of a cow, pig, salmon, or some other animal. This was not entirely satisfactory because those insulins are slightly different from human insulin. Using them resulted in an immune reaction in the blood and certain skin reactions. The preparation was purified, but tiny amounts of impurities always remained. In 1978, researchers were able to trick bacteria called *E. coli* into making human insulin. Almost all insulin is now perfectly pure human insulin. Soon, no insulin besides human insulin will be available.

Previously, insulin came in two different strengths, U40 and U80, which meant 40 units per milliliter or 80 units per milliliter. This system was confusing, especially if the wrong syringe was used — you had to use a U40 syringe for U40 insulin. To eliminate confusion, all insulin commonly used in the United States is now U100, or 100 units per milliliter (there is a U500 form for severe insulin resistance), and all syringes are U100 syringes. This standardization does not necessarily apply in Europe or elsewhere, so check the insulin strength and the markings on the syringe.

Considering insulin options

In the human body, insulin is constantly responding to ups and downs in the blood glucose. In order to avoid having to take many shots a day, forms of insulin were invented to work at different times. The following list explains the various forms of insulin:

- ✔ **Rapid-acting lispro insulin:** Lispro insulin (called *Humalog insulin* by its manufacturer, Eli Lilly) begins to lower the glucose within five minutes after its administration, peaks at about one hour, and is no longer active by about three hours. Lispro is a great advance because it frees the person with diabetes to take a shot just when he or she eats. With the previous short-acting insulin (regular insulin), a person had to take a shot 30 minutes prior to eating. Because its activity begins and ends so quickly, lispro does not cause hypoglycemia as often as the older preparations.

  Novo Nordisk has come out with *insulin aspart* (called NovoLog), which has characteristics indistinguishable from lispro insulin.

  Sanofi-Aventis produces insulin glulisine (trade name Apidra), which is similar in its properties to the other two rapid-acting insulins.

- ✔ **Short-acting regular insulin:** Regular insulin takes 30 minutes to start to lower the glucose, peaks at three hours, and is gone by six to eight hours. Until Humalog, NovoLog, and Apidra came along, patients used this preparation before meals to keep their glucose low until the next meal.

✔ **Intermediate-acting NPH:** This drug begins to lower the glucose within 2 hours of administration and continues its activity for 10 to 12 hours. It can be active for up to 24 hours. The purpose of this kind of insulin is to provide a smooth level of control over half the day so that a low level of active insulin is always in the body, an attempt to parallel the situation that exists in the human body.

✔ **Long-acting insulin glargine and detemir:** Aventis sells an insulin called *insulin glargine,* which goes by the trade name Lantus. Studies have shown that insulin glargine has its onset in 1 to 2 hours after injection, and its activity lasts for 24 hours without a specific peak time of activity, which is exactly what is needed to control the blood glucose over an entire day. Insulin glargine is released in a smooth fashion from the site of injection, and it doesn't matter if you inject the abdomen, the thigh, or the deltoid. Because of its smooth and predictable activity, insulin glargine does not tend to cause low blood glucose at night, which often happens with NPH insulin. However, one disadvantage of insulin glargine is that it can't be mixed with other insulins in one syringe.

I have used this insulin in a number of my patients with type 1 diabetes and have been extremely pleased with the results. I now use it with all new type 1 diabetes patients.

Insulin detemir or Levemir has similar properties to glargine but does not last quite as long. It is a product of Novo Nordisk.

If you do not have good diabetic control (defined as hemoglobin A1c of 7 percent or less) with NPH insulin, ask your doctor to consider using insulin glargine or detemir.

✔ **Premixed insulins:** Several mixtures are available: one with 70 percent NPH insulin and 30 percent regular; one with a 50–50 mix of NPH and regular; one with a 75–25 mix of NPH-like insulin and lispro insulin; and one with a 70–30 mix of NPH-like insulin and insulin aspart. These insulins are helpful for people who have trouble mixing insulins in one syringe, have poor eyesight, or are stable on a preparation that does not change. Insulins that are not premixed are better for young, fairly stable type 2 diabetics.

Whichever type of insulin you take, you need to know a few basic things about its use:

✔ Insulin may be kept at room temperature for four weeks or in the refrigerator until the expiration date printed on the label. After four weeks at room temperature, the insulin should be discarded.

✔ Insulin does not take too well to excessive heat, such as direct sunlight, or to excessive cold. Protect your insulin against these conditions.

✔ You can safely give an insulin shot through clothing.

✔ If you take less than 50 units in a shot, you can use ½-cc syringes that make it easy to measure up to 50 units. If you take less than 30 units, you can use ³⁄₁₀-cc syringes.

✔ Shorter needles may be more comfortable, especially for children, but the depth of the injection helps to determine how fast the insulin works.

✔ You can reuse disposable syringes a couple of times.

✔ Used syringes and needles must be disposed of in a puncture-proof container that is sealed shut before being placed in the trash.

Shooting yourself

Whatever type of insulin you use, you may be taking it by syringe and needle. (I discuss other delivery options later in the chapter, in the sections "Delivering insulin with a pen," "Delivering insulin with a jet-injection device," and "Delivering insulin with an external pump.")

Combining insulin and oral agents in type 2 diabetes

Sometimes the characteristics of the currently available oral agents do not provide the tight control needed to avoid complications. This problem is particularly common after many years of type 2 diabetes. In such cases, insulin may be required. Insulin may be added in a number of ways, but often a shot of glargine insulin at bedtime is all that is needed to start the day under control and continue it with oral agents. For example, metformin may control the daytime glucoses very well after eating, but the first morning glucose may need the overnight shot of glargine insulin. By gradually increasing the dose of glargine, most patients with type 2 diabetes on oral agents can be controlled so that their hemoglobin A1c is 7 or below.

As type 2 diabetes progresses, the oral agents may be less effective, and insulin is taken more often. Two shots a day of intermediate and short-acting insulin may do the trick. Usually you take two-thirds of the dose in the morning and one-third before supper because you need short-acting insulin to control the supper carbohydrates. In this situation, 75 percent protamine lispro (like NPH) and 25 percent lispro insulin may be useful, allowing the patient to measure from only one bottle. This combination is especially valuable in the older person with diabetes, where the tightest level of control is not being sought because the expected lifespan of the patient is shorter than the time necessary to develop complications. In this patient, doctors want to prevent problems like frequent urination leading to loss of sleep or vaginal infections, so they give enough to treat this but not so much that a frail, elderly patient is having hypoglycemia on a frequent basis.

Drawing insulin up is done in the same way no matter which type of insulin is involved. If you look at the syringe in Figure 10-1, you see that it's lined. Starting at the needle end of the syringe, you'll find nine small lines above the needle, followed by a tenth longer line where the number 10 may be found. Each line is one unit of insulin. Above the 10-unit line, you'll find a succession of four small lines followed by a larger line representing 15, 20, 25, and so on.

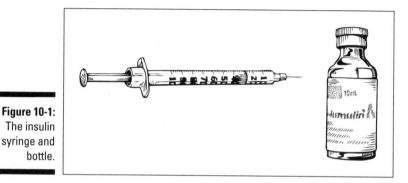

Figure 10-1:
The insulin syringe and bottle.

Illustration by Kathryn Born

If the insulin is short-acting, long-acting, or regular, it should be clear, and you do not have to shake the bottle. The other kinds of insulin are cloudy, and you need to roll the bottle a few times to suspend the tiny particles in the liquid. A new bottle has a cap on the top, which you break off and discard. When you're ready to take insulin, wipe the rubber stopper in the top of the bottle with alcohol.

Pull up the number of units of air that corresponds to the number of units of insulin you need to take. Turn the insulin bottle upside down and penetrate the rubber stopper with the needle of the syringe. Push all the air inside and pull out the insulin dose you need. Because air replaces the insulin, the pressure inside the bottle is unchanged and no vacuum is created. Check to make sure that you have the right amount of the right insulin and no air bubbles in the syringe.

To give the injection, use alcohol to wipe off an area of skin on your arm, chest, stomach, or wherever you're injecting it. Insert the needle at a right angle to the skin and push it in. When the needle has penetrated the skin, push the plunger of the syringe down to zero to administer the insulin.

If you're taking two kinds of insulin at the same time (but not insulin glargine), you can mix them in one syringe, thus avoiding two shots. Here's how you do that:

1. Wipe both bottles with alcohol.

2. Draw up the total units of air corresponding to the total insulin you need.

3. Push the units of air into the longer-acting insulin bottle that corresponds to the number of units of longer-acting insulin you need, and withdraw the needle without drawing any insulin.

4. Push the rest of the units of air into the shorter-acting insulin bottle, and withdraw the correct units of insulin.

5. Go back to the longer-acting bottle and withdraw the correct units of insulin from there.

By doing this, you do not contaminate the shorter-acting insulin with the additive in the longer-acting insulin.

Where you inject the insulin helps determine how fast it works. The site that most rapidly absorbs insulin injections is the abdomen, followed by the arms and legs and then the buttocks. You may use these differing rates of uptake of the insulin to get faster action when your blood glucose is high. If the body part that gets the insulin is exercised, the insulin enters more quickly. If you use the same injection site repeatedly, the absorption rate slows down, so rotate the sites.

The timing of your insulin injections helps to determine the smoothness of your glucose control. The more regular you are in your injections, your eating, and your exercise, the smoother your glucose level.

Conducting intensive insulin treatment

Intensive insulin treatment is essential in type 1 diabetes if you hope to prevent the complications of the disease This treatment means measuring your blood glucose at least before each meal and at bedtime, plus using both short-acting and longer-acting insulin to keep the blood glucose between 80 and 100 before meals and less than 140 after eating. How you do this is the subject of this section.

In a person who doesn't have type 1 diabetes, a small amount of circulating insulin is always present in the bloodstream, and after eating, insulin increases temporarily to control the glucose in the meal. Intensive insulin treatment attempts to mirror the activity of the normal human pancreas as much as possible.

In intensive insulin treatment, you usually take a certain amount of longer-acting insulin at bedtime. I prefer insulin glargine because it produces a smooth basal level of glucose control over 24 hours. In addition, you take a dose of rapid-acting insulin before each meal. I prefer lispro because I have the most experience with it. The dose of lispro is determined by the expected grams of carbohydrates in the meal you're about to eat, as well as by your blood glucose at that moment. Your doctor should provide you with a list of how much insulin to take for a given situation. Each patient is different, and the dosage must be individualized.

Using the carbohydrates in a meal to determine your insulin dose is called *carbohydrate counting*. The key to this system is to know the carbohydrates in your food. Here is where you make use of your friendly dietitian, who can go over your food preferences and show you how many carbohydrates are in them. The dietitian can also show you where to find carbohydrate counts for any other foods that you may eat.

You also need to know how many grams of carbohydrate are controlled by each unit of insulin you take. This number is determined by checking your blood glucose an hour after eating a known amount of carbohydrate. For example, one person may need 1 unit to control 20 grams of carbohydrate, while another person needs 1 unit to control 15 grams of carbohydrate. If both of them eat a breakfast of 75 grams of carbohydrate, the first person might take 4 units of lispro, whereas the second person takes 5 units of lispro. Then additional units are added for the amount that the blood glucose needs to be lowered. A typical schedule is to take 1 unit for every 50 mg/dl that the blood glucose is above 100 mg/dl. Insulin can also be subtracted if the blood glucose is too low. For every 50 mg/dl that the glucose is below 100, subtract 1 unit. (To see how carbohydrate counting works in practice, see the sidebar "Carbohydrate counting to maximum health.")

By measuring your blood glucose frequently, you can find out how different carbohydrates affect your blood glucose. By using the carbohydrate sources that have a low glycemic index, you need less insulin to control them. (See Chapter 8 for more on carbohydrates.)

As you attempt to help your body mirror normal insulin and glucose dynamics, you often have to deal with a greater frequency of hypoglycemia. The best way to handle hypoglycemia is by eating slightly smaller meals and using the unused calories as between-meal snacks. This technique smooths out the ups and downs.

At what point do you adjust your insulin glargine? If you find that several mornings in a row your fasting blood glucose is too high, you might add a unit or two to your bedtime glargine. If it's too low, you might reduce your insulin glargine by a unit or two or try eating a small bedtime snack. A high blood glucose level throughout the day is an indication to raise the glargine. Getting a lot of hypoglycemia at different times of day is a reason to lower the glargine. These adjustments are best done in consultation with your doctor. If, however, you're unable to see your doctor, you can put your knowledge to use and make these adjustments on your own.

ANECDOTE

Carbohydrate counting to maximum health

To find out how you can accomplish carbohydrate counting in everyday life, take a typical type 1 patient. Salvatore Law is a 41-year-old who has had type 1 diabetes for 31 years. He has been well controlled because he follows a good diet, does lots of exercise, and takes his insulin appropriately. He takes 30 units of insulin glargine at bedtime.

Law has a list of dosages of lispro insulin that tells him to take 1 unit of insulin for each 20 grams of carbohydrate he eats. He is about to have breakfast and knows that it will contain 80 grams of carbohydrate. Therefore, he needs four units of lispro insulin. He measures his blood glucose before breakfast and finds that it is 202 mg/dl. His doctor has told him to take an extra unit of lispro insulin for each 50 mg/dl above 100 mg/dl. He adds two more units for a total of six units of insulin taken just before breakfast.

At lunch, his blood glucose measures 58. He is about to have a lunch of 120 grams of carbohydrate, so he needs 6 units for that. However, he reduces it by 1 unit for the glucose measurement that is approximately 50 mg/dl lower than 100, so his final dose is 5 units.

Before supper, Law's blood glucose measures 120. His supper contains only 60 grams of carbohydrate, so he needs 3 units for that. He does not have to adjust the dose because the glucose is close to 100, so he takes only 3 units.

At bedtime, his blood glucose is 108, so he is doing very well. Unless the blood glucose is 200 or greater, he does not need to take any bedtime lispro because he is taking insulin glargine to control his glucose overnight.

Adjusting insulin when you travel

If you're traveling between time zones, you may wonder if you need to change your insulin routine while you're gone. Time changes of less than three hours require no modifications, but changes above three hours require progressively more. You should probably discuss these changes with your physician before you go.

Say that you're taking the red-eye flight at 10 p.m. from San Francisco, arriving at 6 a.m. at Kennedy Airport in New York. If you are taking insulin glargine or detemir, you don't have to change your dose. Just start using lispro (or any other rapid-acting insulin) at the beginning of your meals (which you'll be eating three hours earlier than usual because of the time change).

When you return to California, you add three hours to your day. In this case, you need to take an extra measurement of your blood glucose. If it's around 150, you need do nothing, but if it's 200 or more, take a couple of units of lispro insulin to bring it down. If your blood glucose is much below 100, eat a small snack. Again, you do not have to adjust your insulin glargine.

Delivering insulin with a pen

Several manufacturers, including Eli Lilly, Owen Mumford, Diesetronic, Novo Nordisk, Sanofi-Aventis, and Becton Dickinson, have sought ways to make delivering insulin easier. The insulin pen, shown in Figure 10-2, is one useful tool. The pen doesn't eliminate the need for needles, but it does change the way you measure your insulin. Either the pen comes with an insulin cartridge already inserted, or the cartridge is placed inside the pen just like ink cartridges used to be put in pens and replaced when it runs out.

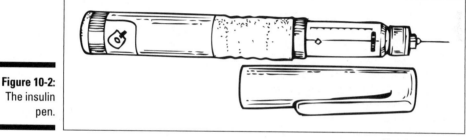

Figure 10-2:
The insulin pen.

Illustration by Kathryn Born

Each cartridge contains 1.5 or 3.0 milliliters of insulin — either NPH, regular, lispro, aspart, glargine, detemir, a mixture of NPH and lispro (such as 75 percent NPH-like lispro and 25 percent lispro), or a mixture of NPH plus aspart. You can then dial the amount of insulin that you need to take. Each unit (sometimes 2 units) is accompanied by a clicking sound so the visually impaired can hear the number of units. The units also appear in a window on the pen. If you draw up too many units, one of the pens forces you to waste the insulin by pushing it out of the needle, while others allow you to reset the pen and start again. Depending on the pen, you can deliver from ½ to 80 units of insulin. You screw on a new needle as needed.

A number of different companies make pens for their own insulin. Available pens include the following options:

- **Autopen:** This pen is available in four different models. Two contain a 1.5-ml cartridge, and two contain a 3-ml cartridge. Within each size, one pen delivers Humalog insulin in 1-unit increments, and the other pen delivers Humalog insulin in 2-unit increments.

- **Humalog Mix 75/25, Humalog Mix 50/50, Humalog KwikPen, Humulin Mix 70/30, and Humulin N:** All these prefilled, disposable pens contain 3 ml of the particular kind of insulin you use.

- **HumaPen Luxura HD:** This pen is used for Humalog insulin when half-unit doses are needed, particularly in children.

- ✔ **HumaPen Memoir:** This pen remembers the 16 most recent doses, their times, and their dates; and is used with 3-ml lispro cartridges.
- ✔ **Levemir FlexPen:** This prefilled disposable pen contains 3 ml of Levemir insulin.
- ✔ **NovoLog FlexPen and NovoLog 70/30 FlexPen:** These prefilled, disposable insulin syringes contain 3 ml of insulin.
- ✔ **NovoPen Junior:** This pen takes NovoLog cartridges containing 3 ml of insulin, and they can be measured in half-unit doses.
- ✔ **NovoPen 3:** This pen holds NovoLog 3-ml cartridges.
- ✔ **SoloStar:** This disposable pen contains 3 ml of Lantus insulin.

Insulin pens require needles, and you must match the pen with the proper needle in order for the pen to work properly. If the needles don't come with the pen, the instructions with the pen tell you which needle to use.

Should you shift from your syringe and needle to a pen? If you're comfortable with the syringe and needle and feel your technique is accurate, you probably have no reason to do so. If you're new to insulin, have some visual impairment, or feel that you're not getting an accurate measurement of the insulin, a pen may be the solution for you.

Delivering insulin with a jet-injection device

Jet-injection devices (see Figure 10-3) are for people who just can't stick a needle into their skin. At around $1,000 or more, they're expensive, but they last a long time and replace the syringe and needle.

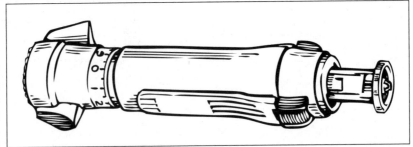

Figure 10-3:
A jet-injection device.

Illustration by Kathryn Born

The only jet injection device that I could verify is still on the market is the Insujet, a device that is made in the Netherlands by the European Pharma Group at www.insujet.com. To contact the company for information about the device, you can e-mail info@insujet.com.

A large quantity of insulin is taken into the injection device, enough for multiple treatments. The amount of insulin to be delivered is measured, usually by rotating one part of the device while the number of units to be delivered appears in a window. The device is held against the skin. With the press of a button, a powerful jet of air forces the insulin through the skin into the subcutaneous tissue, usually with no pain perceived by the patient. The devices come in a lower power form for smaller children. These devices can deliver up to 50 units at one time.

Should you try an insulin jet injector? If you have no trouble with the syringe and needle or find the pen to be an easy substitute, you don't need a jet injector. If you hate needles or need to give frequent shots to a small child who is very resistant to them, a jet injector may solve your problems.

Delivering insulin with an external pump

For some people — and you may be one of them — the external insulin pump (see Figure 10-4) is the answer to their prayers. These devices are as close as you currently can come to the gradual administration of rapid-acting insulin that is normally taking place in the body. They're expensive, costing more than $4,000, but the insulin pump may be the answer for patients who simply cannot achieve good glucose control with syringes, pens, or jet injectors.

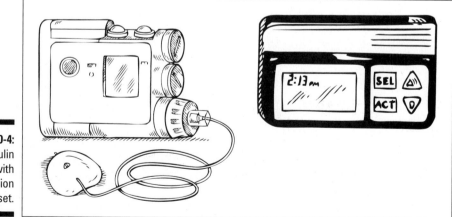

Figure 10-4:
The insulin pump with its infusion set.

Illustration by Kathryn Born

Currently, five companies — Animas, Insulet, Medtronic MiniMed, Roche, and Sooil Development — sell these pumps, which are the size of a pager. Inside the pump is a motor. A syringe filled with short-acting insulin is placed within the pump, with the plunger against a screw that slowly pushes it down to push insulin out of the syringe. The end of the syringe is attached to a short tube, which ends in a needle pushed into the skin of the abdomen. Insulin is slowly pushed under the skin. The Insulet device, called the OmniPod, has the infusion set built in and doesn't require tubing.

The rate at which insulin slowly enters the under the skin is called the *basal rate*. It can be set, by way of computer chips, to vary as often as every half hour to an hour. For example, from 8 a.m. to 9 a.m., the pump may deliver 0.8 units, while from 9 a.m. to 10 a.m., the pump may deliver 1.0 units, depending on the needs of the patient. This amount is determined, of course, by measuring the blood glucose with a meter (see Chapter 7).

When the patient is about to eat a meal, he or she can push a button to deliver extra insulin, called a *bolus* of insulin. (The amount is determined by carbohydrate counting, which I explain earlier in this chapter.) You can get extra insulin if the blood glucose is too high at any time.

Pump usage has its advantages:

- ✔ It's flexible because the bolus is taken just before meals.

- ✔ It often smooths out the swings of glucose during the day because the insulin is administered slowly and in small variable doses, depending on insulin requirements at different times of day.

- ✔ It can be rapidly disconnected and reconnected to take a shower or swim. (However, it can take a little getting used to when worn to bed.) Or insulin delivery can be suspended during exercise to prevent hypoglycemia after exercise.

- ✔ It's safe from overdosage because it has built-in protective devices.

However, pump usage has definite disadvantages besides the high cost:

- ✔ Infections of the skin are frequent because the infusion set is left in place for several days. These infections are usually mild, however.

- ✔ Overall diabetic control is not necessarily better with the pump than with other ways of delivering insulin, especially with the new insulin glargine. The latest proof of this was an article published in *Journal of Diabetes and Its Complications* in November 2010.

- ✔ Because the patient receives only short-acting insulin, if insulin stops entering, ketoacidosis may come on rapidly (see Chapter 4).

> ✔ Some patients are allergic to the tape that holds the infusion set onto the skin.
>
> ✔ Blood glucose must be measured often to adjust the pump for optimal control.

Pump usage is definitely not treatment to be done on your own at the beginning. You need a diabetologist to help with dosages, a dietitian to help you calculate amounts of boluses based on carbohydrate intake, and someone from the manufacturer to teach you how to set the pump and to be available to fix any malfunctions.

If you use a pump and your blood glucose rises above 250 mg/dl, take the following steps:

1. **Take a bolus of insulin with the pump to bring it down. (The amount is determined by your sensitivity to insulin.)**

2. **Recheck your glucose in an hour.**

3. **If the glucose is still above 250 mg/dl, use a syringe to take more insulin.**

4. **Check your infusion set.**

5. **Check the ketones in your urine and report to a doctor if the amount is moderate to large.**

6. **Recheck your glucose every two hours and use more insulin as needed.**

Is an insulin pump for you? If you're willing to invest the time and effort at first, if your schedule is very uncertain, particularly with respect to meals, and if your glucose control has not been good with other means, you should look into this option.

My patients who use the pump have generally had positive experiences. Now that they have it, none of them are willing to give up the pump. Occasionally, they disconnect the pump to allow their skin to heal. They have generally shown improved glucose control and a better hemoglobin A1c.

Do I recommend using an insulin pump? With insulin glargine, you can accomplish a continuous basal control of the blood glucose much like the pump does. The pump proponents say that you need to be able to alter the basal dose for different conditions throughout the day, and you can't do that with a single shot of insulin. However, I am not sure that it makes a great difference in the course of controlling the blood glucose.

Is one pump better than another? All seem to have excellent mechanical features, and all provide you with the ability to adjust your insulin in several ways. They all have alarms for any eventuality like blockage of the tube, an electrical failure, and so forth. They try to differentiate themselves by offering different options for how the insulin is delivered, but you may find that you need the help of a rocket scientist to figure out those differences.

One pump that does deserve special mention, because it is the wave of the future, is the Medtronic MiniMed Paradigm Real Time Revel. This pump is sold with the OneTouch UltraLink Blood Glucose Monitor. Readings taken by the monitor are wirelessly sent to the pump, which uses a software program to calculate the bolus of insulin to be given, taking into account the food about to be eaten, which must be entered into the pump. The wearer must accept the bolus before it is delivered. This product is just short of the so-called *closed loop system,* where the blood glucose determines the amount of insulin to be given, just as the normal pancreas is constantly doing. The pump chooses the boluses, but it does not constantly alter the basal level of insulin, because no continuing information about the current blood glucose level is given. The wearer must test the blood glucose with the meter in order for the pump to know glucose levels.

For an extensive discussion of the various types of insulin pumps that are available, their pros and cons and much more about using a pump to deliver insulin, see my book *Type 1 Diabetes For Dummies* (Wiley).

Utilizing aids to insulin delivery

For those of you still using the old needle-and-syringe method, I want you to be aware of numerous aids that can make taking insulin easier for you:

- ✔ **Spring-loaded syringe holders:** You place your syringe in the holder, hold it against the skin, and press a button. The needle enters and administers the insulin.

- ✔ **Syringe magnifiers:** These magnifiers help visually impaired people administer insulin.

- ✔ **Syringe-filling devices:** You can feel and hear a click as you take up insulin.

- ✔ **Subcutaneous infusion sets:** A catheter is placed under the skin, and injections are made into the catheter instead of the skin to reduce punctures.

- ✔ **Needle guides:** You can use these guides when you can't see the rubber part of the insulin bottle to insert the needle to take up the insulin.

Call your local American Diabetes Association branch or look in the back of the ADA's *Diabetes Forecast* magazine to find sources for these products.

If you take a drug that makes you prone to hypoglycemia, you need to wear a medical bracelet or necklace that identifies you as a person with diabetes who may be hypoglycemic. Numerous companies make these products.

Using Other Medications

Most of this chapter is devoted to medications that lower the blood glucose, but diabetes involves more than elevated blood glucose levels. People with diabetes often have high blood pressure and high cholesterol, and they suffer more sickness when exposed to influenza or pneumonia. You need to consider this fact in the overall management of your disease.

If you have high blood pressure (see Chapter 7), then lifestyle changes, including weight loss and physical activity, may be all you need to control the condition. However, if lifestyle changes alone don't work, numerous medications are available that control blood pressure. See my book *High Blood Pressure For Dummies* (Wiley) for a complete discussion of this subject. Controlling blood pressure is as important as controlling blood glucose in preventing diabetic complications.

Most people with diabetes also have elevated levels of LDL (bad) cholesterol (see Chapter 7). Excellent drugs are available to manage this problem if lifestyle changes don't suffice. See *Controlling Cholesterol For Dummies* (Wiley) by Carol Ann Rinzler and Martin W. Graf for the answers to your questions on this topic. Cholesterol control is another cornerstone of excellent diabetic care. A study published in the *New England Journal of Medicine* in March 2004 indicates that when it comes to LDL cholesterol, the lower, the better. Talk to your doctor about this topic.

Statin drugs are the most frequently used for lowering LDL cholesterol. However, statin use in postmenopausal women is associated with an increased risk for type 2 diabetes, so discuss it with your doctor.

People with diabetes, especially those whose glucose is poorly controlled, are prone to become sicker when they develop influenza or pneumonia. Excellent vaccinations for these illnesses are available. Flu vaccine is given annually, and pneumonia vaccine is given once if you are older than 65 and received a previous vaccination more than five years ago.

Finally, aspirin has been shown to reduce sickness and death due to coronary artery disease (which I discuss in Chapter 5). Because coronary artery disease is such a prominent feature of diabetes, many doctors recommend that all patients with diabetes take a daily aspirin tablet. Diabetics may need more than the usual dose of a baby aspirin to reduce their risk of heart attacks; a full adult pill may be necessary.

Avoiding Drug Interactions

Studies have shown that some patients with diabetes are taking as many as four to five drugs, including their diabetes medications. These drugs often interact, and the results can be harmful. Sometimes (believe it or not) even your doctor is not aware of the interactions of common drugs. You need to know the names of all the drugs you take and whether they affect one another.

Many common medications used for the treatment of high blood pressure also raise the blood glucose, sometimes bringing out a diabetic tendency that may otherwise not have been recognized:

- **Thiazide diuretics** often raise the glucose by causing a loss of potassium. Among these drugs are chlorothiazide (Diuril) and metolazone (Zaroxolyn), which are similar to hydrochlorothiazide.

- **Beta blockers** reduce the release of insulin and include such drugs as propranolol (Inderal), metoprolol (Lopressor), and atenolol (Tenormin).

- **Calcium channel blockers** also reduce insulin secretion. They include nifedipine (Adalat), verapamil (Calan), diltiazem (Cardizem), verapamil (Isoptin), amlodipine (Norvasc), and nifedipine (Procardia).

- **Minoxidil** can raise blood glucose.

Drugs used for other purposes can also raise blood glucose:

- **Corticosteroids,** even in topical use, can raise blood glucose.

- **Cyclosporine,** used to prevent organ rejection, can raise the blood glucose by poisoning the insulin-producing beta cell.

- **Diphenylhydantoin,** known as Dilantin, is a drug for seizures and blocks insulin release.

- **Nicotinic acid and niacin,** used to raise HDL and lower cholesterol, can bring out a hyperglycemic tendency.

- **Phenothiazines,** such as prochlorperazine (Compazine), mesoridazine (Serentil), trifluoperazine (Stelazine), and chlorpromazine (Thorazine), can block insulin secretion and cause hyperglycemia. Many of the newer antipsychotic drugs also cause insulin resistance.

- **Thyroid hormone,** in elevated levels, raises the blood glucose by reducing insulin from the pancreas and increasing the breakdown of insulin.

Oral contraceptives were previously accused of causing hyperglycemia when the dose of estrogen was very high, but current preparations are not a problem.

Many common medications, either on their own or by doing something to make the oral drugs that lower blood glucose more potent, also lower the blood glucose. The most important of these include the following:

- ✔ **Salicylates and acetaminophen,** known as aspirin and Tylenol, can lower the blood glucose, especially when given in large doses.

- ✔ **Ethanol,** in any form of alcohol, can lower the blood glucose, particularly when taken without food.

- ✔ **Angiotensin-converting enzyme inhibitors,** used for high blood pressure, such as quinapril (Accupril), captopril (Capoten), benazepril (Lotensin), fosinopril (Monopril), lisinopril (Zestril and Prinivil), and enalapril (Vasotec), can lower the blood glucose, though the mechanism is unclear.

- ✔ **Alpha-blockers,** another group of antihypertensives that includes prazosin, lower the glucose as well.

- ✔ **Fibric-acid derivatives** like clofibrate (Atromid-S), used to treat disorders of fat, cause a lowering of blood glucose.

If you start a new medication and suddenly find that your blood glucose is significantly higher or lower than usual, ask your doctor to check for the possibility that the new medication has a definite glucose-lowering or glucose-raising effect.

Finding Assistance Obtaining Drugs

Diabetes can be expensive, especially if you need several drugs to control your blood glucose. The pharmaceutical companies understand, and several offer programs to provide medication for a period of time. Table 10-1 tells you what you need to know about these companies.

Table 10-1	How You Can Get Drug Supplies		
Company	**Primary Medication**	**Program Name**	**Phone Number**
Bayer Healthcare Pharmaceuticals	Acarbose	Indigent Patient	866-575-5002
Xubex Pharmacy	Metformin	Free Medication Program	866-699-8239
Eli Lilly	All insulin preparations	Lilly Cares	800-545-6962

(continued)

Table 10-1 *(continued)*

Company	Primary Medication	Program Name	Phone Number
RxOutreach	Glyburide and glimepiride	Rx Outreach	800-769-3880
Novo Nordisk	Insulin preparations	Patient Assistance Program	866-310-7549
Pfizer	Glipizide, glipizide extended release, chlorpropamide	Pfizer Maintain Program	866-706-2400
Sanofi-Aventis	Insulin glargine	Patient Assistance Program	888-847-4877

All these programs require you to get a prescription from your doctor. The doctor usually fills out forms that state that the patient meets the financial requirements and needs the drug. Not all companies give away free drugs for life. But if you cannot afford to buy a drug that you're taking, do not hesitate to call the company and ask whether it has a patient-assistance program.

Chapter 11

Diabetes Is Your Show

· ·

In This Chapter

▶ Preparing for your role as author, producer, director, and star

▶ Tapping into the talents of your physicians

▶ Welcoming other professionals to your crew

▶ Inviting your family and friends — your audience

▶ Making use of the Internet

· ·

Shakespeare said it: "All the world's a stage." That quote applies to diabetes beautifully. You have many roles in life, and one of them is the role of a person with diabetes. But as with any production, you're not expected to do it all alone. You have a large cast and crew who are eager to help you, but you must be willing to ask for their help and know how to use them so that they can give you their best. Believe me, as a member of that crew, everyone wants to give you their best.

The question is, do you want your play to be a comedy or a tragedy? You hold all the major positions, so the choice is entirely up to you. And remember, as with all plays, life goes on offstage. You may also be a brother or sister, mother or father, boss or employee, and so on. Fortunately, the life skills that you discover as someone with diabetes are applicable to all your other roles.

The Internet is a goldmine of information. The resources it offers deserve mention in this chapter on using all the tools available to manage your diabetes.

Your Role as Author, Producer, Director, and Star

Being the author, the producer, the director, and the star may seem like a lot of responsibility — and it is. Unlike many short-term illnesses where the doctor knows what has to be done, instructs you to do it, writes a prescription, and cures you, diabetes is your daily companion for life. No one, not even your mother or spouse, can be with you all of the time. Therefore, you're the one who writes the script and the action. You decide whether you'll take your medication or exercise regularly. You determine whether you'll follow a diet that will control your weight and your blood glucose.

You're the one who needs to gather the resources needed to play the role properly. In this sense, you're the producer. You need your props and your theater, the equipment, the medications, and the environment in which to manage your diabetes. Your environment may be a comfortable home where you can eat the proper diet and a good exercise facility where you can burn up calories while you strengthen your heart. Or it may be the sidewalk where you can safely walk or jog.

After you have the resources, you need to direct your cast and crew to make your play come out the way you envision it. You're the one who sees to it that the primary physician obtains a hemoglobin A1c (see Chapter 7) every three or four months and that you visit the eye doctor at least once a year. The physician is dealing with many patients each day and can easily forget your specific needs, so you must let the doctor know what they are and not expect him or her to read your mind. You may be dealing with other doctors who treat your heart, your lungs, and other parts of you. Each doctor needs to know all the medications you take.

Finally, you're the star of the show. That role is both an honor and a responsibility. Although you may wish that you had never been chosen for this particular role, you have it. You can make of it what you will. You can learn all your lines (understand your disease) and speak them fluently (take your medications, follow your diet, and so on), or not. Obviously, not studying your lines is a lot easier, but in that case, the result can be a tragedy. Take proper care of yourself, and the smile on your face and that of all your fellow cast members and crew will clearly indicate that you have written, produced, directed, and starred in a comedy.

The Primary Physician: Your Assistant Director

In the United States, where you can find numerous specialists, only 8 percent of people with diabetes are regularly seen by a specialist. Because of the large size of the diabetic population and the requirements of a healthcare system with limited resources, the other 92 percent are in the hands of more general doctors, primary physicians, who have to deal with many other illnesses besides diabetes.

Although using a primary physician instead of a specialist may seem not conducive to the best care, I can say many good things about it. Besides diabetes complications, you may have other things go wrong, and the primary physician can handle them as well. After all, if you had only mild heart disease, you might not require a cardiologist, and your primary physician could also manage your bronchitis very well.

 You should expect your primary physician to have a decent working knowledge of diabetes. Chapter 7 describes the proper way to follow a person with diabetes. The various tests are essential to your health, and the primary physician must know which ones to order and when to send you to a specialist because your needs are beyond his or her expertise.

The Diabetologist or Endocrinologist: Your Technical Consultant

One type of specialist, an endocrinologist, should have the most in-depth knowledge of the management of diabetes. She has several years of advanced training (on top of the years of training in general internal medicine) and devotes her practice to taking care of people with diabetes, plus patients with problems of the thyroid, adrenals, or other glands. A *diabetologist* is an endocrinologist who takes care of only diabetic patients.

If you have type 1 diabetes, you will certainly see an endocrinologist sooner or later. If you have type 2 diabetes and get into trouble with complications or control, you'll be sent to an endocrinologist for consultation. You have the right to expect that this physician will be able to answer most questions that arise during the care of diabetes.

This doctor will be up on the newest treatments for diabetes, so if you have questions about the future of diabetes care, ask her. This doctor should also have the best understanding of all the drugs currently used for diabetes, how they interact with each other, their side effects, and other drugs that interact with them.

 If you're not satisfied with the answers you're getting from your primary physician, ask for a referral to a specialist. Many health plans today try to steer you away from the specialist because this doctor orders more expensive tests and costs more to see by virtue of the extra years of specialty training. But do not take no for an answer. If your primary doctor will not refer you, find one who will.

If your endocrinologist or diabetologist makes any changes to your treatment, report those changes to your primary physician. One of the big problems in medicine is the lack of communication between medical-care providers of all types, not just doctors.

For your own sake, make sure that all your medical-care providers know what the others are doing for you. Carry a list of your medications and show it each time you have a doctor visit. You may even want to carry the actual medications so the doctor can verify that you are getting the medications in the strengths that she thinks you are getting.

The Eye Doctor: Your Lighting Designer

The eye doctor (*ophthalmologist* or *optometrist*) ensures that your diabetes does not damage your vision. This doctor has had advanced training in diseases of the eye. Your primary-care physician must see to it (no pun intended) that you have an examination by this specialist at least once a year and more often if necessary.

The eye doctor examines you for the conditions I outline in Chapter 5. He must send a report to your primary physician. He should also take the opportunity to educate you about diabetic eye disease.

An ophthalmologist or optometrist must dilate the pupils of the eyes in order to do a proper examination.

Sometimes the good deed of restoring vision leads to unexpected, negative consequences. One ophthalmologist I talked to told me that he restored the vision of a diabetic patient, only to have the patient buy a gun and nearly shoot someone with whom he had a grievance.

The Foot Doctor: Your Dance Instructor

The foot doctor, or *podiatrist,* is your best source of help with the minor (and some of the major) foot problems that all people suffer. You should go to her if you have such problems as toenails that are hard to cut, corns and calluses, and certainly any ulcer or infection of your foot. It's especially important to visit the podiatrist if you have any neuropathy (see Chapter 5). In that case, you're better off not trying to cut your toenails by yourself.

Foot doctors I spoke with emphasized that the earlier you see a podiatrist, the less likely you are to have a minor problem turn into a major disaster. For example, an infected toe that would respond to soaking by the person without diabetes may need antibiotics, special shoes, and surgical removal of dead tissue in the person with diabetes.

The doctor can tell you which preparations you should not use on your skin. She can show you how important it is that you give lesions time to heal and not rush to put weight on your injured feet. Many podiatrists also give you a list of do's and don'ts for the proper care of your feet, such as conducting daily inspections, avoiding extreme heat, and so on. Chapter 5 details all the things you need to do to preserve good foot health.

The Dietitian: Your Food-Services Provider

This person serves one of the most important roles in your care. Because most diabetes is type 2, and type 2 is greatly worsened by obesity, a good dietitian can really help you to control your blood glucose both by eating the right foods and amounts and helping you to lose weight. The dietitian can also show you which foods belong to which energy source — carbohydrate, protein, and fat. (See Chapter 8 for more on your diet.)

People with type 1 diabetes need to know how food interacts with mandatory insulin injections. The dietitian can teach you to count carbohydrates so that you know how much insulin to take for your meals. (See Chapter 10 for more on carbohydrate counting.)

A good dietitian usually holds up a mirror to you, showing you not only what you eat but how you eat as well. When do you consume most of your calories, and where do they come from? All ethnic foods can be adjusted so that you enjoy the foods you have always eaten while you stay within the bounds of a diabetic diet. A good dietitian is the best source for this kind of information.

The dietitian can also show you what a portion of food really means. This demonstration is an eye-opener in most cases. You usually find that you have been eating portions much larger than necessary. Unfortunately, when it comes to a diabetic diet, you can't have your cake and eat it, too. But you can see in Appendix C, which offers gourmet recipes for people with diabetes, that every culture makes delicious food that is actually good for the person with diabetes. For even more information on this important topic, see my book *Diabetes Cookbook For Dummies* (Wiley).

One thing you want to be sure of is that the dietitian is flexible in her approach to food. You may have to follow a few rules about where your calories come from, but you should have plenty of room for variation within those rules. The diet you are ultimately given should take into account your preferences as well as the fact that the amount of carbohydrate, protein, and fat is different for different individuals. Any dietitian who simply hands you a printed diet and says "Go follow it" is doing you no favor.

The Diabetes Educator: Your Researcher

Every person in your play is actually an educator in addition to his other role, but an actual diabetes educator is specially trained to teach you what you need to know about every aspect of diabetes so that you properly take care of yourself. He should have *CDE* (Certified Diabetes Educator) after his name. A CDE has taken extensive courses in diabetes and has passed an examination.

A diabetes educator teaches you how to take your insulin or pills, how to test your blood glucose, and how to acquire any of the other skills you need. You can find many diabetes educators in a diabetes education program. After you have gotten over the shock of having diabetes, asking your primary physician to refer you to such a program is a good idea. After you have gone through the program, go back and update yourself every few years. New drugs and new procedures are constantly being discovered. A diabetes educator can be a wonderful source of information about these advancements while making sure that you continue in your good diabetic habits.

Although individual education classes may be hard to find and be more expensive than group classes, studies suggest that individual education of people with diabetes is more effective than group education. Glucose control was better and patients' behavior and psychological adjustment were more improved.

The Pharmacist: Your Usher

The role of the usher may not sound important, but how will you enjoy the play if you can't find your seat? The pharmacist is your guide to all the medications and tools required to control your blood glucose and manage any complications that you develop. She ushers you into the use of all these strange and new products. You may see your pharmacist more often than you see any other of your crew who are actually in the medical field.

Each time you start a new medication, a good pharmacist checks to make sure that it does not conflict with other medicines you are taking. The pharmacist tells you about side effects and makes sure that your doctor is checking you for adverse drug reactions or interactions. The pharmacist may give you a printout that you can take home and refer to, telling you all you need to know about your new medication.

Many pharmacists also prepare a list of medications that you take, telling you each drug's strengths and dosage frequency. You can carry this list around in case any doctor ever needs to know what you take.

Modern pharmacists also do a lot of educating. Posters in the pharmacy explain diseases and drugs. Pharmacists can tell you about helpful over-the-counter drugs that your doctor doesn't prescribe. They are also often aware of new drugs and treatments before they become well known. Some pharmacies have blood-pressure devices that you can use for free, as well as glucose meters.

The Mental-Health Worker: Your Supporting Actor

Your mental-health worker may be a psychiatrist, a psychologist, or a social worker, or your primary physician may play this role. This person comes in handy whenever you have days when you feel you just can't cope. (See Chapter 1 for more about dealing with the emotional aspects of diabetes.) The mental-health worker supports you and gets you going again. Diabetes certainly proves the fact that all diseases are both physical and emotional.

Your Family and Friends: Your Captivated and Caring Audience

Your audience is the people you live with, eat with, and play with. Your family and friends can be a tremendous source of help, but you must clue them in to the fact that you have diabetes. If you have type 1 diabetes, you can teach them how to recognize when your glucose is too low, in case you're ever too ill to take care of yourself. If you have type 2, ask them to moderate their diet so that you can follow yours. A diabetic diet is good for anyone. Complying with your diet is difficult enough, and you don't need your family exposing you to high-calorie foods.

A family member or friend can also become your exercise partner. Sticking to a program is a lot easier when a partner is counting on you to show up to work out. Your family and friends can also accompany you when you visit the doctor and remind you to ask the doctor a question or to follow the instructions you received.

Let these people know about your diabetes and buy them a copy of this book so that they better understand what you are going through and how they can best help you.

The Internet: Your Potential Partner in Lifestyle Change

Type 2 diabetes is a lifestyle disease. Some harmful choices for your lifestyle contributed to your development of type 2 diabetes and some helpful choices will help you control it or prevent it if you don't have it yet. Unlike the people in your life, who can hardly be there with you 24 hours a day, the Internet is only a mouse click away at any time. On the Internet you can find help for the two key aspects of your lifestyle that affect diabetes, diet and exercise.

Because weight loss is the main preoccupation of millions of Americans, numerous websites promise incredible results. Probably the single most important feature of a site that will truly help you to succeed is continued feedback. If you get regular new advice (at least weekly) and peer support in the form of message boards where you can interact with others, you will lose three times as much weight as with sites that only provide diet and exercise information on a noninteractive web page.

Sites for diet and weight loss

Following are some of the better sites for diet and weight loss:

- ✔ www.ediets.com: This site gives you a choice of many different diets and provides the food as well as weekly updates and suggestions. You can choose from more than 22 diet plans, and eDiets.com prides itself on the tastiness of its foods, so one of the plans is sure to appeal to you. You can consult with their nutritionists to develop a diet that meets your needs. If, for example, you have a heart issue, the company will tailor your diet for you. Fitness is an important component of their diets.

- ✔ www.diet.webmd.com: This site uses a questionnaire to develop a "diet just for you." The diet, which is called a nutritional plan, is personalized and nutritionally sound. You fill out a daily nutritional journal that the people at WebMD comment on. They analyze your progress and nutritional needs each week. WebMD is filled with useful information for people who must lose weight for any reason. It also emphasizes fitness, as any good diet program should.

- ✔ http://shapeup.org: This is the web address of Shape Up America!, a nonprofit organization founded by former surgeon general C. Everett Koop, MD. It offers lots of free information about nutrition and also advocates for your health. For example, it is working to get the federal government to label beer, wine, and spirits with nutritional information and to classify obesity counseling and treatment as essential health benefits so your insurance has to pay for it.

Sites for exercise programs

Here are some of the better websites for exercise programs:

- ✔ www.freetrainers.com: This site offers individualized fitness programs with individual advice and message boards for reading the experiences of others and offering your own. They have something for everyone from beginning exercisers to established fitness devotees. You can even find a training partner at this site.

- ✔ workoutsforyou.com: At this site, you can get a personalized fitness program, weekly e-mail tips, and unlimited e-mail consultations. There are lots of member testimonials in case you want to read the experience of others. You have to pay for information and a program at this site.

- ✔ www.global-fitness.com: This website for Global Health and Fitness offers a large amount of information on fitness with lots of feedback from trainers. It touts itself as the first weight-loss and fitness program on the Internet, starting in 1996. It is another site where you pay for information and training.

None of these sites tell you about the people who did not do so well or even the ratio of successful to unsuccessful clients. Don't spend a lot of money up front until you are sure the program is what you need and what works for you. Good luck!

Finding reputable websites

Not everything that you find on the Internet is true, let alone reputable. The Health on the Net Foundation has established a set of principles that any site on the Internet can adhere to. From its website at www.hon.ch, you can search for medical sites that follow these HONcode principles:

- ✔ **Principle 1:** Any medical or health advice provided and hosted on this site is only given by medically trained and qualified professionals unless a clear statement is made that a piece of advice offered is from a non-medically qualified individual or organization.

- ✔ **Principle 2:** The information provided on this site is designed to support, not replace, the relationship that exists between a patient/site visitor and his or her existing physician.

- ✔ **Principle 3:** Confidentiality of data relating to individual patients and visitors to a medical/health website, including their identity, is respected by this site. The website owners undertake to honor or exceed the legal requirements of medical/health information privacy that apply in the country and state where the website and mirror sites are located.

✔ **Principle 4:** Where appropriate, information contained on this site is supported by clear references to source data and, where possible, have specific HTML links to that data. The date when a clinical page was last modified is clearly displayed (typically at the bottom of the page).

✔ **Principle 5:** Any claims relating to the benefits/performance of a specific treatment, commercial product, or service is supported by appropriate, balanced evidence in the manner outlined in Principle 4.

✔ **Principle 6:** The designers of this website seek to provide information in the clearest possible manner and provide contact addresses for visitors that seek further information or support. The webmaster displays his or her e-mail address clearly throughout the site.

✔ **Principle 7:** Support for this website is clearly identified, including the identities of commercial and noncommercial organizations that have contributed funding, services, or material for the site.

✔ **Principle 8:** If advertising is a source of funding, the site clearly says so. A brief description of the advertising policy is displayed on the site. Advertising and other promotional material is presented to viewers in a manner and context that facilitates differentiation between it and the original material created by the institution operating the site.

If a site agrees with these principles, you can bet the information on it is very reliable.

Chapter 12

Putting Your Knowledge to Work for You

*I*f you read every word in Part III of this book, you now know as much as the experts. But knowing is often quite a distance from doing. If this fact were not the case, the world would be a much better place to live because most people know what needs to be done. They just don't do it. Things are looking up, however. A study reported at the ADA meetings in San Diego in 2011 showed that the life expectancy for people with type 1 diabetes born after 1964 is almost the same as the general population, 68.8 years compared to 72.4 years.

The key thing is to get going on improving your health now. Don't wait another day to begin to do the things that can prolong your life and increase its quality at the same time. You don't want to regret your life the way poor George Burns did. When a beautiful girl walked into his hotel room and said, "I'm sorry, I must be in the wrong room," he told her, "No, you're not in the wrong room. You are just 40 years too late."

Delaying or Preventing Diabetes

You can do a number of things to delay or prevent your development of diabetes. Among the key things are

✔ **Lifestyle modification:** Lose weight or don't allow yourself to gain weight. Start an exercise program and exercise for 30 to 45 minutes every day. Even without losing weight, a regular program of exercise has been shown to prevent diabetes.

✔ **Monitoring:** Make sure your doctor checks for diabetes with a blood glucose test or a hemoglobin A1c every year, especially if you have pre-diabetes (see Chapter 3).

Although some drugs have been shown to delay the onset of diabetes, they are associated with side effects and aren't currently recommended.

Although the difference between prediabetes and diabetes is based on the level of your blood glucose, some of the complications of diabetes occur even when your blood glucose levels are in the prediabetic range. You want to lower your blood glucose as much as possible. Don't be content with prediabetes.

Developing Positive Thinking

Studies have shown fairly conclusively that if you start with a positive frame of mind, your body can work with you and not against you. Even when things go wrong, if you're optimistic, you can pick yourself up and move forward. If you're pessimistic, you can become depressed and believe that nothing will help you. That kind of attitude is not conducive to good control of your blood glucose and avoidance of complications.

I have a patient who came to me to improve his glucose control just after having a toe amputated. This patient has a good attitude: If he sees a lot of manure, he knows a beautiful horse is in the area. He refuses to believe that a temporary setback is a permanent defeat. I got him on a program of tight diabetic control with the newer oral medications, and his eyes have gotten better and his neuropathy (see Chapter 5) has improved. He believes in his ability to control his blood glucose, and all his actions are directed toward doing just that. The result has been an amazing turnaround in his hemoglobin A1c (see Chapter 7). With his attitude, he is willing to make the changes necessary because he knows they will pay big dividends for his health.

Achieving a positive attitude has a lot to do with how you interpret problems. If you see them as permanent and unchangeable because of a flaw in your own character, you will have trouble being positive. If you see them as temporary and the result of something you can change given enough time, you will be much more optimistic and able to solve most problems. A study in *Diabetes Care* in March 2012 showed clearly the importance of a positive attitude towards diabetes: Among newly diagnosed patients given short-term subcutaneous insulin treatment for two to three weeks after diagnosis, those with a positive attitude remained in remission (did not require medication) significantly longer than those who did not have a positive attitude.

Monitoring and Testing

Many of my patients ask me about a cure for diabetes. One doesn't exist yet, but the future looks very promising. Doctors are working on a portable machine called the *artificial pancreas* that can measure the blood glucose and respond with the right amount of insulin. However, such a gadget is not of much use for the people who take pills. And even if it will be able to help you some day, until the artificial pancreas is available, you have to use your brain to make the calculation that your pancreas would do automatically if it could. The calculation is, of course, how much medicine to take for a given glucose. To make the calculation, you need to know the glucose, which is where monitoring comes in.

Remember, however, that blood glucose tests reflect only a moment in time. What you need to know is whether you are in control 24 hours a day. That is where the hemoglobin A1c comes in. Your doctor should order this test at least every four months if you're stable and every three months if not. If you have close to normal results in this test, you probably don't have to worry about long-term complications (see Chapter 5) and will probably not be suffering from short-term complications (see Chapter 4) either.

Even with near-normal hemoglobin A1c results, you still want to be checked for any sign of complications. You need regular eye examinations, blood and urine tests for kidney damage, and tests for sensation in your feet. Your doctor should do these checks on schedule, and, if not, you have to remind the doctor.

Using Medications

Medications can be tricky. Some of them are very potent, but none of them work if you don't take them. Doctors use the word *noncompliance* when they talk about the tendency of patients not to take their medications. Following are some of the things you need to consider when you take your medications:

- Are you taking the right dose at the right time?
- Are you taking it with or without food according to directions?
- Does it mix with your other medications?
- Are you aware of side effects, and are they being monitored?
- Can the desired effect sometimes be too strong?
- Do you have access to an antidote to its effect if necessary?
- Do you need to adjust the dose when you're not feeling well?

Your doctor, your pharmacist, and your diabetes educator can all help you with your medications, but you're on your own when it comes to taking them. If you have trouble remembering, get yourself a plastic case containing seven sections with a day of the week above each section and fill them with each day's pills so you can easily see whether you took them or not. These cases are available in pharmacies.

Following a Diet

The gourmet recipes in Appendix C should clearly show you that you're not sacrificing very much by following an appropriate diabetic diet, unless you consider avoiding becoming overweight to be a sacrifice. You can enjoy delicious food that provides plenty of energy for your needs.

In years past, people often focused on reducing fat in their diets, especially cholesterol and saturated fat. That reduction is important, but the attention now being paid to carbohydrate intake is especially helpful for diabetics (see Chapter 8). And you can improve your glycemic control even more if you know something about the quality of the carbohydrate as well as the quantity. Try to choose low-glycemic-index carbohydrate, like basmati rice instead of white rice. Any carbohydrate with lots of fiber is a low-glycemic source, and you will have a lower blood glucose as a result and require less insulin to control it. Not only does that mean better diabetic control, but your fats, particularly triglyceride, will also be lower, and that decreases the severity of the metabolic syndrome (see Chapter 5) if you have type 2 diabetes.

Most people can make changes in their diet in the short term, but maintaining these changes over the long term is difficult. The best way to accomplish a long-term change is to have a plan and stick to it. The times when you are in unplanned situations are probably the most damaging to your diabetic control. For example, when you enter a restaurant, you're presented with a menu. The job of the author of that menu is to entice you by the description of the food to order that dish, just as the pictures on the food boxes in stores entice you to buy that food. If you have in mind what is good for your diabetic diet, you tend to order what helps you, not what messes up your control.

I encourage restaurants to devote a section of their menus to delicious diabetic meals so that diabetic diners can more easily avoid temptation, and some restaurants are starting to do so. However, you can't count on that option, so you must go out to eat prepared to order appropriately.

The same holds true when you eat at someone else's home. If the host knows you have diabetes, hopefully he or she will prepare something you can eat. If not, you must select with great care. Do not be afraid to say no. Your friendly dietitian can give you a lot of help on what to select and what to reject.

One thing that helps a lot in diabetes is if you have a fair amount of order in your life. If your life is disorganized, controlling your diabetes will be much more difficult. You must take your medications at about the same time each day and eat at about the same time. You must test at about the same time and exercise at about the same time. But you don't have to eat the same thing all the time. An endless variety of delicious foods is available to you.

Exercising Regularly

The more you exercise regularly, the better you can control your blood glucose. Maintaining a healthy weight helps as well. If you have type 2 diabetes, exercising regularly translates into needing less or no medication. If you have type 1 diabetes, you'll need less insulin.

Your exercise choices are unlimited (see Chapter 9). Yes, even a game of golf is exercise, though most people (who are not professional golfers) do not play the sport more than once or twice a week.

If you're having trouble getting into a regular exercise routine, follow these tips:

- **Do something daily, if possible, but no less than three or four times a week.** If you can't do it regularly on your own, get an exercise partner. You don't need a sports club to find step aerobics. Just walk up a few flights of stairs where you work. Go for a walk outside if the weather permits for at least 20 minutes.

- **Set up a program with goals so that you don't stay stuck in a low level of exercise.** If you don't know how to set good goals for yourself, check with an exercise physiologist or personal trainer. If you're older than 40 and have not exercised and are overweight, check with your doctor before beginning a strenuous program.

- **Don't limit yourself to aerobics.** A little weight lifting a few days a week can make an amazing difference in your strength, your stamina, and your physique. If your sport is tennis, you may find that you can play that third set with much greater ease after you start on a weight program. All other sports benefit from weight lifting in a similar fashion.

Exercise is definitely a way to get high without drugs. It is good for depression or any unhappy state of mind. Don't take my word for it. Get out and find out for yourself. See Chapter 9 for more on exercise.

Using Expertise Available to You

People are usually eager to help you with your diabetic condition. (See Chapter 11 to find out more about your supporting cast.) So much knowledge is out there, just waiting to be tapped. Insurance companies recognize the value of these resources, such as dietitians and diabetes educators, and are usually willing to pay for them.

Diabetes self-management education is another program that you should attend early in your diagnosis and at regular intervals of every three to five years thereafter. Who knows what great advances may have taken place since your last educational program? Sometimes even your doctor is unaware of them.

You can get lots of free information from your friendly pharmacist, the Internet, and other people with diabetes, but be careful of these last two groups. A lot of misinformation is shared on the Internet and among diabetic patients. Before you make a major alteration in your treatment on the basis of uncertain information, check with your physician. (You can find out about some of the most common bits of misinformation in Chapters 17 and 19.)

Every time you have a question about your diabetes, write it down and save it for your next office visit with your doctor, unless it's urgent. If it's urgent, or if you don't know whether or not it is, call your doctor with your question. Let him or her determine whether it needs to be addressed right away.

Having more frequent visits to your primary doctor is associated with quicker achievement of hemoglobin A1c, blood-pressure, and cholesterol targets. In a study in the *Archives of Internal Medicine* in September 2011, patients who visited the doctor every two weeks did significantly better than those who saw the doctor less often. Don't miss your appointments! Another article in the same journal in October 2011 showed that individual education was more effective than group education in improving glucose control.

Don't neglect your family and friends as a helpful source. These people love you and know that you would help them if the tables were turned. The problem is that they can't help you if they don't know what you're dealing with. Tell them the risks that you face (such as hypoglycemia) and ask them how to help you if the need arises. You will find that the result will be a much closer relationship.

Part IV

Special Considerations for Living with Diabetes

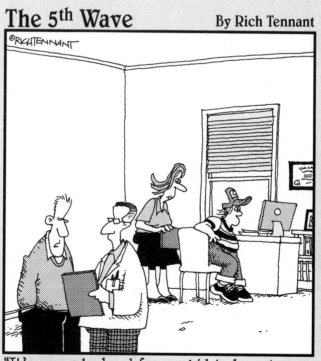

The 5th Wave   By Rich Tennant

"It's gonna be hard for my kid to have type 2 diabetes. He's used to being number 1."

In this part . . .

Two groups of people, children and the elderly, have special needs that the average adult does not have to deal with. Children are growing and developing, and the elderly are often coping with other illnesses as well as diabetes. Both groups have emotional problems that are unique. Children are learning to fit in with peers while separating from parents. The elderly are losing friends and relatives at the same time that their mental processes are declining. This part explains their special problems and how to tackle them.

The middle-aged adult has specific problems to cope with as well, relating to insurance (both life and health) and employment. Fortunately, the barriers for adults with diabetes are rapidly coming down, but you still need to know about possible pitfalls. Discrimination cannot be tolerated, and you can find out what to do about it here.

Finally, I tell you about the huge number of new developments in diabetes, putting them into perspective as to usefulness and appropriateness. I also expose false promises from drug companies and supplement makers. So many things have been proposed for diabetes care without benefit of careful evaluation. The scientific evidence for and against each is presented so that you can make up your own mind.

Chapter 13

Your Child Has Diabetes

*W*hen I wrote the first edition of this book, in 1998, almost all diabetes in children was type 1 diabetes. Since then, a vast change in this situation has taken place. The incidence of type 2 diabetes is rapidly approaching the incidence of type 1 diabetes in children, and the culprits to blame for this huge increase are obesity and lack of exercise. I have a lot more to say about this problem in the section on type 2 diabetes in children later in this chapter.

There are still plenty of new cases of type 1 diabetes in children. This chapter contains basic information about their care, but for a full discussion of type 1 diabetes, see my book *Type 1 Diabetes For Dummies* (Wiley).

Children with diabetes present special problems that adults with diabetes do not have. Not only are they growing and developing from babies to adults, but they have problems of psychological and social adjustment. Diabetes can add complications to a period of time that is not exactly smooth, even without it.

Many doctors believe that if a child has diabetes, the whole family really has the disease because everyone must adjust to it. And because diabetes is the second most common chronic disease in children after asthma, it is no small problem.

In this chapter, you find out how to manage diabetes in your child at each stage of growth and development. You need to remember that your child is first a child and then a child with diabetes. And you also need to remember that no one is to blame for your child's diabetes. Although diabetes is a serious problem, it's nothing you and your child can't handle.

Dealing with Diabetes in Your Baby or Preschooler

If your infant or preschooler is diagnosed with diabetes, you may feel overwhelmed. The information in this section can help you understand that this diagnosis isn't the end of the world — it's the beginning of many years of special care for your child.

Nurturing a diabetic infant

Although type 1 diabetes doesn't usually show up in babies, it can, and you should know what to expect when it does. Obviously, your baby is not verbal and cannot tell you what is bothering him or her. And you may miss the fact that the baby is urinating excessively in his or her diaper. The baby will lose weight and have vomiting and diarrhea, but these symptoms may be ascribed to a stomach disorder rather than diabetes. When the diagnosis is finally made, the baby may be very sick and require a stay in a pediatric intensive care unit. Do not blame yourself for not realizing that your baby was sick with diabetes.

Type 2 diabetes is almost never seen in babies. The current epidemic of type 2 diabetes in children is the result of excessive weight gain, which is rare in babies and toddlers. The treatments described below are for type 1 diabetes.

After the diagnosis of T1DM is made, the hard work begins. You must learn to give insulin injections and to test the blood glucose in a child who will be reluctant to have either one done. You have to learn when and what to feed the baby, both to encourage growth and development and to prevent low blood glucose.

At this stage, you don't need to be as worried about tight glucose control as you will be later on. There are several reasons why not. First, the baby's developing neurological system can be damaged by frequent, severe low blood glucose, so the glucose is permitted to be higher now than later on. Second, studies show that changes associated with high blood glucose leading to diabetic complications do not begin to add up until the prepubertal years, so you have a grace period during which you can allow less tight control.

According to a study in Diabetes Care in June 2011, vitamin D deficiency is associated with increased prevalence of diabetic eye disease in children and adolescents. Make sure your child has sufficient vitamin D. It's available as drops that you can add to your baby's food.

On the other hand, a small baby is very fragile. He or she has less of everything, so small losses of water, sodium, potassium, and other substances lead more rapidly to a very sick baby. If you keep the baby's blood glucose around 150 to 200 mg/dl (8.3 to 11.1 mmol/L), you are doing very well.

Taking care of a toddler with diabetes

Diagnosing diabetes in your preschooler may be just as difficult as it is in the baby. The child may still be preverbal and running around in diapers.

A preschooler is beginning the process of separating from his parents and starting to learn to control the environment (by becoming toilet-trained, for example). This separation process makes it more difficult for you, the parent, to give insulin injections and test the glucose. You must be firm in insisting that these things be done. You'll need to do them yourself because a small child neither knows how to do them nor understands what to do with the information generated by the glucose meter.

Because a toddler's eating habits may not be very regular, the use of very short-acting insulin like lispro is especially helpful (see Chapter 10). Very soon, people with diabetes should have a way of measuring the blood glucose in a painless fashion, which will be of great assistance in monitoring children.

Becoming an educated caregiver

For a time of variable duration in the child with type 1 diabetes — a so-called "honeymoon period" — your child will have seemingly regained the ability to control his or her blood glucose with little or no insulin. (See the nearby sidebar "The honeymoon period.") This period always ends, and it isn't your fault that it does. When it ends, you have to work with your child's doctor, dietitian, and diabetes educator to find out how to control diabetes with insulin.

To give your child appropriate care, you need to know how to do the following things:

- ✔ Identify the signs and symptoms of hyperglycemia, hypoglycemia, and diabetic ketoacidosis (see Chapters 4 and 5). Each child has a particular way of expressing low or high blood glucose, for example, by becoming quiet or loud. Learn the signs for your child, and let anyone else who cares for the child know them.

- ✔ Administer insulin (see Chapter 10). Thanks to rapid-acting insulin, you can wait to see how much the baby is eating before you decide on the amount of insulin.

- ✔ Measure the blood glucose and urine ketones (see Chapter 7). Very frequent blood glucose measurements are essential. The more information you have, the better the control and the less frequent the hypoglycemia. Most children need between four and seven blood glucose measurements a day to achieve excellent control.

Toddlers who are toilet-trained may have accidents when their glucose is high, because high glucose causes a large quantity of urine.

✔ Treat hypoglycemia with food or glucagon (see Chapter 4). Young children require half the adult dose of glucagon. Glucagon may cause a toddler to vomit, but it still raises the blood glucose.

✔ Feed your diabetic child (see Chapter 8).

✔ Set an example for lifelong exercise for your child by exercising with her.

✔ Know what to do when your child is sick with another childhood illness. If your child must go to the hospital, approach it as a positive experience — a chance to get a tune-up.

Your responsibilities as the parent of a diabetic baby or preschooler are extensive and time-consuming. Training your usual helpers to take over, even for a short time, is especially difficult. Unless you hire a professional to take over for a while, you may not get very much time away from your diabetic infant.

Placing your child in preschool is a difficult decision. You can do so only if you are sure that the adult supervisors are fully aware of your child's needs and willing to provide for them.

Your other children may resent the attention that you pay to this one child. If your other children start to misbehave, this may be the reason.

Helping Your Primary-School Child with Diabetes

Around age 10, some children are found to have type 2 diabetes. Important differences exist in the way type 1 and type 2 are recognized and treated. Therefore, I discuss each type separately in this section. In 1990, less than 4 percent of children diagnosed with diabetes had type 2. In 2003, the figure had risen to more than 30 percent. In 2007, almost one of every two children with diabetes had type 2 diabetes. For a discussion of why that number has grown so rapidly, see the section "Preventing and Treating Obesity and Type 2 Diabetes in Children," later in this chapter.

Coping with type 1 diabetes

In some ways, type 1 diabetes care gets a little easier with a primary-school child, but in other ways, it gets more difficult. Your child can finally tell you when he or she has symptoms of hypoglycemia, so that part is easier to recognize and treat. But you must begin to control the blood glucose more carefully because your child is reaching the stage where control really counts.

You still have a child who is growing and developing, so nutrition remains critical. You must provide enough of the right kinds of calories to fuel the growth process. A snack such as 4 ounces of apple juice and a graham cracker between breakfast and lunch, between lunch and supper, and at bedtime can help smooth out glucose control and avoid hypoglycemia.

With age, your child is going to do more to separate from you. He or she may insist on giving insulin shots and doing blood tests. Studies indicate that primary-school years are not a good time for you to give up these tasks, certainly not completely. Your child may not be physically capable of performing them and, in an attempt to hide the disease from peers, may not perform them at all during school. Diet may also suffer at school as the child tries to fit in and not stand out by eating the things that diabetes requires.

Managing hypoglycemia

Because you are beginning to tighten the level of glucose control, hypoglycemia is more of a risk, especially at night. At this stage (and from now on), you can avoid hypoglycemia by taking any or all of the following steps:

- ✔ Give a bedtime snack regularly.
- ✔ Give cornstarch at bedtime. Cornstarch is slowly broken down, so it provides glucose over a longer period of time. One to two tablespoons of uncooked cornstarch can be added to milk (shake well), yogurt, or pudding, or you can try a commercial product such as NiteBite, which can be given before bedtime.
- ✔ Measure and treat low blood glucose before bedtime.
- ✔ Occasionally check the blood glucose at 3 a.m.
- ✔ Ask your child about symptoms of nighttime low blood glucose, such as nightmares and headaches.
- ✔ Be sure your child does not skip meals.
- ✔ Have your child eat carbohydrates before exercising.

At least one member of your family must be able to administer glucagon by injection to treat hypoglycemia should you be unable to get your child to eat or drink.

Handling school issues

When your child goes to school or a daycare setting, you need to address new problems. One issue is that he interacts with other children, wants their approval, and wants to fit in. Your child may consider diabetes a stigma and be very reluctant to share it with other children. A plan of treatment that interferes with school and friendships may be very unwelcome.

Other issues may arise regarding the school's willingness to participate in your child's care. To best handle these issues, you must be aware of your rights.

Federal laws, especially the Diabetes Education Act of 1991, specify that diabetes is a disability and that it's unlawful to discriminate against children with diabetes. If a school receives federal funding or is open to the public, it has to reasonably accommodate the special needs of the diabetic child.

Any school receiving federal funds must develop a Section 504 plan to meet the needs of the disabled child. This plan refers to Section 504 of the Rehabilitation Act of 1973, and it takes every need of the child into account from the moment she is picked up in the morning by a bus driver (who must know how to help the child with a diabetic problem) until she arrives back home at the end of the day. The plan includes the child's self-care abilities, and it lists trained personnel by name and responsibility.

If you plan to send your child to a private school that receives no federal funds, before enrolling, insist on a plan of care for your child identical to a 504 plan.

The law requires that a diabetic child be able to participate fully in all school and after-school activities. Therefore, provisions must be made for blood glucose testing, for treatment with insulin, and for taking snacks or going to the bathroom as needed.

The written Section 504 treatment plan is developed by your doctor, you, and the school nurse, and relevant people in the school have assigned roles. The plan must include

- ✔ Blood glucose monitoring
- ✔ Insulin administration
- ✔ Meals and snacks
- ✔ Recognition and treatment of hypoglycemia
- ✔ Recognition and treatment of hyperglycemia
- ✔ Testing of urine ketones as indicated

As the parent, you are responsible for providing all supplies for testing and treatment. The school provider has a responsibility to understand and treat hypoglycemia, to test the blood glucose and treat it when the level is outside certain parameters, to coordinate meals and snacks, and to permit excused appointments to the doctor as well as restroom use. There is no reason that your child should not participate fully in school.

You have to provide a kit every day for school that contains everything the child needs to test the blood glucose and, if necessary, the urine for ketones. The kit must also include any necessary insulin and syringes. A list of signs and symptoms of high and low blood glucose is another useful addition to this kit. A source of food must be available to the child throughout the school day, both for snacks and prevention of hypoglycemia during exercise. The teachers need to know to remind the child to eat. The child must be free to eat when necessary and not have to request food from the teacher.

These kits and food sources also have to go with the child whenever the child leaves school — for example, for a fire drill or a field trip.

Recognizing and treating type 2 diabetes

A number of clues point to a child having type 2 diabetes rather than type 1:

- ✔ The child is overweight rather than underweight at diagnosis.

- ✔ Symptoms, such as thirst and increased urination, are mild or not present at all; if they are present, they have been going on for a long time (often months).

- ✔ The child has a strong family history of type 2 diabetes.

- ✔ The child's glucose level at diagnosis is usually lower than the glucose of a patient with type 1.

- ✔ The child belongs to an ethnic group at increased risk for type 2, such as African American, Hispanic, Asian, or Native American.

- ✔ The child has acanathosis nigricans, dark or thickened patches on the skin between the fingers and toes, on the back of the neck, and on the underarms. These patches are present in 90 percent of type 2 patients.

- ✔ An older girl may have irregular menses caused by polycystic ovarian syndrome (see Chapter 6).

Despite these clues pointing to type 2, the two types of diabetes can be confused for several reasons. Type 1 diabetic children may be overweight. Type 2 children may have ketones in their urine, just as type 1 patients do. The glucose level at diagnosis in some type 1 children is not very elevated. And the overall occurrence of type 2 is still low enough that the doctor may not think of the possibility.

Some children actually have "double diabetes." These children have type 1 diabetes but were overweight or obese at the time the diagnosis was made. In these children, lifestyle modification plays an important role in the treatment. Weight loss and exercise will help to bring the glucose under control, even though insulin is the primary treatment.

Shifting responsibility to the child

As your child grows and matures, you will constantly be concerned with the question of when to let him or her take over. Tim Wysocki, PhD, looked at 648 children to see when they were able to take over key skills. He found that 50 percent of children had mastered the following tasks at the younger age in the ranges below, whereas 75 percent had mastered the tasks at the older age. You can use these results as a general guide for your child.

✔ Pricking finger with lancet: 5–6

✔ Performing blood glucose test with a meter: 6–7

✔ Stating symptoms of high blood glucose: 7–9

✔ Giving injections to self: 8–10

✔ Drawing up mixture of two types of insulin: 10–11

✔ Stating reasons for need to change insulin dose: 8–12

✔ Testing urine for ketones: 8–14

✔ Adjusting food intake according to blood glucose: 9–14

✔ Adjusting insulin dose according to blood glucose: 13–18

An important thing to remember is that type 2 diabetes responds to treatment with insulin much more rapidly than type 1, and the child may not need insulin at all after a proper diet and exercise are established. No child with type 1 diabetes can live without insulin except possibly during the brief honeymoon period described in the earlier sidebar.

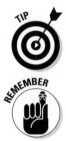

If you have an overweight child — one who is more than 120 percent of his or her ideal weight for height — you should request that your doctor screen him or her for diabetes every two years by using a fasting blood glucose test.

The treatment of type 2 diabetes, both in children and adults, starts with lifestyle change. You, the parent, must make the commitment to exercise with your child every day. You should meet with a dietitian and discuss a diet for the whole family that provides sufficient nutrition for the growing child while allowing for weight loss. If these two things are accomplished, no more steps will be necessary. That means limiting TV and computer time so the child is active rather than passive. You might consider getting a pedometer for your child and encouraging him or her to build up the number of steps taken each day, with prizes for reaching goals.

If diet and exercise do not return the blood glucose to normal, oral hypoglycemic agents (see Chapter 10) are used. Currently, metformin is the only oral drug approved by the FDA for children. If oral agents fail, insulin is given.

Managing Your Adolescent's Diabetes

Until 10 years ago, only 3 percent of cases of diabetes in adolescents was due to type 2 diabetes. Presently 45 percent of new cases of diabetes in adolescents is due to type 2 diabetes. In non-Hispanic blacks, it represents 58 percent of new cases, in Asian/Pacific Islanders 70 percent and in American Indians 86 percent.

If an adolescent or young adult has type 2 diabetes, the information in the previous section applies, because the goal remains the same no matter what the age: Normalize the child's weight and increase exercise in order to achieve normal blood glucose levels. Therefore, I focus my attention in this and the next section on type 1 diabetes roughly corresponding to the teenage years.

Your adolescent or teenager with type 1 diabetes will provide some of your biggest challenges. This is the time period when most childhood diabetes begins. The Diabetes Control and Complications Trial (see Chapter 3) showed that tight glucose control can be accomplished beginning at age 13 and that this control can prevent complications. The higher frequency of severe hypoglycemia that accompanies tighter control was not found to be damaging to the brain of a child at this age. However, children at this age do not think in terms of long-term blood glucose control and prevention of complications. So they're not willing to do many of the tasks required to control their diabetes on a regular basis.

The goal of treatment at this stage is a hemoglobin A1c between 7 and 9 percent (see Chapter 7). A value above 11 percent indicates poor control. (This isn't true for smaller children, who are allowed to have a higher hemoglobin A1c.)

This stage is when your child is most eager to become independent. You don't want to give up all control at this time for several reasons:

- ✔ Your child actually does better if he or she has limits that are clearly stated and enforced.

- ✔ The "shame" of diabetes may cause the child to skip shots and food, especially around friends.

- ✔ The problem of eating disorders (see Chapter 8) may pop up at this time, especially among girls trying to maintain a slim body image. Girls with diabetes know that if they skip their injections, they lose weight. They may ignore the high blood glucose that results.

- ✔ Teenagers with diabetes may still be unable to translate levels of blood glucose into appropriate action.

The hormonal changes that occur in puberty are often associated with insulin resistance. These physical changes may be a source of loss of control rather than any failure of your child to follow the diabetic treatment plan. Upward adjustment of the insulin may overcome this problem.

Strenuous exercise may play an even greater role in the life of your child at this age, and type 1 diabetes is no reason to prohibit exercise. The result will be a significant reduction in the amount of insulin required after exercise. The blood glucose measurements will help you to define your child's need for insulin. If your child plays a team sport, the coach and teammates must be aware of the diabetes and permit your child to eat, go to the bathroom, and take insulin as required.

Make sure that your child snacks regularly; keep snacks readily available no matter where your child may be.

Handing Over the Reins to Your Young-Adult Child with Diabetes

When your child becomes a young adult, you definitely want to give up the control that has helped her to thrive up to this point. Your child should be doing her own testing. She is ready to leave the pediatric level and begin to work with doctors who care for adults, so you will probably be out of the loop. Your child should now have the skill to choose appropriate insulin treatment based on blood glucose levels and calories of carbohydrate consumed (see Chapter 10).

Your child now has new challenges, including finding work, going to college, finding a future mate, and finding a place to live independently. At the same time, the reluctance to admit to diabetes and the desire for a thin body continue to complicate care.

Diabetes care must be intensive at this point (see Chapter 10). Multiple shots of intermediate and short-acting insulin are taken. Your child must follow a diabetic diet (see Chapter 8), and an exercise program is essential (see Chapter 9). The rest of this book really has to do with the tasks that your young adult child with diabetes faces.

Off to college

When your child leaves for college, he or she has all the responsibility for the diabetes. Your job is simply to make sure that all the equipment for testing the blood glucose and administering insulin is available to your child. You should also make the college aware of your child's medical condition. Encourage your child to find one or more people at the college, such as a roommate or sports teammate, who are prepared to help when necessary.

Two issues are particularly important to discuss before the student leaves for school: alcohol use

and sexual activity. Alcohol use may significantly increase in college, which means that your child may consume many empty calories and run the risk of severe hypoglycemia if he or she fails to eat properly. If you have a diabetic daughter, discuss with her the risk of pregnancy when diabetes is not in control. (See Chapter 6 for information.) Young adults of both sexes should know how to prevent sexually transmitted diseases.

College, like the rest of your child's life, can be experienced just as it would be if diabetes were not present. The key is planning.

Preventing and Treating Obesity and Type 2 Diabetes in Children

The epidemic of obesity, which has spread to children in the United States in the past few decades, has led to a much higher prevalence of type 2 diabetes in children than was ever seen before. As many as one-third of all children in the U.S. are overweight or obese. However, only a fraction of these children go on to develop diabetes.

A number of medical conditions can cause obesity in children, but they represent probably 1 percent of the causes. Most of them can be diagnosed during the course of a good physical examination by your child's pediatrician. By far, the major reason for obesity in children is too many calories in and too few burned up by exercise.

Even without diabetes, obesity is a burden for children. The obese child faces severe psychological and social consequences:

✔ Lower respect from peers than other disabled children get

✔ Less comfortable family interactions

✔ Poor body image

✔ Low self-esteem

Defining obesity in children

The definition of obesity in children age 2 to 19 is based on the body-mass index, BMI (see Chapter 7). A child is obese or overweight if his BMI is at the 95th percentile or greater for his age and sex. He is overweight if the BMI is between the 85th and 95th percentile. The growth charts that indicate the percentiles for BMI can be found at www.brightfutures.org/bf2/pdf/pdf/GrowthCharts.pdf.

Obesity is not just responsible for type 2 diabetes. It can also provoke a number of other dangerous medical conditions in children. These include

- Metabolic syndrome, discussed in Chapter 5, leading to an increased tendency for heart attacks and strokes
- Polycystic ovarian syndrome, also discussed in Chapter 5, leading to infertility, abnormal menstrual periods, and hairiness in girls
- Heart disease due to the increased work of the heart
- High blood pressure, which can damage the heart and the kidneys
- Sleep disorders like obstructive sleep apnea with snoring and increased blood pressure
- Fatty liver with abnormal liver enzymes in the blood
- Gallbladder disease
- Bone and joint diseases due to the weight on the bones
- Skin abnormalities like acanthosis nigricans, black velvety patches on the joints and under the arms
- Nervous-system diseases such as increased pressure in the brain with headache and visual disturbances

Preventing obesity in children

Prevention of obesity is much preferred over treating the damage that it does. You can do the following things to prevent obesity in your child:

- Try to have a normal weight before you become pregnant.
- Exercise throughout your pregnancy.
- Breastfeed for at least six months. A study in Diabetes Care in March 2011 showed that it reduces the occurrence of obesity in your child and reduces the increased obesity in your child associated with exposure to your diabetes while in the uterus.
- Eat meals together as a family.

✔ Avoid sugary drinks and fatty foods.

✔ Restrict time for sedentary activities like TV or computers. Adolescent boys with screen time of two hours or more daily have twice the risk of insulin resistance compared to boys with less than two hours.

✔ Don't allow your child to participate in fundraisers that sell candy and cookies.

✔ Insist on exercise daily and do it with your child.

Changes are coming in schools. New federal guidelines set calorie caps on meals in school, gradually reduce the amount of salt in school foods, eliminate trans fats from school food, and reduce the amount of fat in milk and other foods. Food companies are reformulating foods that they sell to schools to meet these guidelines.

Dealing with type 2 diabetes

Adding type 2 diabetes to obesity can be devastating. The consequences of the preceding problems may lead to failure to manage the diabetes because the child wants to avoid any activity that makes him or her even more different from his or her peers.

It is important to separate type 1 diabetes from type 2 because the child with type 2 diabetes has a milder condition and can be treated with pills or diet and exercise alone. However, because children do not appreciate long-term consequences of their actions, you often have the problem of compliance.

You must help your obese child to lose weight because most obese children become obese adults. With the assistance of a dietitian, you can figure out the food that your child can eat to maintain growth and development without gaining more weight. One of the most helpful techniques is to take the child into the supermarket and point out the difference between empty calories and nourishing calories. Another is never to make high-calorie food, such as cake and candy, a reward. Finally, if you keep problem foods out of the house, there is much less likelihood that your child will eat them.

When type 2 diabetes develops, treatment should begin as early as possible to minimize the development of complications. Depending on the severity of the diabetes, the treatment can utilize any or all of the following approaches:

✔ **Lifestyle changes:** Parents must set an example of good dietary and exercise habits. Some studies suggest that if parents go first, children will follow. The best diet is one that emphasizes a variety of vegetables, some fruits, and small amounts of protein with minimal processed carbohydrates like candy and pastries. The best exercise is what you will continue to do regularly.

✔ **Drugs:** The currently available drugs, with the exception of metformin, are either not recommended for children under 16 years of age or not useful for long-term treatment.

✔ **Surgery:** Children with extreme obesity with BMIs of 35 and greater may require bypass surgery or gastric banding. These options have been successful but have complications like infection, deficiency of certain nutrients like vitamins and calcium, pneumonia, and hernia. Surgery should be used especially in children with other risk factors like a strong family history of heart disease, sleep apnea, or high blood pressure. This surgery should only be performed in medical centers with ample experience with children. Be aware that insurance coverage often excludes these options for teenagers.

A recent paper from New York-Presbyterian Hospital, presented at meetings of the Endocrine Society, showed that lap-band surgery in adolescents between 14 and 17 years caused a safe and significant drop in BMI and blood levels of C-reactive protein, an indicator of inflammation often found elevated in diabetes. Blood levels of glucose and fats also fell.

The Endocrine Society has published bariatric surgery recommendations for children and adolescents. Essentially, the recommendations exclude children who have not attained final or near-final adult height. The BMI must be greater than 50 kg/m^2 or greater than 40 kg/m^2 if other diseases such as diabetes or heart disease are present. A trial of lifestyle change has been unsuccessful. The family unit should have a psychological evaluation and be stable. The surgeon should be experienced and have a team that can do long-term follow-up. The adolescent will adhere to healthy dietary and exercise habits after surgery.

Surgery in preadolescents or in people planning to become pregnant within two years is not recommended. Adolescents with eating disorders are also excluded.

Taking Special Care of Sick Children

The comments in this section apply primarily to a child with type 1 diabetes, because children with type 2 diabetes do not lose diabetic control to nearly the same extent.

Any child is susceptible to all the usual childhood illnesses, but diabetes complicates your child's care during these times. An illness can affect diabetes in opposite ways. An infection may increase the level of insulin resistance so that the usual dose of insulin is not adequate. Or it may cause nausea and vomiting so that no food or drink can stay down, and the insulin may cause hypoglycemia. For this reason, you need to measure the blood glucose in your sick child every two to four hours. If the glucose is over 250 mg/dl (13.9 mmol/l), you need to give extra short-acting insulin (see Chapter 10). If it's under 250, you give more carbohydrate-containing nutrients.

You also need to test ketones in your child's urine or blood once or twice a day (see Chapter 7) while he or she is sick, especially if the glucose is over 300 mg/dl. If the ketones become elevated, you need to discuss the situation with your doctor.

You should probably feed your child with clear liquids like tea and soda during the sick days. Don't offer your child milk, because it upsets the stomach. As long as your child can hold down clear liquids, you can continue to take care of him or her. If clear liquids cannot be held down, you must contact your doctor and bring your child to the hospital.

While the blood glucose remains over 250 mg/dl, use tea, water, and diet soda so as not to add calories of carbohydrate. When the blood glucose is less than 250 mg/dl, you can use regular soda or glucose drinks.

Checking for Thyroid Disease in Type 1 Children

Because type 1 diabetes is an autoimmune disease (see Chapter 2), it is not surprising that children with type 1 have other autoimmune diseases more commonly than unaffected children. The disease that is found most commonly in association with type 1 diabetes is autoimmune thyroiditis. This condition is discovered by obtaining a blood test that shows an abnormal increase in proteins in the blood called thyroid autoantibodies. In a study of 58 patients with type 1 diabetes (Diabetes Care, April 2003), 19 were found to have autoimmune thyroiditis.

Autoimmune thyroiditis usually results in no symptoms, but occasionally it causes low thyroid function (hypothyroidism), and even more rarely it causes high thyroid function (hyperthyroidism). Autoimmune thyroiditis is found mostly in girls between 10 and 20 years of age. This condition is easily treated, as I explain in my book *Thyroid For Dummies* (Wiley).

Autoimmune thyroiditis is so common in type 1 diabetes that patients are recommended to be screened yearly for thyroid disease with a simple blood test that checks the level of thyroid-stimulating hormone (TSH).

Appreciating the Value of Team Care

When your child is first diagnosed with diabetes, the stress can be overwhelming. The guilt that comes with this diagnosis may leave you unable to help your child much at first and certainly unable to learn all that you need to know to master the areas of importance to the health of your child.

Therefore, you must depend on the help of a diabetes care team throughout the duration of his or her childhood, and especially when the diagnosis is first made.

Another resource that can be tremendously valuable for you and your child is a diabetes summer camp. These camps are located all over the country and provide a safe, well-managed place where your child can go and be in the majority. He or she can learn a great deal about diabetes while enjoying all the pleasures of a summer camp environment. (Certainly not a minor benefit is the opportunity for you to have time off for perhaps the first time in years.)

You can find an extensive list of camps for diabetic children throughout the United States by going to the website `www.childrenwithdiabetes.com/camps/index.htm`. It's one of the many services of the website "Children with Diabetes."

In Chapter 11, I compare diabetes to a stage play. There, the person with diabetes was the author, the producer, the director, and the star. When you have a child with diabetes, he or she is the star, but you take on the roles of author, producer, and director. You obviously have a great responsibility, but it's one that I feel certain you can handle. Just don't try to do it alone. Use your medical experts as well as your family and friends to make it manageable.

Chapter 14

Diabetes and the Elderly

. . . .

In This Chapter

▶ Diagnosing and managing diabetes in the elderly

▶ Minimizing the risk of heart disease

▶ Eating and taking medications properly

▶ Focusing on unique eye problems of the elderly

▶ Anticipating urinary and sexual problems

▶ Understanding Medicare coverage

. . . .

*E*veryone wants to live a long time, but no one wants to get old. Nevertheless, getting old is better than the alternative. Woody Allen says the one advantage of dying is that you don't have to do jury duty. I think I would rather do jury duty.

The first issue I have to tackle in this chapter is defining *elderly*. Every year my definition seems to change, but I think it's fair to talk about the age of 70 as the beginning of being elderly. Using that definition, by the year 2020, more than 20 percent of the United States population will be elderly. As much as one-fifth of that elderly population will have diabetes.

Elderly people with diabetes have special problems. Because of those special problems, they're hospitalized at a rate that is 70 percent higher than the general elderly population. In this chapter, you find out about those problems and the way to handle them.

Diagnosing Diabetes in the Elderly

The incidence of diabetes in the elderly (which is almost always type 2 diabetes) is higher for many reasons, but the main culprit seems to be increasing insulin resistance with aging. A study in *Diabetes Care* in August 2008 suggests that the increased insulin resistance associated with aging is due to exactly the same causes as that found in younger people, namely physical inactivity and obesity. The pancreas seems to be able to make insulin at the usual rate. The fasting blood glucose actually rises very slowly as you get older. The glucose after meals, however, rises much quicker and leads to the diagnosis.

Because the fasting blood glucose is usually normal, the hemoglobin A1c (see Chapter 2) is used to help to make the diagnosis in the elderly population. A hemoglobin A1c that is above 6.5 percent is considered diagnostic of diabetes. Results that fall between normal and that value are in a gray zone that probably indicates prediabetes (see Chapter 2).

The Diabetes and Aging Study (*Diabetes Care,* June 2011) showed that a hemoglobin A1c of 8 percent was associated with the lowest rates of complications and death in older diabetic patients while a level of less than 6 percent was associated with higher death rates.

Elderly people with diabetes often do not complain of any symptoms. When they do, the symptoms may not be the ones usually associated with type 2 diabetes, or they may be confusing. Elderly people with diabetes may complain of loss of appetite or weakness, and they may lose weight rather than become obese. They may have incontinence of urine, which is usually thought of as a prostate problem in elderly men or a urinary-tract infection in older women. Elderly people with diabetes may not complain of thirst because their ability to feel thirst is altered.

Evaluating Intellectual Functioning

You need to evaluate the intellectual function of an elderly person with diabetes because managing the disease requires a fairly high level of mental functioning. The patient has to follow a diabetic diet, administer medications properly, and test the blood glucose. Studies have shown that elderly people with diabetes have a higher incidence of *dementia* (loss of mental functioning) and Alzheimer's disease than nondiabetics, making it much harder for them to perform these tasks.

A study in *Diabetes Care* in October 2010 indicated that some loss of intellectual function in the elderly was due to large changes in blood glucose during each day. Treatment that moderates these changes may be helpful. Another study in *Diabetes Care,* in November 2008, showed that microalbuminuria (see Chapter 7) was predictive of loss of intellectual function and drugs that reversed microalbuminuria (ACE inhibitors or angiotensin receptor blockers) were protective.

The patient can take *cognitive screening tests* to determine his or her level of function. Testing helps determine whether the patient can be self-sufficient or will need help. Many older people who are living alone with no assistance really require an assisted-living situation or even a nursing home.

Considering Heart Disease

The major cause of death in elderly people with diabetes is a heart attack. Strokes and loss of blood flow in the feet are also much more common in diabetics than nondiabetics. Usually, elderly diabetics not only suffer from diabetes but also have high blood pressure and high cholesterol, are overweight or obese, and do little exercise.

After the diagnosis of diabetes is made, it is too late for prevention, but a major effort should be made to control the glucose, the blood pressure, and the cholesterol in order to postpone the onset of vascular disease.

Aspirin has been shown to protect against blood clots in the heart and in the vessels that provide blood to the legs and brain. If another drug isn't being used to prevent clotting — like clopidogrel (Plavix), warfarin, or heparin — aspirin should be used in all elderly people with diabetes. Low-dose aspirin, 75 to 162 mg a day, is as effective as higher doses. Check with your doctor before you start it!

If you have been smoking for decades, although you can't do much about cancer or emphysema, you can prevent sudden death associated with cigarette smoking. That complication of smoking disappears in a few days of no cigarettes.

Diabetics are at the same high risk of having a first heart attack as nondiabetics are of having a second heart attack. Blood-pressure drugs called *beta blockers* have been shown to reduce second heart attacks in nondiabetics. Along with aspirin, beta blockers should be considered as standard treatment for diabetics before a heart attack ever occurs. Talk to your doctor about getting on these drugs.

Preparing a Proper Diet

Diet and exercise are the foundations of good diabetic care for the elderly just as they are in the younger population. The information I provide in Chapter 8 (on diet) and in Chapter 9 (on exercise) should be used to create a wellness plan to manage diabetes as well as to help the elderly patient feel good and ward off any other health issues.

Diminishing intellectual function can have a negative effect on the diet of elderly people with diabetes, because they may not understand or be able to prepare a proper diabetic diet. The elderly have other problems when it comes to proper nutrition:

✔ They may have poor vision and be unable to see to read or cook.

✔ They may have low income and be unable to purchase the foods that they require.

✔ Their taste and smell may be decreased, so they lose interest in food.

✔ They often have a loss of appetite.

✔ They may have arthritis or a tremor that prevents cooking.

✔ They may have unhealthy teeth or a dry mouth.

Any one of these problems may be enough to prevent proper eating by the elderly person, with the result that the diabetes is poorly controlled.

Anyone over the age of 65 who has Medicare Part B insurance coverage is covered for the services of a dietitian for *medical nutrition therapy*. Be sure to take advantage of this benefit. The dietitian can analyze the elderly person's current intake and make recommendations to insure a balanced diet that will help with control of the blood glucose.

Avoiding Hypoglycemia

The elderly, who are already somewhat frail, are especially hard-hit by the consequences of hypoglycemia and are especially prone to it because of several factors:

✔ Their food intake may be uncertain.

✔ They may be taking multiple medications.

✔ They may sometimes skip medications.

✔ They often live alone.

✔ Their mental state may not permit them to recognize when they are becoming hypoglycemic.

✔ Their kidney function is often impaired, causing many diabetic medications to last longer than in a younger person.

The hemoglobin A1c goal for healthy elderly adults is 7 percent. However, if the life expectancy is less than five years, the elderly person is frail, or the risks of intensive therapy outweigh the benefits, the goal is 8 percent. This decreased level of control will help to avoid hypoglycemia.

Using Medications

Medications that may lower blood glucose to abnormally low levels, such as the sulfonylureas and insulin, are not the drugs of first choice in the elderly. As I explain in the previous section, hypoglycemia hits elderly patients particularly hard and should be avoided if at all possible. With that goal in mind, I explain the proper order of drug usage for elderly diabetics in this section. Each of these medications is discussed in detail in Chapter 10.

Elderly people are often on several medications, and the monthly expense for drugs may be great enough to cause them to skip doses or not buy the drug. As I explain many times in this book, compliance with your treatment routine is essential to good health. If you are not taking your diabetes medication(s) as prescribed, you must let your doctor know.

✔ Metformin is probably the first drug to try because it does not increase insulin secretion (which can lead to hypoglycemia) and because it is inexpensive. Kidney function, which is decreased in the elderly, must be checked when using this drug. The doctor should measure the level of creatinine in the blood. If it is greater than 1.4 mg/dl in women or 1.5 mg/dl in men, it should not be used. The drug should be started at a low dose of 500 mg and gradually raised over several weeks to avoid stomach and intestinal problems.

✔ Sulfonylureas are added when a second drug is needed. However, sulfonylureas can cause hypoglycemia — especially the older drug chlorpropamide. The newer drugs in this category, such as glyburide and glipizide, are preferred; glipizide may not cause hypoglycemia as often. Your doctor should start you on half the usual dose and raise it slowly over a number of weeks.

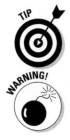

The sulfonylurea-like drugs called the *meglitinides* (repaglinide and nateglinide) may have an advantage in the elderly because they do not last as long. Nateglinide is also available in a generic form.

Drugs like acarbose (Precose), in the class called alpha-glucosidase inhibitors (see Chapter 10), have a very limited effect on the blood glucose and a lot of intestinal side effects. I do not recommend their use in the elderly.

If pills fail to provide reasonable control of the blood glucose so that the hemoglobin A1c is lower than 9, the patient must use insulin. A shot of glargine at bedtime, combined with taking a pill during the day, often accomplishes the desired level of control. Two drugs that are beginning to have a greater role in diabetes in the elderly are the GLP-1 agonists and the DPP-4 inhibitors (see Chapter 10). Two daily injections of exenatide (Byetta) or the new once-a-week preparation may be very helpful in achieving some weight loss and lowering of the blood glucose. Sitagliptin (Januvia) or the other DPP-4 inhibitors may provide all the extra glucose control needed by the patient.

Dealing with Eye Problems

Elderly people with diabetes are at risk for the eye problems brought on by the disease, and these problems can affect all aspects of proper diabetes care. Older patients often get cataracts, macular degeneration, and open-angle glaucoma in addition to diabetic retinopathy.

Fortunately, the risk of developing eye diseases associated with diabetes has been found to decrease as people age, at every level of hemoglobin A1c. For example, a 70-year-old with a hemoglobin A1c of 11 is at much lower risk than a 60-year-old with the same hemoglobin A1c.

An annual eye examination is recommended. One of the biggest failures in diabetes care is that as many as one-third of the elderly never have an eye examination at all. If no examination is done, how can disease be found when it is early enough to treat? When problems are detected, they can be treated, and the patient's vision can be saved.

Coping with Urinary and Sexual Problems

Urinary and sexual problems are common in elderly people with diabetes and greatly affect quality of life. An older person with diabetes may experience paralysis of the bladder muscle so that urine is retained; when the bladder fills, overflow incontinence is the result. Also, an older person may be unable to get to the bathroom fast enough. Or, spasms in the bladder muscle may lead to incontinence. The result may be frequent urinary-tract infections. A urologist may be able to help.

Almost 60 percent of all men over the age of 70 are impotent, and 50 percent have no *libido* (the desire to have sex). The percentages are even higher for diabetic men. These problems can have many causes (see Chapter 6), but older men are especially likely to have blockage of blood vessels with poor flow into the penis. The elderly take an average of seven medications daily, many of which affect sexual function.

To have sex at any age, you need sexual desire and the physical ability to perform, you need a willing partner, and you need a safe, private place. Any or all of these factors may be missing for the elderly.

Treating sexual dysfunction may not be necessary if the male and his partner are okay with the situation. If they aren't, Chapter 6 points out a number of treatments for potency problems.

Monitoring Foot Problems

The risk of foot problems is much higher in elderly patients because they have diminished circulation. It is essential that you examine your feet with your eyes to check for foot problems, or if your parent or loved one has diminished intellectual function, that you examine his feet daily. Make sure the doctor checks his feet at every visit. Almost half of elderly patients can't see or reach their feet, so it must be done by someone else.

Most foot problems are reversible if found early. Regular foot doctor visits may be as routine as visits to the dentist. See Chapter 5 for more information on prevention and treatment of foot problems.

Considering Treatment Approaches

When deciding on treatment for an elderly patient with diabetes, you first have to consider the individual. Does this person have a low life expectancy? Or is this person physiologically young, with the possibility of living for 15 or 20 more years? If the patient is only 65 years old and in relatively good health, he or she has a life expectancy of at least 18 more years — plenty of time to develop complications of diabetes, especially macrovascular disease, eye disease, kidney disease, and nervous system disease. That person may require more intensive diabetes care than someone who is older and has worse overall health.

The level of care provided to an elderly patient may be basic or intensive:

- **Basic care** is meant to prevent the acute problems of diabetes like excessive urination and thirst. You can accomplish this goal by keeping the blood glucose under 200 mg/dl (11.1 mmol/L). Basic care is used for an elderly person with diabetes who is not expected to live very long, either because of the diabetes or other illnesses.

- **Intensive care** is meant to prevent diabetic complications in an elderly person expected to live long enough to have them. The goal here is to keep the blood glucose under 140 mg/dl (7.7 mmol/L) and the hemoglobin A1c as close to normal as possible while avoiding frequent hypoglycemia.

The benefits in terms of preventing complications of diabetes are much greater when the hemoglobin A1c is lowered from 11 to 9 than when it is lowered from 9 to 7. The goal of treatment for many elderly people can be set higher in order to avoid hypoglycemia.

Treatment always starts with diet and exercise. Education about both can be of great value, especially if the patient's spouse is also involved. I discuss diet in the section "Preparing a Proper Diet," earlier in this chapter, and in Chapter 8.

Exercise may be limited in the elderly person with diabetes. Recent studies have shown that exercise is helpful even in the very old because it reduces the blood glucose and the hemoglobin A1c. However, because elderly patients have more coronary artery disease, arthritis, eye disease, neuropathy, and peripheral vascular disease, exercise just may not be possible. (See Chapter 9 for more on exercise.)

If an elderly patient can't walk at all, he or she may still be able to do resistance exercises sitting in a chair. These exercises increase strength and lower the blood glucose.

When diet and exercise are inadequate to control an elderly patient's diabetes, medications must be added. I discuss medications in the section "Using Medications," earlier in this chapter, and in Chapter 10.

Understanding the Medicare Law

In 1998, the federal government began to offer benefits for the 4.2 million people with diabetes who are eligible for Medicare (over age 65). Under the policy, all people with diabetes enrolled in Medicare Part B or Medicare Managed Care are eligible to receive coverage of glucose monitors, test strips, and lancets. It does not matter which method they use to control their disease.

If you're enrolled in Medicare, you can get these benefits by having your physician prescribe the supplies and document how often you use them.

The Health Care Financing Administration, which administers Medicare, has also passed regulations that permit people with diabetes to get reimbursed for education programs. In addition, if you have Medicare insurance and have type 1 diabetes, you are eligible for Medicare to pay for your insulin pump.

To find out more about Medicare, call the Medicare Hotline at 800-633-4227. The government provides a hotline for the hearing-impaired at 877-486-2048. For a complete rundown of Medicare coverage of diabetes supplies and services on the Internet, go to www.medicare.gov/publications/pubs/pdf/11022.pdf.

Chapter 15

Occupational and Insurance Problems

*A*fter we got his diabetes under control, one of my patients wrote to his mother, "Dear Mom, I'm not working, but my pancreas is." Most people need to work, and some people even want to work. People need to work for the same reason that a certain man did not turn in his brother-in-law who thought he was a chicken: We need the eggs (though not too many).

As a person with diabetes, when you try to get a job, you may run into various forms of discrimination. Part of the problem is the fear that the company will have to pay higher insurance premiums if it hires a person with a chronic illness. Part of the problem is a lack of understanding of the great strides that have been made in diabetes care so that a person with diabetes often has a better record of coming to work than a nondiabetic.

In this chapter, you find out what you need to know when you apply for work, health insurance, and life insurance. You discover how to work the healthcare system so that you derive the greatest benefits possible at the lowest cost.

Traveling with Diabetes

Whether you travel for your job or for pleasure, if you need insulin injections and must carry syringes and needles, you have to follow the rules of the Transportation Security Administration (TSA) if you fly within the United

States. Airlines outside the U.S. may have different rules; check with your airline before you travel overseas.

The TSA instructs that you should "make sure injectable medications are properly labeled (professionally printed label identifying the medication or a manufacturer's name or pharmaceutical label). Notify the screener if you are carrying a hazardous waste container, refuse container, or a sharps disposable container in your carry-on baggage used to transport used syringes, lancets, etc." Updated information is available at the TSA website, www.tsa.gov/311. You can also call the TSA call center at 866-289-9673.

The TSA permits prescription liquid medications and other liquids needed by persons with disabilities and medical conditions. These items include

- ✔ All prescription and over-the-counter medications (liquids, gels, and aerosols) including K-Y jelly, eye drops, and saline solution for medical purposes

- ✔ Liquids including water, juice, or liquid nutrition or gels for passengers with a disability or medical condition

- ✔ Life-support and life-sustaining liquids such as bone marrow, blood products, and transplant organs

- ✔ Items used to augment the body for medical or cosmetic reasons, such as mastectomy products, prosthetic breasts, bras or shells containing gels, saline solution, or other liquids

- ✔ Gels or frozen liquids needed to cool disability or medically related items used by persons with disabilities or medical conditions

If the liquid medications are in volumes larger than 3 ounces each, they may not be placed in the quart-size bag used for personal liquids of less than 3 ounces. They must be declared to the Transportation Security Officer.

Specifically with respect to medications for diabetes, notify the Security Officer that you have diabetes and are carrying your supplies with you. (Medication and supplies you are going to use should be in your carry-on luggage.) The following diabetes-related supplies and equipment are allowed through the checkpoint after they have been screened:

- ✔ Insulin and insulin-loaded dispensing products (vials or box of individual vials, jet injectors, biojectors, epipens, infusers, and preloaded syringes)

- ✔ Unlimited number of unused syringes when accompanied by insulin or other injectable medication

- ✔ Lancets, blood glucose meters, blood glucose meter test strips, alcohol swabs, meter-testing solutions

- ✔ Insulin pump and insulin-pump supplies (cleaning agents, batteries, plastic tubing, infusion kit, catheter, and needle; insulin pumps and supplies must be accompanied by insulin)

- ✔ Glucagon emergency kit

- ✔ Urine ketone test strips

- ✔ Unlimited number of used syringes when transported in sharps disposal container or other similar hard-surface container

- ✔ Sharps disposal containers or similar hard-surface disposal container for storing used syringes and test strips

Here are some suggestions for managing your diabetes if you're changing time zones:

- ✔ Obtain a list of doctors in the countries you will visit who speak your language. To find English-speaking doctors, you can contact the U.S. embassy in each country or go to the website of the International Association for Medical Assistance to Travelers, `http://iamat.org/doctors_clinics.cfm`.

- ✔ If using an insulin pump, change the basal hourly rate to the same dose every hour so that whether it's 8 a.m. or 8 p.m., the same dose is given. When you arrive in the new time zone, you can adjust the basal rate back to your usual doses.

- ✔ If you use long-acting insulin, change a single dose to two half doses 12 hours apart.

- ✔ Stick to your regular schedule using local time for any oral medications.

Wherever you go, make sure you wear a bracelet or necklace that identifies you as a person with diabetes.

Knowing Where You Can't Work

You may have grown up watching Eliot Ness on television and had your heart set on being a member of the Federal Bureau of Investigation. If you require insulin, forget it. The FBI has a policy called a *blanket ban* on hiring certain groups of people, including people with diabetes who take insulin. A blanket ban does not take into account the condition of the individual, the past employment history, the way the person manages his or her diabetes, or the responsibilities of the position. It simply says, in effect, "You've got the disease, so you can't work here." This policy is a throwback to the days before 1980, when a person with diabetes could never be sure what his blood glucose was doing.

Another important institution that has a blanket ban in place is the United States military. If you have any kind of diabetes, you are not eligible to serve. If you develop diabetes after you've been in the military, you will probably be discharged. This policy doesn't make a lot of sense because many countries have people with diabetes in their military forces and have no difficulty with them, but so it goes.

Fortunately, blanket bans in the United States are falling faster than Alex Rodriguez home runs. For example, the Department of the Treasury lifted a blanket ban on becoming a member of the Bureau of Alcohol, Tobacco, and Firearms if you have insulin-requiring diabetes. Recently, several states lifted a ban on hiring people with diabetes to be school-bus drivers. This action resulted from lawsuits against several school districts that fired drivers with spotless driving records just because they had diabetes. (This reversal doesn't mean that no safeguards against risky drivers exist. Drivers are being evaluated on a case-by-case basis before they are accepted to drive children, which is fair.)

Previously, commercial drivers with diabetes could drive within a state but could not cross state lines. Now the Department of Transportation (DOT) looks at people with diabetes on a case-by-case basis to determine if they're fully able to drive commercially from state to state. As long as the person has no history of hypoglycemia with unconsciousness, the DOT grants an exemption that permits the individual to drive between states, with reconsideration taking place every two years.

At one time, people with diabetes who took insulin were banned from becoming firefighters. Now they are permitted to serve in this work, too, on a case-by-case basis. However, the rule says they must have a hemoglobin A1c of less than 8 percent. I believe this policy needs to be changed because people function perfectly well at higher levels of hemoglobin A1c, even at 10 or 11 percent.

Another blanket ban that is falling is the ban on piloting airplanes. For 37 years, a person who took insulin could not fly a plane. In 1996, the Federal Aviation Administration (FAA) reconsidered its ban based on the great advances in controlling diabetes. The FAA decided to permit people to fly privately but not for commercial airlines. Even if they have a private license, however, they can't use it outside the airspace of the United States. Applications for a pilot's license are evaluated on a case-by-case basis.

Is there ever a justification for a blanket ban? The answer is no, and it has been proved in a number of studies. In one study of accidents of all kinds, people with diabetes actually had fewer accidents, including automobile accidents, than groups of people without diabetes. In another study of people over age 65 with diabetes, the rate of automobile accidents was no greater than that of the nondiabetic groups.

Flying a plane: It's not easy, but it's worth it

Getting a pilot's license is not easy but is well worth the effort for the person who loves to fly. To be successful, you must have no other disqualifying conditions, such as arteriosclerotic disease of the heart or brain, diabetic eye disease, or severe kidney disease (see Chapter 5). You must have had no more than one hypoglycemic reaction with loss of consciousness in the last five years and have had at least a year of stability after that. You must be evaluated by a specialist every three months after you get the license and measure your blood glucose multiple times a day. You must carry a glucose meter and meter supplies in flight, along with supplies for rapid treatment of hypoglycemia. Your blood glucose must be between 100 and 300 mg/dl (5.5 to 16.6 mmol/L) a half hour before takeoff, every hour of the flight, and a half hour before landing. However, you're not expected to measure your blood glucose in flight if doing so interferes with properly flying the plane. Phew! If Lindbergh were diabetic, he never would have made it to Paris.

Becoming Familiar with Workplace Law

A number of laws protect you in the workplace if you work in the United States, but the most important is probably the Americans with Disabilities Act (ADA) of 1990. This act states,

> *The determination that an individual poses a "direct threat" shall be based on an individualized assessment of the individual's present ability to safely perform the essential functions of the job.*

In 1998, the U.S. Court of Appeals ruled that the ADA protects Americans with diabetes. The act applies to employers with 15 or more employees. What the ADA means is that you are qualified for a particular job if you can perform the essential functions of the job as determined by the employer, with or without reasonable accommodation. Therefore, you can't be discriminated against in hiring, firing, promotion, training, pay, or any other aspect of employment because you have diabetes. Your boss cannot ask whether you have diabetes but can expect you to pass a physical examination to verify that you are well enough to do the job.

The Federal Rehabilitation Act of 1973 is an important law that protects you when you apply for a federal job or a job in a company that receives federal assistance. A person with diabetes is specifically protected under this law. The most important provision states,

No otherwise qualified handicapped individual in the United States shall, solely by reason of his handicap, be excluded from the participation in, be denied the benefits of, or be subjected to discrimination under any program or activity conducted by the Executive agency. . . .

To exclude you, federal agencies have to prove that you will not be able to perform safely if given the job. That proof is hard to come by and puts the burden on them, not you. They must decide on a case-by-case basis. As I note earlier in the chapter, the FBI and the military are exempt from this law.

Curiously, a problem arose in the Americans with Disabilities Act when diabetes began to respond so well to treatment. Only a person with a disability could sue under this act. In a perfect example of a Catch-22 (where you can't avoid a problem because of contradictory rules), people with diabetes were no longer considered disabled, so even though they were discriminated against, they couldn't sue. In 2008, President George Bush signed the Americans with Disabilities Act Amendments Act, bringing diabetics again under the act.

What can you do if you run into discrimination on the job due to your diabetes? You can contact the U.S. Equal Employment Opportunity Commission (EEOC). You can find your nearest EEOC office on the web at www.eeoc.gov/field/index.cfm or call 800-669-4000. You may have only 180 days from the alleged discriminatory act to file the charge.

Navigating the Health-Insurance System

You can get insurance for your medical care several ways. This section describes the most common forms.

Private insurance

If you or your child has diabetes, you can count on several things being true when you interact with the medical insurance system in the United States: You may be denied coverage more often, and you will pay more out-of-pocket than families without diabetes, even when you have coverage.

If you are an older adult with diabetes, your bill will be one and a half times as much for medical care as a person without diabetes, although Medicare pays for much of it. You want to be sure that you are not medically short-changed in an effort to save money.

The good news is that you can get health insurance, although you may be turned down more often. The type of insurance you can get is the same as the nondiabetic population: Blue Cross/Blue Shield, health maintenance organizations (HMOs), CHAMPUS, and so on.

Currently, there are two major forms of payment for medical care — fee-for-service and capitated payment — with a lot of hybrids in between. The old *fee-for-service* method pays the medical provider — whether a physician, a lab, or a hospital — based on the number of services provided. More services and procedures mean more profit for the provider. So the incentive is to do more in order to make more money. (Not that providers would ever do more than is necessary for the money.)

The other main method of reimbursement is *capitation*. Here the provider gets a fixed amount of money for each patient. The risk is divided among many patients so that if one costs more, ideally another will cost less. This system is the basis of the health maintenance organization (HMO), which hires physicians to provide the care. HMOs look to enroll people who cost as little as possible for their medical care. The incentive is to do less in order to save money, which is then kept by the provider. (Not that providers would ever do less than is necessary for the money.)

Because they seem to end up costing less money overall, capitation plans are growing while fee-for-service plans are declining. The government is even encouraging HMOs to enroll Medicare recipients in order to reduce costs. At the same time, the government requires HMOs to enroll people who cost more, like most people with diabetes.

As a healthcare consumer, you want to look for a large group containing many patients because such a group can spread out your extra expenses among many people who don't consume as much medical care. Before you sign up, ask several questions:

- ✔ What is your total annual cost, and how often is a payment required?

- ✔ Will you have a *deductible,* meaning that you have to pay the first so-many dollars before the insurance starts paying?

- ✔ Will you have a *copayment,* meaning that every time you use a provider, you have to pay some dollars?

- ✔ Does your plan pay for durable medical equipment, like an insulin pump (see Chapter 10), which can be very expensive? (You want to ask this even if, when you sign up, you may not foresee a need for it.)

- ✔ Will your plan pay for your diabetes medication and diabetes supplies, and to what extent?

- ✔ Can your physician order any medications you need, or is he or she restricted to certain medications?

- ✔ How often will you need to travel to the pharmacy to pick up medications? (Some plans make you go back every 30 days.)

- ✔ Are you covered for specialists, particularly eye doctors and foot doctors?

> ✔ Are you limited to certain hospitals, certain physicians, and certain laboratories? (If so, this restriction may be much more inconvenient for you, not to mention possibly requiring you to change from a physician with whom you are very comfortable.)
>
> ✔ Is home healthcare included in the plan, and to what extent?

Each state has its own laws concerning the way medical insurance is offered in that state. Some states allow *medical underwriting,* through which a company can refuse to insure a person with a particular medical condition. Other states forbid this practice. To learn the rules and regulations in your state, go to the site of the Georgetown University Health Policy Institute at www.healthinsuranceinfo. net. You can also get a copy of its publication "A Consumer Guide for Getting and Keeping Health Insurance." Unfortunately, the site no longer provides up-to-date information, but it still offers links to insurance policies in many states.

After you sign up for a plan, you need to be vigilant to be sure you are getting what you paid for. You and your physician may need to make many phone calls to get what you need, but if you persist you can often come away with a "Yes." Even goods and services that are excluded in your original contract may be provided by the insurance company if you're persistent.

Big changes on the horizon

The Patient Protection and Affordable Care Act signed by President Obama in March 2010 will have profound effects on the ability of the person with diabetes to get affordable medical care. Beginning in 2010, insurers could no longer deny insurance coverage to children because of preexisting conditions. In 2014, adults will have the same right through the new American Health Benefit Exchanges. Also beginning in 2010, insurers could no longer drop people who are diagnosed with a new condition such as diabetes or its complications.

Here are some other important provisions of the new law:

✔ Creating the Cures Acceleration Network to finance research into cures for diseases

✔ Creating a new National Diabetes Prevention Program to fund grants for community efforts to help people with diabetes

✔ Allowing young adults to remain on their parents' plan until age 26

✔ Requiring restaurant chains with 20 or more locations to post calorie counts for every item they sell

✔ Allowing employers to use workplace wellness programs to reward employees

✔ Permitting no annual limit on benefits after January 1, 2014

✔ Allowing no coverage waiting periods greater than 90 days after January 1, 2014

✔ Reducing and eventually eliminating the amount that Medicare patients have to pay for their medications (the doughnut hole) by 2020

✔ Providing more payment for preventive medical care

Insurance for low-income patients

In the United States, you may be eligible for health insurance for low-income patients, called Medicaid, if your income falls below certain levels that are listed at this website: `www.medicaid.gov/Medicaid-CHIP-Program-Information/By-Topics/Eligibility/Eligibility.html`.

Each state sets its own guidelines and administers the program for itself. You obtain a card that shows you are eligible and take it to your doctor, lab, or hospital. Many doctors do not currently accept Medicaid patients because of the low level of reimbursement. Another provision of the Act signed by President Obama is reimbursement of primary care doctors at the same level as Medicare reimburses them beginning in 2013.

High-risk pools

About 45 percent of the U.S. population gets its health insurance through their employer in a group health program. Another 27 percent gets its insurance through government programs like Medicare, Medicaid, military healthcare, and Native American care. People who don't get insurance through one of those sources can get insurance at a high premium, usually, but some people have had a chronic medical condition and can't find insurance at any price.

For those people, about 34 states have formed pools of clients who can't get insurance anywhere else. The premium is usually higher than private insurance, but at least the members can get insurance. President Obama's Health Act helps these people as well by lowering the premium for these pools. By 2014, the insurance exchanges will take over from the high-risk pools.

To find out if you qualify and where the locations of the state high-risk pools are on the Internet, go to the Health Insurance Research Center at `www.healthinsurance.org/riskpoolinfo.lasso`.

Changing or Losing a Job

One of the major reasons why people with diabetes used to stay in jobs they didn't care for was their fear of losing their health insurance. These days, this worry doesn't have to stop you, because several laws protect you from the loss of health insurance if you change or lose your job.

The Consolidated Omnibus Budget Reconciliation Act (COBRA) stipulates that your employer must keep you on your current health insurance for as long as 18 months after your job ends and longer if you are disabled. If your child is at the age when he or she is no longer covered under your policy, the child's coverage can continue for up to three years. You, rather than your employer, have to pay the premiums for this continued insurance.

If you are leaving work because of retirement at age 65, sign up for Medicare without fail. It is a generous program (which you supported while you were working) that recognizes the specific needs of people with diabetes. Since 1998, Medicare has expanded its coverage to include blood glucose monitors and test strips after your physician certifies the need. It also offers payment for specific types of outpatient diabetes education programs, as long as they are considered necessary by your physician. And recently it has begun to pay for nutrition counseling and eye examinations. Most plans pay for an insulin pump, insulin, and syringes. To find out more about Medicare, call the Medicare Hotline at 800-633-4227. The government provides a hotline for the hearing-impaired at877-486-2048.

Some employers have conversion policies that allow you to stay with your insurance company if you leave work, but with individual rather than group coverage. These policies can be pretty expensive.

Some states offer "Pooled Risk" health insurance for people who have lived in the state a certain number of months but can't get group or individual coverage. Check with your state insurance office.

Considering Long-Term Care Insurance

People with diabetes are living longer and longer, and you're going to need a way to pay for your care when you can no longer pay health-insurance premiums. When you're 90, your 88-year-old wife will most likely not be in a position to pay for your insurance, nor will your 65-year-old daughter. Medicare doesn't cover most of your long-term care expenses. Medicaid does cover some long-term care, but not everything you may need. This is where long-term insurance may help, if you can afford it. Obama's Healthcare Act steps in here by allowing payment of monthly premiums through payroll deduction to buy long-term care as of January 2011.

If you have plenty of money and want to protect it from the financial hit of a long-term illness, long-term insurance is for you. If you have little money, then the years of premiums are going to wipe out your savings, and you may end up needing to drop the policy before you even use it.

One big problem is that many companies that sell long-term insurance don't cover people with diabetes. If you can get this type of insurance coverage while you're still working, you may be able to get into a large group where your particular illness is not considered and the premiums may be relatively low. However, you'll obviously be paying those premiums for a longer time than if you start coverage when you are older.

Before you buy, you should check several important features of a long-term care insurance policy:

✔ What are the *benefit triggers,* the physical limitations that trigger coverage? To make this determination, generally insurance companies look at activities of daily living, such as the ability to bathe yourself, dress yourself, eat without help, go to the bathroom, and get out of bed. When you can't perform one or more of these tasks, benefits begin.

✔ How much of the cost of care does the insurance pay, some or all?

✔ What levels of care does the policy provide? Your policy may offer coverage only for adult day-care services or may cover anything up to and including living in a nursing facility.

✔ Is a waiver of premiums built in so that you don't have to pay premiums when you are disabled?

✔ Is the policy guaranteed renewable so you can renew no matter whether you use it, although the premiums will be higher?

Whatever you do, if you buy long-term care insurance, make sure you take good care of yourself so you live long enough to get some benefit from it.

Shopping for Life Insurance

As you may expect, the situation with life insurance and people with diabetes is in a state of flux. Insurance companies like to calculate your chance of dying and charge you (or turn you down) based on those calculations. Many companies are using calculations based on the life span of people with diabetes in 1980 or before. Using those statistics, diabetics clearly died earlier than their nondiabetic friends. Thus, the cost of life insurance is greater for people with diabetes than nondiabetics.

As new studies are done, they should indicate that the life spans of people with diabetes and nondiabetics are approaching equality. In some cases, people with diabetes, who take better care of themselves than people without a chronic illness, are living even longer. So the situation is improving, and insurance companies will catch up sooner or later. Can you imagine the surprise if insurance companies were ever to charge people with diabetes less than others because of their good habits?

Insurance companies look at levels of blood glucose and the hemoglobin A1c. Try to get yourself in excellent control before you apply. You may be able to save a bundle or get your insurance much more easily.

With the Internet, you can quickly find and compare the cost of insurance at numerous companies based on your age; your habits (warning: If you smoke, you pay through the nose); and the presence of conditions such as diabetes, high blood pressure, and high cholesterol. Many companies take a standard rate for a healthy person with no diseases and add 50 percent more if you have diabetes. Of course, your actual cost depends on your specific circumstances, including your age when you first buy the insurance.

Chapter 16

What's New in Diabetes Care

In This Chapter

▶ Choosing the right medications

▶ Exploring studies that may someday lead to changes in treatment

▶ Investigating the link between heart disease and diabetes

*I*n previous editions of *Diabetes For Dummies,* I have enthusiastically spoken about the great efforts of pharmaceutical companies to provide you with the best drugs to lower your glucose, reduce your blood pressure, and lower your cholesterol. In this edition I have the sad responsibility to warn you about these same pharmaceutical companies.

As a consequence of my skepticism, I am not going to talk about new drugs in this chapter but rather about how to make informed choices about medications and new products that may make managing your disease easier. In addition, you find out about major efforts to get cells that don't usually make insulin to turn into the insulin-producing beta cells. I also tell you about some possible links between diabetes and other medical conditions.

Protecting Yourself from the Dangers of New Drugs

In an effort to instantly gratify their stockholders and find the next "billion dollar drug," drug companies seem to have lost sight of their major goal, which is to find drugs that are both effective and safe for the treatment of diabetes. Although some drug companies continue to pursue this goal, many of them are guilty of the following misconduct:

✔ Withholding studies that they have paid for that show that their drugs are not as effective as they claim. A study in the *New England Journal of Medicine* in January 2008 showed that the companies that make antidepressants allowed 94 percent of positive studies to be printed but only 14 percent of negative studies. Even the positive studies, if carefully evaluated, were not nearly as positive as the companies claimed. This behavior is not limited to companies that make antidepressants.

✔ Strongly advertising the one study that shows positive effects when many others show negative effects.

✔ Withholding studies that indicate their drugs may have dangerous side effects.

✔ Promoting their drugs for purposes that are not permitted by the FDA.

✔ Advertising their drugs as though they are the best or only treatment when older and better treatments exist.

✔ Providing catered lunches and samples to doctors to convince them to use their drugs. A basic conflict of interest exists in the relationship between doctors and pharmaceutical companies.

✔ Paying large sums of money to private doctors to do "studies" of their drugs that rarely find negative things about the drugs.

✔ Paying rebates to private doctors to use their drugs, whether or not they are the best choice for the patient.

These problems are not limited to doctors and the pharmaceutical industry. Any time "advisors" are also salespeople, they advise the purchase of what they sell. But just because this practice takes place in every industry doesn't make it right. And in the medical industry, it's often a matter of life or death.

What steps can you take to avoid the dangers I outline above? Here are a few suggestions:

✔ **Do not ask your doctor to prescribe new drugs that are heavily promoted by advertising.** Too few people have used them and too little time has passed to truly know the potential of these new drugs.

✔ **Don't take samples from your doctor.** Drug companies use samples to get you and your doctor hooked on their drug.

✔ **Don't ask for a drug just because a key organization like the American Heart Association, the American Diabetes Association, the Endocrine Society, or others promotes the drug.** These organizations have become big and fat from the money provided by those drug companies.

✔ **Do wait several years before trying a new drug.** The drugs that are currently available are more than adequate to control your blood glucose, your blood pressure, and your cholesterol *if you take them as prescribed.*

Checking the Role of Infection in Type 2 Diabetes

Ever since a bacterial organism was found to be the cause of stomach ulcers, scientists have looked for other diseases that bacteria may play a role in. Although most specialists agree that the current epidemic of type 2 diabetes is due to increasing obesity and lack of exercise, looking for the possible role of infection in this disease is reasonable. A group from the University of California at Davis investigated the link and published the results in *Diabetes Care* in March 2012.

The group studied 782 elderly Latino subjects and looked for evidence of infection by checking for antibodies to various viruses and bacteria in their blood. They checked for herpes simplex, varicella virus, cytomegalovirus, *Toxoplasma gondii,* and *Helicobacter pylori.* With the exception of *H. pylori* (the same organism associated with ulcers), people who had evidence of infection with the other organisms did not have a higher rate of type 2 diabetes. However, people who had that infection had a 2.7 times greater likelihood of developing diabetes at any time than people who had no evidence of infection with *H. pylori.* This study leads me to believe that there may be a role for antibiotics in the treatment of type 2 diabetes.

Finding that Insulin Production Persists in Type 1 Diabetes

Doctors and scientists previously thought that shortly after the onset of type 1 diabetes, all production of insulin by the beta cells of the pancreas ceased. A group at Massachusetts General Hospital decided to test this assumption, and it published the results in *Diabetes Care* in March 2012.

The group studied 182 subjects with type 1 diabetes. They performed an ultrasensitive assay for C-peptide, a protein that is a product of the synthesis of insulin by the human pancreas. The study found measureable, though very small, levels of C-peptide in 10 percent of individuals between the ages of 31 and 40, decades after the onset of clinical type 1 diabetes.

The authors of the study suggest that such patients may benefit from efforts to preserve beta cell function and prevent complications. The presence of C-peptide means insulin is still being produced, which means there are some live beta cells in the pancreas. Efforts to increase these cells or cause them to make more insulin will make the diabetes much easier to control.

Connecting a Bone Hormone to Diabetes

Osteoblasts, cells in bone that increase bone formation, produce a number of proteins. One of them is osteocalcin, which plays a role in bone mineralization and calcification. Animal studies suggested that osteocalcin may also play a role in glucose metabolism. Scientists have been looking for the role of osteocalcin in human metabolism.

A group from Japan published its finding in the *Journal of Clinical Endocrinology and Metabolism* in January 2009. By studying 179 men and 149 postmenopausal women with type 2 diabetes, it found a negative correlation between levels of osteocalcin and fasting blood glucose and hemoglobin A1c. People in the study with lower levels of osteocalcin had evidence of poorer diabetic control than those with higher levels. Men (but not women) with lower levels of osteocalcin also had higher levels of fat mass.

Measures that improve bone formation may also improve glucose metabolism in men and women.

Marking the Importance of a Hormone in Type 2 Diabetes

Adiponectin is a hormone made in adipose (fat) tissue that plays an important role in type 2 diabetes. Adiponectin has been shown to reduce inflammation (which plays a role in type 2 diabetes) and increase insulin sensitivity. As adipose tissue increases, production of adiponectin decreases. In a study in the *Journal of the American Medical Association* in July 2009, the level of adiponectin was found to be negatively associated with the presence of type 2 diabetes. The study was a meta-analysis, which combines the results of several other studies. (Sometimes single studies may not include enough patients to make them statistically significant, but when combined with others, the studies may reach significance.)

A total of 14,598 people were included in this meta-analysis. Among those people were 2,623 cases of type 2 diabetes. Higher levels of adiponectin were consistently associated with a lower risk of diabetes.

A second study in the *Journal of Clinical Endocrinology and Metabolism* in June 2010 provided further evidence of the positive role of adiponectin. The authors looked at levels of adiponectin compared with levels of pathology in major arteries. Patients with less pathology, which would be found in nondiabetics and well-controlled diabetics, had higher levels of adiponectin.

The way to raise your adiponectin level is to lower your body fat. Higher adiponectin levels will be just one of many benefits.

Lowering Blood Glucose in Pregnancy

As explained in Chapter 6, prevention of gestational diabetes is important in preserving the health of the growing fetus and the mother and avoiding complications of birth. Controversy has been continuing as to whether higher-than-normal blood glucose levels that did not reach the level of diabetes posed a danger to mother and child.

A large number of medical centers combined to form the Hyperglycemia and Adverse Pregnancy Outcomes Study Cooperative Research Group to answer this question, among others. They published their results in the *New England Journal of Medicine* in May 2008.

The group evaluated blood glucose levels in 23,316 pregnant women. They looked at the birth weight of the newborns and their levels of C-peptide. Higher levels of C-peptide indicate that the fetuses were exposed to higher levels of glucose and had to make more insulin, which tends to cause fat accumulation in the babies.

The study found that birth weight and C-peptide levels have a continuous association in the babies even though the mothers' glucose level didn't reach that diagnostic of diabetes. Even at these lower levels of maternal blood glucose, the rate of necessary cesarean sections at delivery (because of a large baby) was higher, and newborns had a higher rate of low blood glucose (a consequence of too much insulin production in the newborn when the maternal supply of glucose is cut off at birth).

A later study from the same group (in *Diabetes Care* in March 2012) showed that the hemoglobin A1c was not a useful alternative to an oral glucose tolerance test in predicting complications in the pregnancy.

If you have been tested for gestational diabetes and don't reach the criteria for that diagnosis, the outcome of your pregnancy will still be improved by careful diet and regular exercise.

Developing Parkinson's Disease as a Consequence of Diabetes

Diabetes has been associated with a number of neurological diseases (see Chapter 5), including neuropathy (pain or loss of movement due to nerve damage), dementia (loss of memory and language, and abnormal behavior), and specifically Alzheimer's disease. For some time, scientists have also questioned the link between diabetes and Parkinson's disease (which causes shaking, rigidity, and slowness of movement, among many other symptoms).

A publication in *Diabetes Care* in April 2011 looked at the association. Among 288,662 participants in the National Institutes of Health-AARP Diet and Health Study, 1,565 people were diagnosed with Parkinson's disease. The authors found that the risk of Parkinson's disease was 40 percent higher in people with diabetes than it was in nondiabetics. This increased risk was mostly in people who had diabetes for at least ten years.

Another study in *Diabetes Care* in May 2011 confirmed this relationship. The authors looked at the nationwide Danish Hospital Register and identified 1,931 patients with Parkinson's disease. They found that having diabetes resulted in a 36 percent increase in the risk of Parkinson's disease.

Because insulin is a key hormone in normal brain function, it's not surprising that a disease associated with abnormal sensitivity to insulin (type 2 diabetes) would also be associated with abnormal brain function. Scientists are investigating insulin in Parkinson's disease at this time.

These findings suggest that avoiding diabetes and controlling diabetes if you can't avoid it may help to prevent Parkinson's disease.

Eating Slowly May Prevent Diabetes

It has often been suggested that obese individuals eat more rapidly than normal-weight individuals and that the result is more obesity and more diabetes. A group in Athens, Greece, decided to find out the truth behind this narrative, and it published its findings in the *Journal of Clinical Endocrinology and Metabolism* in January 2010. They observed 17 healthy adult males as they consumed a test meal of 300 milliliters of ice cream in 5 minutes or 30 minutes. After consuming the test meal, the participants were tested for hormones that increased hunger and hormones that decreased hunger. Hormones that decreased hunger were found to be significantly higher after the 30 minute consumption than after the 5 minute consumption. The participants reported less hunger after the 30 minute consumption.

The authors conclude that slowing down your rate of eating will make you less hungry in the end and that you'll therefore consume less food.

Understanding the Importance of the ACCORD Trial

The ACCORD (Action to Control Cardiovascular Risk in Diabetes) trial is a study of 10,250 people who have had T2DM and are at high risk to have a heart attack. The average hemoglobin A1c was 8.2 percent, which is higher than the average patient with T2DM. The patients were randomized into two treatment arms, a standard treatment arm that had a goal of an A1c target between 7 and 7.9 percent and an intensive treatment arm that had a goal of an A1c target less than 6 percent.

All patients already had known heart disease, diabetes, and at least two of the following additional risk factors:

✔ High blood pressure

✔ High cholesterol

✔ Obesity

✔ Smoking habit

When patients with these characteristics are allowed to maintain their usual A1c of 8.2 percent, their death rate is 50 per 1,000 patients per year.

The study was due to be completed in 2010, but in early February 2008, the researchers announced that they were closing the part of the study that attempted to get the A1c down to 6 percent because there was a higher death rate among the intensively treated patients than the other group. Here were the results up to that point:

✔ The intensive group had an average A1c of 6.4 percent.

✔ The standard group had an average A1c of 7.5 percent.

✔ The standard group had a death rate of 11 per 1,000 patients per year.

✔ The intensive group had a death rate of 14 per 1,000 patients per year.

Therefore, although the death rate for both groups was far below the level for these people with an A1c of 8.2 percent initially (11 or 14 versus 50 per 1,000), the intensively treated group that reached their goal had a slightly greater death rate than the standard group that reached their goal.

Subsequent papers from this study published in the *New England Journal of Medicine* in April 2010 have shown the following information:

✔ The use of combination therapy with a statin drug and a fibrate (see Chapter 10) did not reduce the rate of fatal heart or nonfatal heart attacks or strokes compared with a statin alone in these high-risk patients.

✔ Targeting a blood pressure of less than 120 mm Hg did not reduce the risk of fatal and nonfatal major heart attacks compared to a blood pressure target of 140 mm Hg in these high-risk patients.

The moral of this story is not that intensive treatment is dangerous in T2DM, but that intensive treatment is dangerous in this population of high-risk patients with heart disease and other risk factors.

Note that the death rate for both groups is much lower than that of the poorly treated patients. These patients are so sick that the difficulties associated with trying to keep their blood glucose at a level of 100 mg/dl all the time may be too great.

The more you control your blood glucose early in diabetes, the less chance that you will get to the point of the patients in this study.

Taking Advantage of Metabolic Memory

The Diabetes Control and Complications Trial, the results of which were published in 1993, showed that tight control of the blood glucose in type 1 diabetes substantially reduces the occurrence of complications of diabetes. Although the formal study ended in 1993, researchers continued to follow 90 percent of the participants. They called the follow-up the Epidemiology of Diabetes Interventions and Complications. Their results were published in the *New England Journal of Medicine* in December 2005 and December 2011.

Although the intensively treated group had only 6.5 years of intensive treatment, the long-term risk of complications, particularly kidney disease, was significantly reduced, even after 18 years during which the two groups had essentially the same level of treatment. This phenomenon is called *metabolic memory,* the tendency of the body to remember the very good treatment, resulting in a decrease of complications over time compared with the group not treated intensively.

Very good control of the blood glucose early in the disease has benefits that last for decades. Maintain that level of control, and you reduce the chance of complications enormously.

Chapter 17

What Doesn't Work When You Treat Diabetes

In This Chapter

▶ Recognizing the signs that a treatment won't work

▶ Identifying drugs, diets, and other treatments that don't help

---

*E*veryone wants a quick and easy solution to their problems. For every problem, five people offer a quick and easy answer. Just send in the money. These cheats have got what it takes to take what you've got.

Being fooled by these claims may be a lot more serious for you than for the person who walked up to the man dressed as a polar bear who was promoting soft drinks in a shopping center. The first man said: "Don't you feel foolish, dressed like a bear?" The "bear" replied: "Me, foolish? You're the one talking to a bear."

This chapter tells you as much as I know about diabetes tests and treatments that don't work. Don't expect to find every "wonder cure" for diabetes that you've read or heard about. As soon as this book is published, new, more seductive claims will be made. I hope that you will remain skeptical, use the information in this chapter to test claims out, and check with your doctor before you try something that may do more harm than good.

Developing a Critical Eye

Many clues can alert you that a treatment may not work. Here are a few:

✔ **If a treatment is endorsed by a Hollywood star or a sports figure, be highly skeptical.** Always consider the source and make sure that it's reputable. In this case, the fame of the star is being used to convince you, not any special knowledge that he or she possesses.

✔ **If the treatment has been around for a long time but is not generally used, don't trust it.** If a treatment has been around for a while and really works, it will have been tried in an experimental study where some people take it and some don't. Doctors and medical texts recommend drugs that pass that test.

✔ **If it sounds too good to be true, it usually is.** An example would be the claims about chromium improving blood glucose levels. The study that "proved" it was done on chromium-deficient people, a situation that does not exist in the United States.

✔ **Anecdotes are not proof of the value of a treatment or test.** The favorable experiences of one or a few people are not a substitute for a scientific study. Perhaps those people did respond to the drug (or supplement or miracle cure), but it may have been for entirely different reasons.

A lot of information about diabetes is available on the web. In Appendix A, I provide the best resources currently available for diabetes from this amazing source. The same rules apply when you consider the validity of claims made on the web, with a few extra rules thrown in:

✔ **Don't rely on search engines for validity.** Search engines do not check claims for validity.

✔ **Go to the site of the claim and see whether most of the information there makes sense.** If you find a lot of silly information, that should be a red flag. If you still feel the treatment might work, ask the webmaster (the person who develops the site) for references. If none are forthcoming, forget about the idea.

✔ **Go to sites that you know are reliable to see whether you can find the same recommendations.** The treatments discussed on sites like the American Diabetes Association (ADA) and the Diabetes Monitor (see Appendix A) can be relied on. When a treatment's value is uncertain, these sites can usually tell you the truth.

✔ **Go to medical conferences put on by reputable experts.** You will be given web addresses that are reliable.

Identifying Drugs and Supplements That Don't Work

In the past decade, so many drugs have been touted as the cure for diabetes that you would think everyone would be cured by now. The fact is, as I say again and again, you *do* have the tools right now to control diabetes, but the solution is not as simple as taking a pill. If it were, this book would not be necessary. In this section, I tell you about some drugs that have received unwarranted hype because they "worked" in a few people.

How the ADA labels new drugs

The American Diabetes Association evaluates new therapies and places them in one of four categories:

✔ Clearly effective

✔ Somewhat/sometimes effective or effective for certain categories of patients

✔ Unknown/unproven but possibly promising

✔ Clearly ineffective

If you're about to try a new therapy that has not been recommended by your doctor and is not discussed in this book, you may want to contact the ADA and find out its position on the treatment. Of course, if you're involved in a clinical trial that is trying to determine the effectiveness of a therapy, no one will know whether it works or not.

The Federal Trade Commission is concerned with all the phony "cures" for diabetes. They have set up a phony website called "Glucobate" that promises to be a cure for diabetes. When you click on "Order Now" they tell you about the hoax and offer tips to avoid being scammed, most of which you will find in this chapter.

If you participate in a clinical research study of a new drug, a system is in place to protect you. Make sure that the study has been approved by a review board in an institution that has been approved to do the research. Such institutions are usually accredited by an established organization like the Association for the Accreditation of Human Research.

See the sidebar "How the ADA labels new drugs" for information on how the American Diabetes Association evaluates new treatments.

Chromium

You can find articles singing the praises of chromium for controlling the symptoms of diabetes in all kinds of magazines and newspapers and on the Internet. Should you take supplements of chromium?

The strongest case for chromium comes from a study of people with type 2 diabetes in China. They were given high doses of chromium and were found to improve their hemoglobin A1c, blood glucose, and cholesterol while reducing the amount of insulin they had to take. However, these people were chromium deficient in the first place. People in the United States and other countries where the diet is sufficient in chromium do not have this deficiency and do not show improvement in glucose tolerance when they take chromium. In addition, chromium is present in such small amounts normally that it is hard to measure even in people without chromium deficiency.

The exact amount of chromium you need in your diet is uncertain but is estimated to be 15 to 50 micrograms daily. People who take much more than that tend to accumulate it in their livers, where it can be toxic. Some studies suggest that chromium can cause cancer in high doses.

For now, the evidence does not support the use of chromium in diabetes except for people who are known to be chromium deficient.

Aspirin

People who take the sulfonylurea drugs (see Chapter 10) sometimes have a greater drop in blood glucose when they take aspirin. This drop is because aspirin competes with the other drug for binding sites on the proteins that carry sulfonylureas in the blood. When they're bound to protein, the sulfonylureas are not active; when they're free, they are. Aspirin knocks the sulfonylureas off so that they're free. As a result, aspirin has been recommended as a drug to lower blood glucose.

By itself, aspirin has little effect on blood glucose. Its effect with sulfonylureas is so inconsistent that it can't be reliably depended on to lower the blood glucose.

Cinnamon

A number of articles in the medical literature since 2001 have suggested that cinnamon lowers the blood glucose in type 2 diabetes and improves fat levels as well. To verify these claims, a study called a meta-analysis was done and published in *Diabetes Care* in January 2008. In a meta-analysis, an analysis is done of all studies that are randomized so that the subjects don't know if they are getting the drug or a placebo. In this case, none of five studies showed that cinnamon had a positive effect either on the blood glucose or blood fats. You may have noticed the same thing if you were taking a daily dose of a teaspoon of cinnamon. You can cease and desist!

Pancreas formula

Pancreas formula is sold on the Internet as a mixture of herbs, vitamins, and minerals that help diabetes. No clinical or experimental evidence shows that pancreas formula does anything of value in the human body. The claims that are made for this "treatment" are not supported by factual evidence.

Fat Burner

You may hear and read a lot of advertising for the Fat Burner product in reputable newspapers and on reputable radio stations. Advertisements claim that you can "burn fat without diet or exercise," and they will even throw in, ABSOLUTELY FREE, a bottle of Spirulina to enhance your Fat Burner weight-control program. If you believe this is possible, I have a bridge I would like to sell you, *cheap.* In order to burn fat, you must exercise and stop taking in large amounts of carbohydrates or other sources of calories.

Ki-Sweet

The literature for Ki-Sweet offers another lesson in being skeptical. The creators of this "miracle" sweetener claim that it has a "special designation from the American Diabetes Association." The ADA denies the claim, but how many people will buy something when they see ADA approval and not bother to see whether it's true? No evidence exists that Ki-Sweet, made by squeezing the juice of kiwi, has any advantages over other sweeteners (which I discuss in Chapter 8).

Gymnema silvestre

Gymnema silvestre is a plant found in India and Africa that is promoted as a glucose-lowering agent as part of an alternative medical treatment called *Ayurvedic medicine.* Gymnema silvestre has never been tested in a controlled study in humans. One statement in its advertising is, "For most people, blood sugar lowers to normal levels." No evidence exists that this is the case.

The facts about aspartame

Many news sources report that aspartame (see Chapter 8) causes cancer. Because so many people eat and drink products that contain aspartame, I want to clarify the facts.

Aspartame is an acceptable artificial sweetener with no known dangers to human beings.

No evidence shows that aspartame causes cancer when used in normal amounts. The Food and Drug Administration has an acceptable daily intake for food additives, including a 100-fold safety factor. It is inconceivable that anyone would use more aspartame than that.

Avoiding Illegal Drugs

Drugs like cocaine, heroin, speed, and marijuana are not just illegal; they are especially harmful for the person with diabetes for several reasons:

- ✔ Some make you excessively hungry, and you take in too many calories.
- ✔ All cause you to lose your awareness of hypoglycemia, so you don't treat it.
- ✔ All cause a loss of judgment that results in the failure to take medications, eat properly, and exercise.
- ✔ Some cause a reduced insulin response to food, so you become hyperglycemic.
- ✔ Some cause you to lose your appetite, so you become hypoglycemic and malnourished with vitamin deficiencies.

Not a lot of valid information is available about each illegal drug's impact on diabetes, because we cannot do studies where these drugs are given to one group of diabetics while a control group takes a placebo. But we do know the following:

- ✔ Marijuana (grass, weed, bud, cannabis) causes increased appetite, which results in taking in too many calories.
- ✔ Amphetamine (speed, Dex, crank) and ecstasy (derived from amphetamine and also called MDMA, E, X, adam, bean, and roll) increase the body's metabolic rate, resulting in hypoglycemia because the user often does not eat properly and is unaware of the onset of low blood glucose.
- ✔ Cocaine (coke, snow, nose candy, dust, toot) and freebase cocaine (crack, rock) lead to food deprivation, increased metabolism and caloric needs, and vitamin deficiency.
- ✔ Heroin (dope, junk, smack) is similar to cocaine but has additional risks associated with injections, such as infection.

Do you need any more reason to get high on exercise rather than drugs?

Knowing the Dangers of Some Legal Drugs for Other Purposes

Just because a drug is legal does not mean it has no undesirable side effects. Several classes of drugs need to be used with caution. They may cause weight gain, prevent normal metabolism, and have many other effects that negatively affect your diabetes. This list is not exhaustive. One of the first places to look if you are doing everything right but still have poor control of your blood glucose is among the medications you take for other reasons.

Antipsychotics

In an issue of *Diabetes Care* (February 2004), four major medical associations warned that second-generation antipsychotic drugs, used to treat a variety of severe mental illnesses, can cause rapid weight gain, most of which is fat, leading to prediabetes, diabetes, insulin resistance, and abnormal blood fats.

The drugs differ in their risks, but clozapine (Clozaril, made by Novartis) and olanzapine (Zyprexa, made by Eli Lilly) appear to be the worst offenders. Other drugs named include risperidone (Risperdol, made by Johnson & Johnson), quetiapine (Seroquel, made by AstraZeneca), ziprasidone (Geodon, made by Pfizer), and aripiprazole (Abilify, made by Bristol-Myers Squibb).

If you are taking one of these drugs, ask your doctor to screen and monitor you for evidence of weight gain and insulin resistance. The benefits of taking the drug may outweigh the risks. In the article, the panel suggests that baseline screening consisting of a medical history and physical examination along with fasting glucose and blood fats be done before using the drug.

If you are overweight or obese, you should receive nutritional and physical activity counseling if you take one of these drugs. If you are at risk of developing diabetes, your doctor should use the drug that is least associated with this problem.

AIDS medications

Certain drugs that control AIDS, called *protease inhibitors,* block the body's ability to store glucose, so people who use them may develop diabetes. More than 80 percent of the people who use them develop excess stomach fat, and half develop glucose intolerance. More than 10 percent develop diabetes. Table 17-1 shows the specific drugs with their brand names and manufacturers.

Table 17-1	Protease Inhibitors That Affect Glucose Metabolism	
Generic Name	*Brand Name*	*Manufacturer*
Saquinavir (hard gel)	Invirase	Hoffman–La Roche
Saquinavir (soft gel)	Fortovase	Hoffman–La Roche
Ritonavir	Norvir	Abbott Laboratories
Indinavir	Crixivan	Merck
Nelfinavir	Viracept	Pfizer
Amprenavir	Agenerase	GlaxoSmithKline
Lopinavir and ritonavir	Keletra	Abbott Laboratories
Atazanavir	Reyataz	Bristol-Myers Squibb
Fosamprenavir	Levixa	GlaxoSmithKline

You should be screened before starting these drugs, and your doctor should monitor you carefully for weight gain and glucose intolerance. If diabetes does develop, the protease inhibitors are continued and the diabetes is treated. So far, none of the protease inhibitors stands out as more likely to cause diabetes.

Recognizing Diets That Don't Work

For the overweight person with type 2 diabetes, any diet that causes some weight loss helps for a time. But you have to ask yourself these questions:

- ✔ Am I prepared to stay on this diet indefinitely?

- ✔ Is this diet healthy for me in the long run?

- ✔ Does it combine all the features I need — namely weight loss, reduction of blood glucose, and reduction of blood fat levels — with palatability and reasonable cost?

If you can say yes to all these questions, the diet will probably work for you.

So how do you know which diets are healthy and effective, and which aren't? First, take a close look at Chapter 8, where I discuss diet in much more detail. Next, develop a discerning eye for defects in the latest diet fads.

When you walk into a reasonably large bookstore, you may be overwhelmed by the number of diet books. But the more books that are written about this subject, the less we seem to know for certain. Why would authors bother to write dozens of new books on dieting each year if the solution rested in some older book? You can bet that word of mouth would have made that book the all-time bestseller in any category.

The diet books in print these days are way too numerous to list here, but they can be grouped into a few categories:

- **Diets that promote a lot of protein with little carbohydrate:** The trouble with these diets is that they're not a healthy and balanced approach. Unless you use tofu as your source of protein, you will be getting a lot of fat in your diet, much of it saturated fat, which is not good for you. The diet is lacking in vitamins that a supplemental vitamin pill may or may not provide. Few people stay on such a diet for long. How many people can eat chicken for breakfast, lunch, and supper? The diet is also lacking in potassium, an essential mineral.

  People who do follow this kind of diet for a long time also find that they have problems with hair loss, cracking nails, and dry skin. Their breath and their urine smell of acetone because of all the fat breakdown. They become very dry and need to drink large quantities of beverages.

  I see a place for this diet as a starter. Some people with type 2 diabetes who have high blood glucose levels show rapid improvement when started on a diet like this. As the glucose comes under control, the diet can be changed to a more balanced one.

- **Diets that promote little or no fat:** The people who can follow a diet that is less than 20 percent fat deserve a new designation — *fatnatics*. This kind of diet is extremely difficult to prepare and perhaps even more difficult to eat unless you're a rabbit. In order to make up the calories, people on this diet eat large amounts of carbohydrates. Chapter 8 makes it clear why this is not a good idea for people with diabetes.

  Like the protein diet, this diet may be lacking in essential vitamins and minerals, especially the fat-soluble vitamins. Rarely do people stay on such a diet after they leave the confines of a spa or other sanctuary where the diet is promoted. However, this approach may also be a good way to start a dietary program for a person with type 2 diabetes, as long as the total calories are not greater than the daily needs of that individual.

- **Very-low-calorie diets:** These diets require taking in food and drinks that contain less than 800 kilocalories daily (and generally do not taste very good). They are lacking in many essential nutrients and must be supplemented by vitamins and minerals. This approach cannot form the basis of a permanent diet because the dieter would eventually become emaciated. Most dieters who start this kind of program do not last on it and regain every ounce they have lost and then some. (There are always exceptions, of course.)

  I do not like this kind of diet even as a starter diet because it is so unlike usual eating habits that people rapidly find it to be intolerable. Eating is a basic part of human existence, and it's a source of great pleasure for people and other animals. A diet that takes away this fundamental activity cannot be tolerated for very long.

What about hypnosis?

The National Institutes of Health, a very respected source, has listed hypnosis as a treatment for "stabilization of blood sugar in diabetes." Although it has a disclaimer that says that publishing this statement does not imply endorsement of the treatment, the fact that the statement comes from the NIH gives this treatment credibility. The only trouble is that no experimental evidence exists that proves the usefulness of hypnosis. So you have to be wary, even when the advice comes from the most respected of sources.

The transition from a very-low-calorie diet to a balanced diet is very difficult and rarely succeeds.

Part V
The Part of Tens

The 5th Wave   By Rich Tennant

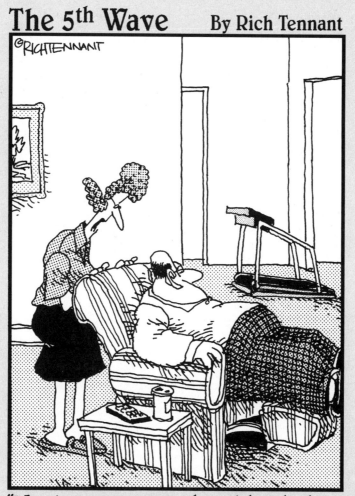

"You know, anyone who wishes he had a remote control for his exercise equipment is missing the idea of exercise equipment."

In this part . . .

The Part of Tens puts it all together and gives the most valuable techniques for thriving with diabetes. With just a little background from the other parts, you can use this section to really fine-tune your diabetes care. You find the ten commandments of excellent care, along with ten major myths about diabetes that you can discard. Finally, you find out how to utilize the skills and knowledge of the people around you, both the diabetes experts and your friends and family.

Chapter 18

Ten Ways to Prevent or Reverse the Effects of Diabetes

. . . .

In This Chapter

▶ Understanding the importance of monitoring, dieting, testing, and exercising

▶ Solidifying prevention with medication, the right attitude, and planning

. . . .

*W*hen I originally wrote this chapter, I came up with 20 things you had to do in order to prevent or reverse the effects of diabetes. I decided that was too much to ask of you, so I reduced the list to ten essentials. Surely you can do everything in this chapter when you consider that it is only half as difficult!

Can you pick and choose what you will do? No. Everything here is essential to living a long and high quality life with diabetes. You wouldn't want to save your sight and lose your kidneys. So read this chapter very carefully and practice every recommendation. And if you think I should have left any of the other ten behaviors in, let me know.

Major Monitoring

You have this incredibly compact and accurate glucose meter. Now you want to use it to find out how your blood glucose is doing at any time of day or night under any circumstances. You don't feel well. Is it low blood glucose or the beginning of a cold? Test! You just ate a large portion of pasta. Did it raise your blood glucose too much? Test! You can monitor your glucose in so many ways, almost without pain, that you have no excuse for not doing so. And you don't have to do it with a finger stick every time. Most meters allow you to do it in other parts of your body — your arm, leg, or abdomen for example — especially when the blood glucose would not be expected to change rapidly as it would during or after exercise or after a meal. At those times, you should only use your finger.

People with type 1 diabetes need to test at least before meals and at bedtime because their blood glucose level determines their dose of insulin. People who have stable type 2 diabetes may test once a day at different times or twice a day. If you're sick or about to start a long drive, you may want to test more often because you don't want to become hypoglycemic — or hyperglycemic for that matter. The beauty of the meter is that you can check your blood glucose in less than ten seconds any time you feel it's necessary.

Devout Dieting

If you are what you eat, then you have the choice of being controlled or uncontrolled depending on what you put into your mouth. If you gain weight, you gain insulin resistance, but a small amount of weight loss can reverse the situation. The main point you should understand about a "diabetic diet" is that it's a healthy diet for everyone, whether they have diabetes or not. You should not feel like a social outcast because you're eating the right foods. You don't need special supplements; the diet is balanced and contains all the vitamins and minerals you require (although you want to be sure you're getting enough calcium and vitamin D).

You can follow a diabetic diet wherever you are, not just at home. Every menu has something on it that's appropriate for you. If you're invited to someone's home, let them know you have diabetes and that the amount of carbohydrate and fat that you can eat is limited. If that fails, limit the amount that you eat. (See Chapter 8 for more on your diet.)

A person with T2DM who follows a careful diet can reduce his hemoglobin A1c by 1 percent or more. This translates into a reduction in the occurrence of complications like eye disease, kidney disease, and nerve disease of more than 25 percent. Is that benefit worth your effort?

Tenacious Testing

The people who make smoke detectors recommend that you change the battery without fail each time you have a birthday. You should use the same simple device to remember your "complication detectors." Make sure that your doctor checks your urine for tiny amounts of protein and your feet for loss of sensation every year around the time of your birthday. It takes five to ten years to develop complications of diabetes. When you know the problem is present, you can do a lot to slow it down or even reverse it. Never has it been truer that "an ounce of prevention is worth a pound of cure." (For more on complications that may develop, see Chapters 4 and 5.)

I make it very easy for you to get the tests you need at the time you need them. The online cheat sheet for this book gives you the current testing recommendations. Make a copy for your doctor if he or she does not already have such a list. Demand that you get the tests when they are due. A doctor with a busy medical practice may forget whether you have had the tests you need, but you don't have an excuse for forgetting. Make sure she tests your hemoglobin A1c, your blood pressure, and your cholesterol among other things.

Enthusiastic Exercising

When you take insulin (as opposed to pills), controlling your diabetes is a little harder because you have to coordinate your food intake and the activity of the insulin. But I have patients who have had diabetes for decades and have little trouble balancing their food and insulin. They are the enthusiastic exercisers. They use exercise to burn up glucose in place of insulin. The result is a much more narrow range of blood glucose levels than is true of the insulin takers who do not exercise. They also have more leeway in their diet because the exercise makes up for slight excesses.

I am not talking about an hour of running each day or 50 miles on the bike. Moderate exercise like brisk walking can accomplish the same thing. The key is to exercise faithfully. (For more on exercise, see Chapter 9.) Thirty minutes of moderate exercise every day will not just improve your diabetes. It will also reduce the possibility of a stroke, a heart attack, and many cancers, and just keep you feeling generally good. Exercise can reduce your hemoglobin A1c by 1 percent or more, just like diet.

Lifelong Learning

When I see a patient new to me who has had diabetes for some time, I am amazed at the lack of knowledge of many fundamental areas of their disease. You would think that they would want to know anything that might help them to live more comfortably and avoid complications.

So much is going on in the field of diabetes that I have trouble keeping up with it, and it's my specialty. How can you expect to know when doctors come up with the major advances that will cure your diabetes? The answer is lifelong learning. After you get past the shock of the diagnosis, you are ready to learn. This book contains a lot of basic stuff that you need to know. You can even take a good course in diabetes. Then you need to keep learning. Go to meetings of the local diabetes association. Become a member of the American Diabetes Association and get its terrific magazine called *Diabetes Forecast,* which usually contains the state-of-the-art developments. You can also occasionally go to the websites that I discuss in Appendix A.

Remember that a lot of misinformation is available on the web, so you must be careful to check out a recommendation before you start to follow it. Even information on reliable sites may not be right for your particular problem.

Above all, never stop learning! The next thing you learn may be the one that will cure you.

Meticulous Medicating

Compliance, which means treating your disease in accordance with your doctor's instructions, is a term that has special relevance for the patient with a chronic disease like diabetes who must take medications day in and day out. Sure, it's a pain (even if you could take insulin by mouth and not by injection). But the basic assumption is that you're taking your medication. Your doctor bases all his or her decisions on that assumption. Some very serious mistakes can be made if that assumption is false.

Check with your pharmacist to make sure that your pills don't interfere with one another. Some pills are taken with food; others are taken with no food for a period before and after that medication. Taking them correctly is just as important as taking them at all.

Every time a study is done on why patients' health conditions do not improve, compliance is high up or leads the list of reasons. Do you make a conscious decision to skip your pills, or do you forget? Whatever the reason, the best thing to do is to set up a system so that you're forced to remember. Keeping your pills in a dated container quickly shows you if you have taken them or not. You can even divide the pills by time of day.

Appropriate Attitude

Your approach to your disease can go a long way toward determining whether you will live in diabetes heaven or diabetes hell. If you have a positive attitude, treating diabetes as a challenge and an opportunity, managing your disease is easier and your body actually produces chemicals that make it happen. A negative attitude, on the other hand, results in the kind of pessimism that leads to failure to diet, failure to exercise, and failure to take your medications. Plus, your body makes chemicals that are bad for you when you are depressed.

Diabetes is a challenge because you have to think about doing certain things that others never have to worry about. It brings out the quality of organization, which can then be transferred to other parts of your life. When you're organized, you accomplish much more in less time.

Diabetes is an opportunity because it forces you to make healthy choices for your diet as well as your exercise. You may end up a lot healthier than your neighbor without diabetes. As you make more and more healthy choices, you feel and test less and less like a person with diabetes.

Preventive Planning

Life is full of surprises (like the sign on a display of "I Love You Only" Valentine cards: Available in Multipacks). You never know when you will get more than you bargained for. That is why having a plan to deal with the unexpected is so important. Say you're invited to someone's home, and she serves something that you know will raise your blood glucose significantly. What do you do? Or you go out to eat and are given a menu of incredible choices, many of which are just not for you. How do you handle that? You run into great stress at work or at home. Do you allow it to throw off your diet, your exercise, and your compliance with your doctor's orders?

A little advance planning can overcome any eating challenge. Discuss good foods with the people who regularly cook for you. Check out the calorie breakdown of the foods you eat at fast food places, usually available on the Internet. Many restaurants provide the nutritional breakdown on their websites. Make a diet for yourself and follow it.

The key to these situations is the realization that it's not possible for everything to go right all the time. In the case of the friend who cooked the wrong thing for you, you can at least eat a small portion to limit the damage. At the restaurant, you should come prepared with the food choices you know will keep you on your diet. It may be better not to look at the menu and simply discuss with your waiter what is available from your list of correct foods.

Fastidious Foot Care

A recent headline read: "Hospital sued by seven foot doctors." I would certainly not like to treat any doctor with seven feet or even a doctor who is seven feet tall. Whether you have two feet or seven feet, you must take good care of them. The problem occurs when you can't feel with your feet because of neuropathy (see Chapter 5). You can easily know when this problem exists just by checking with a 10-gram filament. If your feet cannot feel the filament, they will not feel burning hot water, a stone, a nail in your shoe, or an infected ulcer of your foot.

When you lose sensation in your feet, your eyes must replace the pain fibers that would otherwise tell you there is a problem. You need to carefully examine your feet every day, keep your toenails trimmed, and wear comfortable shoes. Your doctor should inspect your feet at every visit.

Diabetes is the primary cause of foot amputations, but this drastic situation is entirely preventable if you pay attention to your feet. Test bath water by hand, shake your shoes out before you put them on, wear new shoes only a short while before checking for pressure spots, and get a 10-gram filament and see whether you can feel it. If you smoke, you are especially at a high risk for an amputation of your toes or foot. The future of your feet is in your hands.

The other aspect of fastidious foot care is making sure the circulation in the blood vessels of your feet remains open. This test is done by your doctor performing an ankle-brachial index once a year (see Chapter 5). It quickly tells you and your doctor if you're experiencing a problem with your circulation.

Essential Eye Care

You're reading this book, which means you are seeing this book. So far, there are no plans to put out a Braille edition, so you had better take care of your eyes or you will miss out on the wonderful gems of information that brighten every page.

Caring for your eyes starts with a careful examination by an ophthalmologist or optometrist. You need to have an exam at least once a year (or more often if necessary). If you have controlled your diabetes meticulously, the doctor will find two normal eyes. If not, signs of diabetic eye disease may show up (see Chapter 5). At that point, you need to control your diabetes, which means controlling your blood glucose. You also want to control your blood pressure because high blood pressure contributes to worsening eye disease, as does high cholesterol.

Although the final word is not in on the effects of excess alcohol on eye disease in diabetes, is it worth risking your sight for another glass of wine? Smoking has definitely been shown to raise the blood glucose in diabetes. Even at a late stage, you can stop the progression of the eye disease or reverse some of the damage if you stop smoking now.

Chapter 19

Ten (Or So) Myths about Diabetes That You Can Forget

*M*yths are a lot of fun. They're never completely true, but you can usually find a tiny bit of truth in a myth. The trouble is that some myths can hurt you if you allow them to determine your medical care. This chapter is about those kinds of myths — the ones that lead you to fail to take your medication or stay on your diet, or even lead you to take things that may not be good for you.

Perfect Treatment Yields Perfect Glucoses

Doctors are probably as responsible as their patients are for the myth that perfect treatment results in perfect glucose levels. For decades, doctors measured the urine glucose and told their patients that if they would just stay on their diet, take their medication, and get their exercise, the urine would be negative for glucose. Doctors failed to account for the many variables that could result in a positive test for glucose in the urine, plus the fact that even if the urine was negative, the patient could still be suffering diabetic damage. (The urine becomes negative at a blood glucose of 180 mg/dl [10 mmol/L] in most people, a level that still causes damage.)

The same thing is true for the blood glucose. Although you can achieve normal blood glucose levels most of the time if you treat your diabetes properly, you can still have times when, for no apparent reason, the glucose is not normal. So many factors determine the blood glucose level at any given time that this should hardly be a surprise.

Pregnancy Is Not an Option for Women with Diabetes

Perhaps the myth that diabetic women shouldn't become pregnant was true when the current tools for managing diabetes weren't around, more than 30 years ago. Now we know that a woman with diabetes can have a normal pregnancy if she follows a few precautions. One is that she should not become pregnant unless she has good control of her glucose, because conception when she is out of control has been shown to lead to congenital malformations in her growing fetus.

Frequent testing of the blood glucose is a must during pregnancy, as is a very careful diet and regular exercise. Frequent visits to the diabetes specialist and the obstetrician are also essential. So a pregnancy in a woman with diabetes is not as carefree as one in a disease-free woman, but the new baby and the new mother can be perfectly healthy. Diabetes is almost never a reason not to have a family.

You Can't Enjoy Your Food

I hope you will not become a victim of this myth after reading this book. I provide recipes from great restaurants and chefs that clearly deserve the designation "gourmet" throughout Appendix C. If you want more info on the great food you can enjoy, see my book *Diabetes Cookbook For Dummies* (Wiley). Hopefully you learned in Chapter 8 that no food is forbidden to the person with diabetes. The key is moderation and not allowing yourself to gain weight.

Diabetes is not caused by sugar or fat or any other specific food. Type 2 diabetes typically occurs when the total food consumption leads to weight gain (weight gain is not always present) in a person who is genetically inclined to develop diabetes. Even then, regular exercise may postpone or prevent diabetes. Eating together is one of the most common social events, and by using the information in Chapter 8, you can continue to enjoy food despite diabetes.

You Can Tell the Level of Your Blood Glucose by How You Feel

Many of my patients have claimed that they can tell their blood glucose level by how they feel, and I have challenged them to prove it. Guess who wins every time, with the exception of significant hypoglycemia? Sure, if your blood glucose is below 50 mg/dl and you are sweaty and have palpitations and a headache, you know that you are low — but even then, you don't know how low. Therefore, you don't know how much treatment to give yourself to bring it back up but not too high.

 Patients with high blood glucose rarely can tell within 50 mg/dl what their level is. Less than half of patients who guess come close to the correct answer. People who don't test but who instead rely on the way they feel will suffer one or several of the short-term and long-term complications described in Chapters 4, 5, and 6.

You Have to Be Overweight to Get Diabetes

Although the current wave of new cases of diabetes mostly occurs in overweight people, plenty of people with diabetes have a normal weight. First of all, 1 of every 20 people with diabetes has type 1 diabetes, which is usually associated with normal or even reduced weight. Secondly, up to 10 percent of people with type 2 diabetes are normal or subnormal in weight.

It's important to realize this myth of having to be overweight because so many people with diabetes (up to one third) are undiagnosed. They may assume that they can't be diabetic because they are slim. If they happen to have a parent with diabetes, their risk of the diagnosis increases.

On the other hand, if you developed type 2 diabetes when you put on weight, there's a good chance the diabetes will regress if you lose weight. It will also improve your blood pressure and cholesterol. Plus, you will like what you see in the mirror.

If You Need Insulin, You're Doomed

Many people with type 2 diabetes believe that once they have to take insulin, they're on a rapid downhill course to death. This is not so. If you're using insulin, it probably means that your pancreas has pooped out and cannot produce enough insulin to control your blood glucose, even when stimulated by oral drugs. But taking insulin is no more a death sentence for you than it is for the person with type 1 diabetes.

Some people believe that insulin itself causes complications like impotence or other damage. No evidence supports this theory. One study suggested that using insulin to lower the blood glucose so the hemoglobin A1c was less than 6 percent caused more deaths than lowering it to a more modest level like 7 percent.

This study examined patients who had already had a heart attack and were quite sick when the study began. Even so, the doctors could not get the patients' hemoglobin A1c to the level they wanted with insulin. The goal was set too low. It does not take lowering to 6 percent to prevent complications in new patients with diabetes; 6.5 percent will accomplish this. First of all, using insulin is often a temporary measure for when you're very sick with some other illness that makes your oral drugs ineffective. When the illness is over, your insulin needs end.

Secondly, you may be on insulin because oral agents you tried failed to control your glucose. I see many people in this situation who can be taken off the insulin and given one of the newer oral agents, which actually control their glucose better than the insulin.

One typical patient came to me on 60 units of insulin weighing 180 pounds with a hemoglobin A1c of 7.4. I gradually lowered his insulin as I added rosiglitazone (now I would add metformin instead; see Chapter 10) to his treatment. He lost 22 pounds, came off insulin entirely, and now has a hemoglobin A1c of 6.

Thirdly, elderly people with diabetes may need insulin to keep their blood glucose at a reasonable level but do not need very tight control because their probable life span is shorter than the time it takes to develop complications. Their treatment can be kept very simple. The insulin is being used to keep them out of immediate trouble, not to prevent complications.

Finally, people with type 2 diabetes who truly need to be on insulin intensively need to check their blood glucose more often and live more like a person with type 1 diabetes. I hope you realize that with today's methods, this level of intensive treatment means a much higher quality of life than it used to.

People with Diabetes Shouldn't Exercise

If any myth is really damaging to people with diabetes, it is this one: People with diabetes shouldn't exercise. The truth is exactly the opposite. Exercise is a major component of good diabetes management — one that, unfortunately, all too often gets the least time and effort on the part of the patient as well as his or her care providers.

And I'm not just talking about aerobic exercise where your heart is beating faster. Some form of muscle strengthening needs to be a part of your lifestyle. (See Chapter 9 to find out the benefits of muscle strengthening.) If you have a muscle that you can move, move it!

I Can't Have Diabetes, Because I Have No Symptoms

In Chapter 3, I discuss the symptoms of both type 1 and type 2 diabetes and point out there that many patients have no symptoms or their symptoms may mimic those of other common conditions such as menopause and aging. For exactly this reason, the American Diabetes Association recommends screening for diabetes every three years beginning at age 45. If screening produces a false negative (the person has diabetes but the test doesn't show it), three years is not enough time to develop complications, and, hopefully, the next test will be positive if diabetes is present.

If I Am Sick and Can't Eat, I Can Skip My Diabetes Medications

When you get sick, you make more of the hormones that tend to raise the blood glucose. So even though you don't feel like eating, you probably need to take your medications, and maybe even more than usual, particularly if you are on insulin.

How can you know what to do? Test your blood glucose! That handy meter will help you decide if things are okay, if your control is a little off, or if you need to contact your doctor for advice. Even if you don't do much testing because your blood glucose is generally so good, you may want to test every four to six hours during illness if you find that your glucose is high, low, or unstable.

Diabetes Wrecks Your Sense of Humor

After the initial stages of accepting diabetes, your sense of humor should return. (See Chapter 1 for more on dealing with diabetes.) If your humor doesn't return, it's no laughing matter.

Dr. Joel Goodman, director of The HUMOR Project, pointed out in a lecture I attended that you "jest for the health of it." Numerous scientific studies have shown the health benefits of laughter.

The comedian Steve Allen pointed out in an interview (performed by Dr. Goodman) that there is humor in every aspect of life — you just have to look for it. The saying goes, "Someday we'll laugh about this." The question is, "Why wait?"

My diabetic patients have been the source of many funny stories, some of which I tell in this book. I want to give you the assignment of coming up with *at least* one funny story from your diabetic past. Send me an e-mail at drrubin@drrubin.com or write me a note about it. Of course, what you think is funny may not be funny to someone else. This is clearly shown by our individual preferences in comedians. Ask ten of your friends who their favorite comedian is and see if you don't come back with 12 answers.

Soak Your Feet Daily if You Have Diabetes

Here's an eleventh myth since you just gave me a standing ovation for writing this book. A standing ovation deserves a brief encore.

This myth causes more damage than it prevents. Soaking the feet tends to dry them. The skin can crack and infection can occur, which is, of course, the opposite of what you are trying to accomplish. Protect your skin by using a moisturizing lotion on a regular basis.

Make sure you inspect your feet every day, particularly if there is any question about your ability to feel abnormalities in your feet. Washing your feet with a good soap containing a moisturizing lotion is a good time to do that inspection.

Follow that up by applying a thick (not a thin or watery) moisturizing lotion to your feet. They will continue to give you good service for many years to come.

Chapter 20

Ten Ways to Get Others to Help You

In This Chapter

▶ Teaching friends and loved ones about hypoglycemia

▶ Making sure your primary physician is following the standards of care

▶ Finding an exercise partner

▶ Enlisting other types of help

Diabetes is a social disease. No, I don't mean that you catch it like herpes. I mean that you can't continue very long with diabetes without calling on the help and expertise of others. Asking for help is not such a bad thing. People who regularly interact with others seem to live longer and have a higher quality of life.

Diabetes has become so pervasive in the United States that practically everyone either knows someone who has diabetes or has it himself. There is a huge, growing body of knowledge about all aspects of diabetes, but you have to be willing to share your diagnosis with others so they can help you. These days I even get new patients when people who know they have diabetes share their diagnosis and symptoms with someone else and that person realizes that he has diabetes as well.

In this chapter, you discover how to make use of the great resources that are available to people with diabetes. So many knowledgeable people are out there — it would be a shame not to utilize their information. (Why, even I use my colleagues' knowledge on very rare occasions!)

Explain Hypoglycemia

If you take either insulin or one of the sulfonylurea medications (see Chapter 10), you may become hypoglycemic. Occasionally, hypoglycemia can be so severe that you're unaware of the problem. At that point, someone in your environment needs to know the symptoms of hypoglycemia and how to treat it. Chapter 4 contains all that information.

You may want to make a list of the signs and symptoms of hypoglycemia and pass it around to your family and friends. You should keep that list and an emergency kit to treat hypoglycemia at home and at work. You may even want to wear a medical alert bracelet so someone can identify your problem when none of these people are around.

Follow the Standards of Care with Your Doctor

Decades of following diabetes patients, along with increasing scientific knowledge, has led to the establishment of "standards of care" for people with diabetes. These recommendations usually appear in a supplement to the January issue of *Diabetes Care,* a journal of the American Diabetes Association. I outline these standards in Chapter 7 and on the cheat sheet for this book, which you can find online. By following the standards of care, you have a good chance of avoiding the short- and long-term complications of diabetes. If these complications have already occurred, you have a good chance of having them diagnosed while they are still treatable.

You are the one who needs to make sure that you get an annual eye examination, get your urine tested for microalbumin and your nerves tested for sensation, and get all the other tests that must be done regularly and routinely. (See Chapter 7 for more on these tests.) You can't do these tests alone, however. You need your physician to order the tests and send you to the eye doctor. Don't expect your physician to remember all these details. Just as you have trouble keeping to a program of care over a lifetime, your physician does much better with acute illnesses than chronic ones.

Find an Exercise Partner

Few people continue a regular exercise program completely on their own; I have trouble with that, myself. However, when you know that someone is waiting for you, you tend to perform the exercise much more regularly. I have many patients who are regular exercisers because I emphasize exercise so much. All of them exercise with a partner.

If you belong to a club, finding an exercise partner is easy. First, you select the sport, and then you hang out in the place where the sport is played. If the sport is a racket sport, you will soon find others at about your level. If the sport is something like running, you have to be a little forward and ask whether you can join someone or a group about to run. The people you can keep up with are your natural exercise partners.

If you're not a member of a club, finding an exercise partner is a little more difficult. You may have to approach people with whom you work, or you may need your significant other to commit to exercising with you. Most people are happy to walk with you, and some will run and bike with you. Cyclists seem to like group activity, and you can check out listings at a local bike shop or the Sunday newspaper in the activities section to find a group. If you can't seem to find an exercise partner, try a personal trainer.

Use Your Foot Doctor

Your foot doctor is your first line of defense against lesions of the foot. He or she knows what the foot should look like and will notice problems very early, when they're still reversible. Your doctor probably has a foot doctor that he likes to work with.

One of the most useful things the foot doctor can do is to cut your nails. It is too easy to accidentally cut your skin when you try to cut your own nails. If you have diabetes, the consequences can be serious.

Should you notice an abnormality, you must get to the foot doctor immediately. In this situation, you are much better off erring on the side of too much rather than too little medical care. In my practice, I ask the patients about their feet at every visit and examine the feet of those who have been found to have neuropathy (see Chapter 5) in the past. If I discover a foot problem, the foot doctor sees it that day.

Doctors have performed the first hand transplantation, which seems to be going well, but as far as I know, no plans exist to do a foot transplantation. Take good care of your feet because they have to last a lifetime. Your foot doctor can be your major ally in this endeavor.

Enlist Help to Fight Food Temptation

Ever since Adam and Eve, the problem of temptation has been on the front burner. For a diabetic, the constant temptation is to eat foods that do not further your major diabetic goal, which is to control your blood glucose. The opportunities for screwing up your diet are boundless. Just like your exercise partner, your "food partner" — your significant other — can make staying on your diet a lot easier for you.

If your partner cooks most of the meals in your household, he or she has a responsibility to prepare the right kinds of foods. To do so, your partner must know what to make and what to avoid (see Chapter 8). If you go to the dietitian, take your partner along.

Numerous books of recipes and meals are written specifically for people with diabetes. The first cookbook you should look at is *Diabetes Cookbook For Dummies* (Wiley), which I wrote with Cait James. That book would not have been written if it didn't offer a special feature — the recipes of some of the finest chefs in the United States and Canada. I include a number of good recipes in Appendix C of this book. You can also go on the Internet to find good recipes; see Appendix A for a list of great websites to check out.

I believe that one big problem in diabetes (as well as the nondiabetic obese population) is large portions of food. One of the simplest of diets is to eat the same foods but half as much. As I worked with the chefs in the various restaurants represented in Appendix C, again and again they remarked to me that Americans eat much more food in a portion than Europeans. Americans have learned to avoid fat, but they eat too much carbohydrate.

When it comes to eating out, your loved one can steer you to restaurants where you can choose foods that work for you. When you're in the restaurant, he or she can point out the healthy choices. The best way to direct you is to set an example of appropriate eating for you.

If you're asked to dinner in someone's home, your partner can help by telling your host in advance that you have diabetes and need to avoid eating certain foods. It is unwise, however, to turn your loved one into a nag. Asking to be reminded each time you stray from your diet will lead to hostility.

Expand Your Diabetes Knowledge

The person who serves as your diabetes educator is the source of a huge amount of necessary and sometimes critical information. Every person with diabetes ought to go through a program of education after the initial shock of the diagnosis is past (see Chapter 1). Never hesitate to ask a question, no matter how basic you think it may be. You will be surprised by how many others want the same information. Insurance will generally pay for yearly education, but check your insurance to be sure.

Of course, every caregiver should be a diabetes educator as well. When you are past the formal diabetes education program, don't hesitate to ask questions of your physician, your dietitian, or any of the other people in your team (see Chapter 11).

Knowledge about diabetes is expanding so fast that great advances are arriving almost daily. Some of these advances may be just what you need.

Fit Your Favorite Foods into Your Diet with a Dietitian

Years ago, a diagnosis of diabetes meant that you had to make enormous changes in your diet. This adjustment was hard enough for people who ate the usual American diet but much harder for people who came from another culture and had an entirely different diet. Fortunately, this situation has changed dramatically.

The dietitian's job is to come up with a diabetic diet plan based on *your* food choices, not those of the dietitian. If you have special dietary needs because of your culture, a dietitian must be able to accommodate those needs if they are reasonable.

 Members of your culture ate the foods that you like for generations without developing diabetes in large numbers. The main reasons they didn't develop diabetes in large numbers are that they did not eat the large portions you eat and they were much more physically active than you are. If you want to keep enjoying "your" foods, eat and exercise like your great-grandparents.

 Do not be satisfied with a printed sheet of paper with the heading "Diabetic Diet." The key word in diabetic diets is *individualization*. You probably won't stay on a diet that you do not enjoy.

Seek Out Appropriate Specialists

The specialist who knows the most about diabetes is the *diabetologist* (or endocrinologist), a physician with advanced training in diabetes care who maintains his or her edge by attending diabetes meetings regularly and keeping up with the literature by reading the most important clinical diabetes journals. In addition, these days an up-to-date specialist has to be aware of what is on the Internet and how to differentiate reality from hype. This person can explain the latest advances in diabetes to you.

Not only do you want to find a diabetes specialist, but should you develop a complication of diabetes, you also want to use a specialist in that area. At the first sign of kidney disease associated with diabetes, ask your doctor to refer you to a nephrologist. You should already be examined by an eye doctor on an annual basis. If there is any question of loss of sensation or abnormal muscle movements, see a neurologist. If there is any indication of heart trouble, get a referral to a cardiologist.

The pace of advances in diabetes is amazing. A general physician cannot keep up with it. The diabetes specialist concentrates on diabetes and the other specialists concentrate on their fields, and that is to your benefit.

Discuss Your Medications with the Pharmacist

One of your most valuable and least utilized resources is your pharmacist. He or she is loaded with information about drug actions, interactions, side effects, proper dosage and administration, and contraindications, as well as what to do in case of an overdose. Every time you get a new medication, you can have your pharmacist run it against the medications you're already taking and see whether any problems might occur. Thanks to computers, this comparison should take only a few minutes. If you work with one drug store, you should be able to get a printout of your entire list of medications, which you can carry with you in case you ever need medical care.

The pharmacist can also save you money by recommending generic equivalents to the brands that your doctor prescribes. The doctor may have good reason to prescribe them, so the pharmacist will check with him before giving you a different medication.

The information in the computer tends to be all-inclusive. If a drug has ever had a side effect, no matter how rare, it will probably be in the computer. The drug manufacturer wants to be able to say that it warned you about every possibility. If a side effect or drug interaction is serious, discuss it with your physician before you start the new medication.

Share This Book with Everyone

If you really want your friends and loved ones to understand what you're going through, why not give them a copy of this book and ask them to read it? You can select the chapters that are most important to you. Your family and friends will probably be delighted to have a resource they can understand, and you can expect a lot more help from them.

When I began writing this book, I did so because I saw a need for information that could be understood by most people without the benefit of a medical-school education. At the same time, I wanted you to have a little fun because "a spoonful of sugar helps the medicine go down." But I did not want to trivialize diabetes, and hope I have not done so. If you believe I have succeeded in what I set out to do, share this book with others.

Part VI
Appendixes

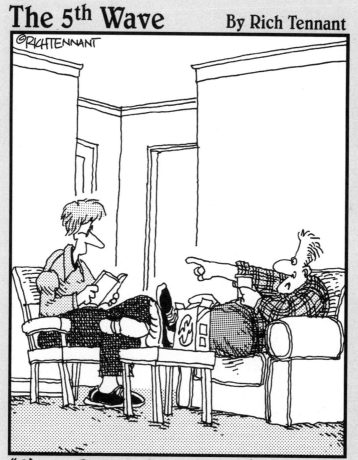

The 5th Wave   By Rich Tennant

"C'mon, Darrel! Someone with diabetes shouldn't be lying around all day. Whereas someone with no life, like myself, has a very good reason."

In this part . . .

You can check out various online resources provided in Appendix A and a glossary of important diabetes-related drugs and terminology in Appendix B. Appendix C gives you tasty, diabetes-friendly recipes courtesy of chefs from some of my favorite restaurants.

Appendix A

Dr. W. W. Web

· ·

*T*he World Wide Web hosts more information about diabetes than anyone can digest. This appendix presents the best sites for you to check. You should be able to get answers online to just about any questions that you have, but you must be cautious about the source of the advice. Don't make any major changes in your diabetes care without checking with your physician.

As I note in Chapter 19, to determine whether information you find on a website is really useful, you need to discuss it with your physician, your diabetes educator, or other members of your team (see Chapter 11). Any website I discuss in this appendix can be relied on, but sometimes free advice is worth no more than you pay for it. Remember that the web is constantly changing and growing, so these addresses are valid at least on the day I listed them.

Getting Started at My Website

You can start your search for information at my web page:

www.drrubin.com

You can find general information and advice about diabetes, daily tips, new developments, and answers to questions. You also find all of the sites listed in this appendix, so you need only click on them to see them for yourself.

Perusing General Sites

These sites tell you about diabetes from A to Z. The site sponsors run the gamut from well-known organizations to individual doctors who specialize in diabetes. Sometimes the sites get a little technical, in which case you can return to this book for clarification.

The American Diabetes Association

The huge website for the American Diabetes Association has just about everything you need to know about diabetes and then some. If the information becomes a little technical in places, you've probably gotten into the professional section by mistake. You can order all the ADA's publications from here.

www.diabetes.org

Online Diabetes Resources by Rick Mendosa

Rick Mendosa, who has diabetes himself, has cataloged just about everything there is on the web concerning diabetes. Collecting all this info is a huge project, and he manages to bring it off beautifully. He also has some excellent articles that he has written on various topics in diabetes.

www.mendosa.com

National Diabetes Education Program

The federal government sponsors the National Diabetes Education Program to improve treatments and outcomes for people with diabetes, to promote early diagnosis, and to prevent the onset of diabetes. It is a vast undertaking.

http://ndep.nih.gov

National Diabetes Education Initiative

Through the National Diabetes Education Initiative, the federal government is determined to teach physicians about the importance of meeting the standards of diabetes care and how to go about doing so. You can learn a lot by looking at its programs.

www.ndei.org

Medscape Diabetes and Endocrinology Home Page

At this site you can find numerous articles about diabetes from medical literature, as well as free access to the files of the National Library of Medicine.

www.medscape.com/diabetes-endocrinology

The Diabetes Monitor

The Diabetes Monitor is the creation of diabetes specialist Dr. William Quick. He discusses every aspect of diabetes, including the latest discoveries.

www.diabetesmonitor.com

Juvenile Diabetes Research Foundation

The Juvenile Diabetes Research Foundation prides itself on its contribution to research in diabetes. At its website you can find what you want to know about the latest government programs that emphasize finding a cure for diabetes.

www.jdf.org

Children with Diabetes

The site Children with Diabetes is the creation of a father of a diabetic child. It has an enormous database of information for the parents of children with diabetes.

www.childrenwithdiabetes.com

Joslin Diabetes Center

The Joslin Diabetes Center has been one of the world's leading pioneers in diabetes care, and the information on this site reflects that fact. The site also tells you how you can join Joslin, do research, or go to diabetes camp.

www.joslin.org

Canadian Diabetes Association

If you're Canadian, you want to visit this site because a lot of its information (obviously) pertains to the special needs of Canadians with diabetes. However, much of the information is general and of use to everyone. A major benefit is that the information is in French as well as English.

```
www.diabetes.ca
```

The International Diabetes Federation

This organization, representing more than 100 countries, meets every three years and can be a source for knowledgeable diabetes experts around the world.

```
www.idf.org
```

Ask NOAH About Diabetes

This site provides a large amount of information in both English and Spanish. It comes from the New York Online Access to Health, a partnership of New York institutions.

```
www.noah-health.org/en/endocrine/diabetes/
```

Behavioral Diabetes Institute

If you have a psychological issue relating to your diabetes, you may find help at this site, which claims to be the "first organization dedicated to tackling the unmet psychological needs of people with diabetes."

```
http://behavioraldiabetesinstitute.org
```

Contacting Companies That Make Diabetes Products

This section helps you find the companies that make the products you need to control your diabetes. If you have questions about the proper use of a drug or a device, you can usually find answers here. But keep in mind that the companies are very limited (by the FDA) with respect to the uses of their products. Often doctors use drugs in ways that have proven to be successful but have not yet received FDA approval.

Glucose meters

The following companies make the meters used by the largest number of people with diabetes. You can expect that these companies will still be around if you start having problems with your meter after a year or two of use.

- ✔ **Abbott Laboratories:** www.abbott.com/index.htm
- ✔ **AgaMatrix:** www.wavesense.info/company
- ✔ **Bayer:** www.bayercontour.com
- ✔ **Diagnostic Devices:** http://prodigymeter.com
- ✔ **LifeScan:** www.onetouch.com
- ✔ **Nipro Diagnostics:** www.niprodiagnostics.com
- ✔ **Roche:** www.accu-chek.com/us

If you want more information on glucose meters, flip to Chapter 7.

Lancing devices

A company that has a very large share of the market for lancing devices is Owen Mumford, which you can find at www.owenmumford.com/en. (I discuss lancing devices in Chapter 10.)

Insulin pumps

Five companies dominate the market for insulin pump devices (which I talk about in Chapter 10). They are

- ✔ **Animas:** www.animascorp.com
- ✔ **Insulet Corp:** www.myomnipod.com
- ✔ **Medtronic MiniMed:** www.medtronicdiabetes.net/products
- ✔ **Roche:** www.accu-chekinsulinpumps.com/ipus/
- ✔ **Sooil Development:** www.sooilusa.com/m2_01.html

Insulin

These three companies dominate the insulin market in the United States:

- ✔ **Eli Lilly and Company:** www.lilly.com/products/Pages/products.aspx
- ✔ **Novo Nordisk:** www.novonordisk.com
- ✔ **Sanofi-Aventis:** http://en.sanofi.com/products/diabetes/diabetes.aspx

Insulin syringes

If you want to find the major company for syringes, go to the website for Becton, Dickinson, and Company at www.bd.com/us/diabetes.

Insulin jet-injection devices

Jet-injection devices provide "painless" insulin injection. The only company that seems to still be making this device is in the Netherlands. It is called the European Pharma Group and can be found at www.insujet.com.

Oral medications

I include only six companies in this list, but the market for oral medications is heating up, so if you read about diabetes advancements or talk to your doctor or specialist, you'll likely hear about several more.

- ✔ **Amylin** (Byetta): www.amylin.com
- ✔ **Bristol-Myers Squibb** (Glucophage, Glucovance, Glucophage XR, Onglyza): www.bms.com
- ✔ **Eli Lilly** (Tradjenta): www.lilly.com
- ✔ **Merck** (Januvia): www.merck.com
- ✔ **Pfizer** (Glucotrol): www.pfizer.com
- ✔ **Sanofi-Aventis** (Amaryl): http://en.sanofi.com/products/diabetes/diabetes.aspx

Getting Info from Government Websites

These sites provide lots of authoritative information in their many online publications about diabetes. They also tell you about the latest government programs to eradicate the disease.

National Institute of Diabetes and Digestive and Kidney Disease

This site is loaded with great publications about diabetes.

    http://diabetes.niddk.nih.gov

Centers for Disease Control and Prevention

If you want to know all the latest statistics about every aspect of diabetes, the CDC has you covered.

    www.cdc.gov/diabetes

Healthfinder

Healthfinder is a service of the U.S. Department of Health and Human Services. It has information about many important diseases and has a large section about diabetes.

    www.healthfinder.gov

PubMed search service of the National Library of Medicine

This website is where you go to use the National Library of Medicine. The site is easy to use and gives you (for free) a large number of the latest scientific papers on any medical topic of interest.

    www.ncbi.nlm.nih.gov/PubMed

Nongovernment website for searching the National Library

Although not a government site, MedFetch is excellent for creating repeated searches of the National Library on a topic like diabetes over time. The information arrives by e-mail, and the results are delivered in one of six languages: English, Spanish, French, Italian, German, or Portuguese.

www.medfetch.com

Obtaining Diabetes Information in Other Languages

At this site for Diabetes UK, a charity based in the United Kingdom, you find diabetes educational information in numerous languages.

www.diabetes.org.uk/Other_languages

Visiting Sites for the Visually Impaired

Diabetes has a major impact on vision when the disease is not controlled (see Chapter 5). You can find huge quantities of information on every issue relating to visual impairment at the sites listed in this section.

American Foundation for the Blind

The American Foundation for the Blind has resources, information, reports, talking books, and limitless facts and wisdom about dealing with visual impairment.

www.afb.org/default.aspx

Blindness Resource Center

This site for the Blindness Resource Center points you in the right direction for information on every aspect of blindness. It is a guide to other sites about visual impairment.

    www.nyise.org/text/blindness.htm

The Diabetes Action Network (National Federation of the Blind)

This national organization is another major source of information about every aspect of blindness.

    www.nfb.org/diabetics

Helping Animals with Diabetes

Yes, your dog and cat and many other animals can get diabetes, and websites exist that can help.

Dogs and other pets

This site tells you everything you need to know to manage your canine with diabetes.

    www.diabetesindogs.net

Cats

This site is packed with helpful information for the pet owner who has a diabetic cat.

    www.felinediabetes.com

Finding Recipes for People with Diabetes

You can find a number of excellent recipes on the web, but approach them with caution. Although you can generally count on the recipes in books to contain the nutritional information they list, when you find a recipe on the web, you need to evaluate its source to be sure the listed nutritional information is accurate.

You can trust the sites that I list here. These are the best of the currently available websites that provide recipes appropriate for a person with diabetes. Things change so frequently on the web that it's difficult to keep up to date, so check back often. And in addition, be sure to check out Chapter 8 and Appendix C for advice on healthy eating and good recipes to try.

- ✔ The nutrition section of the American Diabetes Association website begins at www.diabetes.org/food-and-fitness/food/what-can-i-eat. Here you find discussions of nutrition as well as lots of recipes.

- ✔ "Children with Diabetes" includes a large amount of information on meal planning, sugar substitutes, and the food guide pyramid, as well as many recipes, at www.childrenwithdiabetes.com/d_08_000.htm.

- ✔ The Joslin Diabetes Center points out that "There is no such thing as a diabetic diet." That's one of many statements about nutrition you can find at www.joslin.org/info/Diet_and_Nutrition.html.

- ✔ "3 Fat Chicks on a Diet" has complete calorie counts for most fast food restaurants at www.3fatchicks.com/.

- ✔ The Vegetarian Resource Group maintains a large site filled with information for vegetarians who have developed diabetes at www.vrg.org.

- ✔ *Diabetic Gourmet Magazine* offers a valuable site that contains information about diagnosis and treatment, as well as numerous recipes that you can use, at http://diabeticgourmet.com.

Appendix B

Glossary

Acarbose: An oral agent that lowers blood glucose by blocking the breakdown of carbohydrates in the intestine.

ACE inhibitor: A drug that lowers blood pressure but is especially useful when diabetes affects the kidneys.

Acetone: A breakdown product of fat formed when fat rather than glucose is being used for energy.

Advanced glycated end-products (AGEs): Combinations of glucose and other substances in the body. Too much may damage various organs.

Algorithm: In diabetes care, a step-by-step plan for determining how much insulin to use for the blood level of glucose and the intake of carbohydrates.

Alpha cells: Cells in the Islets of Langerhans within the pancreas that make glucagon, which raises blood glucose.

Amino acids: Compounds that link together to form proteins.

Amyotrophy: A form of diabetic neuropathy causing muscle wasting and weakness.

Angiography: Using a dye to take pictures of blood vessels to detect disease. In diabetes, angiography is often used in the eyes.

Antibodies: Substances formed when the body detects something foreign, such as bacteria.

Antigens: Substances against which an antibody forms.

Artificial pancreas: A large machine that can measure blood glucose and release appropriate insulin.

Atherosclerosis: Narrowing of arteries due to deposits of cholesterol and other factors.

Autoimmune disorder: Disease in which the body mistakenly attacks its own tissues.

Autonomic neuropathy: Diseases of nerves that affect organs not under conscious control, such as the heart, lungs, and intestines.

Avandia: Brand name for rosiglitazone. *See Rosiglitazone.*

Background retinopathy: An early stage of diabetic eye involvement that does not reduce vision.

Beta cells: Cells in the Islets of Langerhans in the pancreas that make the key hormone insulin.

Blood urea nitrogen (BUN): A substance in blood that reflects kidney function.

Body-mass index (BMI): A number derived by dividing your weight (in kilograms) by your height (in meters), and dividing that number by your height (in meters) again. Your BMI is an indicator of your appropriate weight for your height.

Borderline diabetes: A term formerly used to mean mild or early diabetes; it is no longer used.

Carbohydrate: One of the three major energy sources — the one usually found in grain, fruits, and vegetables, and the one most responsible for raising the blood glucose.

Carbohydrate counting: Estimating the amount of carbohydrate in food in order to determine insulin needs.

Cataract: A clouding of the lens of the eye often found earlier and more commonly in people with diabetes.

Charcot's foot: Destruction of joints and soft tissue in the foot leading to an unusable foot as a result of diabetic neuropathy.

Cholesterol: A form of fat that is needed in the body for production of certain hormones. It can lead to atherosclerosis if present in excessive levels. Butter and egg yolks are high in cholesterol.

Continuous subcutaneous insulin infusion (CSII): Continuous delivery of insulin under the skin, usually by an insulin pump, to mimic the way the body provides insulin.

Conventional diabetes treatment: Usually refers to treatment in type 1 diabetes where only one or two shots of insulin are given daily.

Creatinine: A substance in blood that is measured to reflect the level of kidney function.

Dawn phenomenon: The tendency for blood glucose to rise early in the morning due to secretion of hormones that counteract insulin.

Detemir insulin: A long-acting insulin that provides a constant basal level for 24 hours.

Diabetes Control and Complications Trial (DCCT): The decisive study of type 1 diabetes that showed that intensive control of blood glucose would prevent or delay complications of diabetes.

Diabetic ketoacidosis: An acute loss of control of diabetes with high blood glucose levels and breakdown of fat leading to acidification of the blood. Symptoms are nausea, vomiting, and dehydration. This condition can lead to coma and death.

Diabetologist: A physician who specializes in diabetes treatment.

Dialysis: Artificial cleaning of the blood when the kidneys are not working.

Endocrinologist: A physician who specializes in diseases of the glands, including the adrenal glands, thyroid, pituitary, parathyroid glands, ovaries, testicles, and pancreas.

Euglycemia: A state in which the blood glucose remains in the normal range.

Exchange plan: A dietary plan where foods that are similar in type are grouped together so that a diet can substitute any one for any other within that group. The seven groups are starches and breads, meats and meat substitutes, fruits, milks, vegetables, fats, and other carbohydrates.

Exenatide: An injectable medication that improves diabetic control by inducing weight loss, slowing absorption of carbohydrates, and helping the pancreas to release insulin when blood sugars are high.

Fiber: A substance in plants that can't be digested. It provides no energy but can lower fat and blood glucose if it dissolves in water and is absorbed, or it can help prevent constipation if it does not dissolve in water and remains in the intestine.

Fructose: The sugar found in fruits, vegetables, and honey. It has calories but is more slowly absorbed than glucose.

Gastroparesis: A form of autonomic neuropathy involving nerves to the stomach, causing the stomach to hold food.

Gestational diabetes mellitus: Diabetes that occurs during a pregnancy, usually ending at delivery.

Glargine insulin: A long-acting form of insulin that provides a constant basal level for 24 hours.

Glimepiride: An oral agent that lowers glucose by raising insulin levels.

Glucagon: A hormone made in the alpha cell of the pancreas that raises glucose and can be injected in severe hypoglycemia.

Glucose: The body's main source of energy in the blood and cells.

Glycemic index: The extent to which a given food raises blood glucose, usually compared to white bread. Low-glycemic-index foods are preferred in diabetes.

Glycogen: The storage form of glucose in the liver and muscles.

Glycosuria: Glucose in the urine.

Hemoglobin A1c: A measurement of blood glucose control reflecting the average blood glucose for the last 60 to 90 days.

High-density lipoprotein (HDL): A particle in blood that carries cholesterol and helps reduce atherosclerosis.

Honeymoon phase: A period of variable duration, usually less than a year, after a diagnosis of type 1 diabetes when the need for injections of insulin is reduced or eliminated.

Humalog insulin: *See Lispro insulin.*

Hyperglycemia: Levels of blood glucose greater than 100 mg/dl fasting or 140 mg/dl in the fed state.

Hyperinsulinemia: More insulin than normal in the blood; often found early in type 2 diabetes.

Hyperlipidemia: Elevated levels of fat in the blood.

Hyperosmolar syndrome: Very high glucose in type 2 diabetes associated with severe dehydration but not excessive fat breakdown and acidosis. It can lead to coma and death.

Hypoglycemia: Levels of blood glucose lower than normal, usually less than 60 mg/dl.

Impaired glucose tolerance (IGT): Levels of glucose between 140 and 200 mg/dl after eating; not normal but not quite high enough for a diagnosis of diabetes.

Impotence: Loss of the ability to have or sustain an erection of the penis.

Insulin: The key hormone that permits glucose to enter cells.

Insulin glargine: An insulin that provides a constant basal level 24 hours a day.

Insulin pump: Device that slowly pushes insulin through a catheter under the skin but also can be used to give a larger dose before meals.

Insulin reaction: Hypoglycemia as a consequence of too much injected insulin for the amount of food or exercise.

Insulin resistance: Decreased response to insulin; found early in type 2 diabetes.

Insulin-dependent diabetes: Former name for type 1 diabetes.

Intensive diabetes treatment: Using three or four daily insulin injections based on measurement of blood glucose, along with very careful diet and exercise, to approximate the normal range of glucose.

Islet cells: The cells in the pancreas that make insulin, glucagon, and other hormones.

Juvenile diabetes mellitus: Previous term for type 1 diabetes.

Ketones or ketone bodies: The breakdown products of fat metabolism.

Ketonuria: Finding ketones in the urine with a test strip.

Lancet: A sharp needle to prick the skin for a blood glucose test.

Laser treatment: Using a device that burns the back of the eye to prevent worsening of retinopathy.

Lipoatrophy: Indented areas where insulin is constantly injected.

Lipohypertrophy: Nodular swelling of the skin where insulin is constantly injected.

Lispro insulin: A very rapid-acting form of insulin that's active within 15 minutes of injection.

Low-density lipoprotein (LDL): A particle in the blood containing cholesterol and thought to be responsible for atherosclerosis.

Macrosomia: The condition of a fetus growing very large when the mother's diabetes is not controlled.

Macrovascular complications: Heart attack, stroke, or diminished blood flow to the legs in diabetes.

Metabolic syndrome: A combination of hypertension, increased visceral fat, high triglycerides, low HDL cholesterol, often obesity, and high uric acid associated with increased heart attacks.

Metformin: An oral agent for diabetes that lowers glucose by blocking release of glucose from the liver.

Microalbuminuria: The loss of small but abnormal amounts of protein in the urine.

Microvascular complications: Eye disease, nerve disease, or kidney disease in diabetes.

Miglitol: An oral hypoglycemic drug that lowers blood glucose by blocking the breakdown of complex sugars and starches.

Monounsaturated fat: A form of fat, from vegetable sources like olives and nuts, that does not raise cholesterol.

Morbidity rate: The rate at which sickness occurs compared with those who remain well.

Mortality rate: The rate at which death occurs compared with the total population.

Nateglinide: A drug similar to repaglinide that is given before a meal to stimulate insulin for that meal.

Neovascularization: Formation of new vessels, especially from the retina of the eye.

Nephropathy: Damage to the kidneys.

Neuropathic ulcer: An infected area, usually on the leg or foot, resulting from damage that was not felt.

Neuropathy: Damage to parts of the nervous system.

Non-insulin-dependent diabetes: Former name for type 2 diabetes.

NPH insulin: An intermediate-acting insulin, which starts to work in 4 to 6 hours and ends by 12 hours.

Ophthalmologist: A doctor who specializes in diseases of the eyes.

Oral hypoglycemic agent: A glucose-lowering drug taken by mouth.

Pancreas: The organ behind the stomach that contains the Islets of Langerhans where insulin is produced.

Periodontal disease: Gum damage, which is more common in uncontrolled diabetes.

Peripheral neuropathy: Pain, numbness, and tingling, usually in the legs and feet.

Pioglitazone: An oral agent that lowers glucose by reducing insulin resistance.

Podiatrist: A person who specializes in treating the feet.

Polydipsia: Excessive intake of water.

Polyunsaturated fat: A form of fat from vegetables that may not raise cholesterol but does lower HDL.

Polyuria: Excessive urination.

Postprandial: After eating.

Proliferative retinopathy: Undesirable production of blood vessels in front of the retina.

Protein: A source of energy for the body made up of amino acids and found in meat, fish, poultry, and beans.

Proteinuria: Abnormal loss of protein from the body into the urine.

Receptors: Locations on cells that bind to a substance like insulin to permit the substance to do its job.

Regular insulin: A fast-acting form of insulin, active in one to two hours and gone by four to six hours.

Repaglinide: An oral drug that lowers glucose by causing insulin secretion.

Retina: The part of the eye that senses light.

Retinopathy: Disease of the retina.

Rosiglitazone: One of a class of oral antidiabetic agents that lowers glucose by reducing insulin resistance. Not recommended.

Saturated fat: A form of fat from animals that raises cholesterol.

Secondary diabetes: Diabetes caused by some other disease, which raises glucose or blocks insulin.

Sitagliptin: A once-daily pill that reduces blood glucose.

Somogyi effect: A rapid increase in blood glucose in response to hypoglycemia.

Sulfonylureas: The earliest class of glucose-lowering agents, which work by stimulating insulin secretion.

Synthetic: Produced by artificial means.

Triglycerides: The main form of fat in animals.

Troglitazone: The first of the class of glucose-lowering agents that reverses insulin resistance. Liver problems have caused its removal from the drug market.

Very-low-density lipoprotein (VLDL): The main particle in the blood that carries triglyceride.

Visceral fat: The fat accumulation that results in increased waist measurement.

Vitrectomy: Removal of the gel in the center of the eyeball because there has been leakage of blood and formation of scar tissue.

Appendix C

Mini-Cookbook

This appendix should make it clear to you that you can have great food from every ethnic corner of the world and still stay within the requirements of a diabetic diet. In a short appendix like this, I could not include every possible type of food, but I tried to select foods that most people enjoy either at home or in a restaurant. I chose the restaurants from among the best in the country, with an emphasis on San Francisco because that is where I reside and (happily) get to try them. I've also included a sampling of delicious salad recipes from my book *Diabetes Cookbook For Dummies* (Wiley). If you like what you see, pick up a copy for even more delectable diabetic-friendly recipes.

Getting to Know the Contributing Restaurants and Chefs

The chefs and restaurants who contributed recipes were a pleasure to work with and deserve great praise for their willingness to accommodate the needs of diabetic diners. Some restaurant recipes were altered slightly to keep them appropriate for a diabetic diet, but changes were never done without the approval of the chefs who created them. Some of their recipes may take a little longer than others to prepare, but all are worth the time and the effort. In any case, you can go to the restaurant that provided the recipe, order that meal, and know that you are on your diabetic diet.

Border Grill

Situated in Santa Monica, California, the critically acclaimed Border Grill restaurant features the bold foods of Mexico. The original restaurant is joined by Border Grill Downtown LA and Border Grill Las Vegas, as well as the Border Grill Truck, a gourmet taco truck on the cutting edge of the street-food scene in Los Angeles.

The restaurants and truck are the inspiration of two women who are chefs, restaurateurs, cookbook authors, and television personalities: Mary Sue

Milliken and Susan Feniger. They are well known from Bravo's *Top Chef Masters* and Food Network's *Two Hot Tamales* and are natural teachers who enjoy sharing their passion for bold flavors and strong statements through many media. If you find, as I did, that their recipes make you hunger for more, look for their book *Mexican Cooking For Dummies* (Wiley).

Border Grill, 1445 Fourth St., Santa Monica, California. 310-451-1655.

Gaylord India Restaurant

A bit of India in San Francisco, Gaylord is synonymous with delicious and authentic Indian food, served with true Indian hospitality. At Gaylord, master chefs specialize in North Indian cuisine including centuries-old techniques of tandoori cooking. Head chef Rajah Giri was trained in the home of North Indian cooking.

Gaylord India Restaurant, One Embarcadero Center, San Francisco, CA. 415-397-7775. www.gaylords1.com.

Greens

When residents of the San Francisco Bay area think of great vegetarian food, Greens is the first name that comes to mind. Greens uses the freshest ingredients, many of which come from the Zen Center's Green Gulch Farm, across the Golden Gate Bridge in Marin County. This brief trip results in no loss of freshness for the fine seasonal organic produce.

Chef Annie Somerville came to Greens in 1981 and became executive chef in 1985. She continues to create outstanding dishes with a balance of colors and flavors and contrast of textures. In addition to the Green Gulch and Start Route Farms in Marin County, she uses artisan cheeses from West Marin and Sonoma counties. She has authored the award-winning book *Field of Greens: New Vegetarian Recipes from the Celebrated Greens Restaurant* (Bantam).

Greens, Fort Mason, Building A, San Francisco, CA. 415-771-6222. www.greensrestaurant.com.

Gerald Hirigoyen

Gerald Hirigoyen is the chef and owner of several San Francisco restaurants, including Piperade and Laubaru. By whatever designation, his food is straightforward and flavorful, and the social atmosphere is full of character and energy. The high quality of the food is in contrast to the moderate prices of everything on the menu. Much of the menu can be enjoyed not only for taste but also for the healthful qualities of the food.

Gerald Hirigoyen trained in the Basque region of France and in Paris with some of the great names in French cuisine. He came to San Francisco in 1980 and ran the kitchens of several fine restaurants, but in 1991, he decided to go out on his own and start his restaurant. He has received numerous awards and much recognition for the quality of his food. *Food and Wine* magazine called him one of 1994's "Best New Chefs in America."

Paulette Mitchell

Paulette Mitchell, the author of 13 cookbooks, is known for her quick-to-prepare recipes with gourmet flair. She is the author of the award-winning *15-Minute Gourmet* cookbook series. She also is a video producer of Telly Award–winning travel and culinary videos as well as a media spokesperson, freelance writer, culinary speaker, cooking instructor, and television personality. As an avid world traveler, Paulette is most inspired by flavors from diverse cultures both near and far.

Paulette's most recently published cookbook is *The Complete 15-Minute Gourmet: Creative Cuisine Made Fast and Fresh* (Thomas Nelson).

Grilled Romaine Caesar Salad

Prep time: 10 min plus chilling time • **Cook time:** 5 min • **Yield:** 4 servings

Ingredients	Directions
½ sheet toasted nori	**1** Grind nori sheet in a blender or food processor to a fine powder. Add the tofu, 2 tablespoons olive oil, lemon juice, garlic, Worcestershire, salt, and pepper and puree until smooth. Refrigerate the dressing for 30 minutes.
1 package silken tofu	
3 tablespoons olive oil, divided	
1½ ounces lemon juice	**2** Meanwhile, wash the romaine hearts and slice off the ends. Cut each romaine heart in half. Drizzle each half with the remaining olive oil and season with salt and pepper.
2 cloves garlic	
1 teaspoon vegan Worcestershire sauce	
Salt and pepper to taste	**3** Place each romaine heart face down on hot grill (or grill pan) for 45 seconds or until lightly charred. Remove and serve on chilled plate with drizzled Caesar dressing. Garnish with grilled bread or croutons.
6 romaine hearts	
Grilled bread or croutons as garnish	

Per serving: Calories 104; Fat 7g (Saturated 1g); Cholesterol 0mg; Sodium 134mg; Carbohydrate 5g (Dietary Fiber 1g); Protein 6g.

Note: This delicious recipe is Vegetate's (Washington, D.C.) take on a classic Caesar salad; they replace the anchovies with toasted ground nori (seaweed sheets often used for making sushi rolls), and instead of eggs, they use silken tofu, a high-protein, cholesterol-free improvement.

Summer Tomato Salad

Prep time: 10 min • **Cook time:** 0 min • **Yield:** 4 servings

Ingredients	*Directions*
4 medium tomatoes, diced small	**1** Combine all the ingredients in a large bowl and serve the salad at room temperature.
1 garlic clove, minced	
6 leaves basil, chiffonaded	
2 tablespoons olive oil	
1 tablespoon balsamic vinegar	
Salt and pepper to taste	

Per serving: Calories 99; Fat 7g (Saturated 1g); Cholesterol 0mg; Sodium 152mg; Carbohydrate 8g (Dietary Fiber 1g); Protein 1g.

Tip: Try a combination of tomatoes in this salad to add color and flavor. Look for Green Zebras, Yellow Teardrops, pear tomatoes, grape tomatoes, and everyone's first favorite tomato, the cherry. So many choices, so little time!

Note: This dish, courtesy of Paley's Place in Portland, Oregon, is low in saturated fat and contains no cholesterol but still remains intense in flavor from the fresh basil and garlic.

HOW TO SEED AND DICE TOMATOES

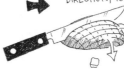

Figure AC-1: How to seed and dice a tomato.

1. USE A CUTTING BOARD. SLICE THE TOMATO IN HALF. SLICE OFF THE ENDS.

2. SCRAPE OUT THE SEEDS WITH A SMALL TOOL OR YOUR FINGER.

3. WITH THE FLAT SIDE DOWN, SLICE THE TOMATO HALF IN ONE DIRECTION, THEN IN THE OTHER DIRECTION, TO DICE.

Illustration by Liz Kurtzman

Blood Orange, Beet, and Avocado Salad

Prep time: 25 min • **Cook time:** 1 hr or more • **Yield:** 6 servings

Ingredients	Directions
1 bunch yellow beets	**1** Preheat the oven to 400 degrees. Cut the leaves and roots from the beets. Rub the beets with about 1 tablespoon of olive oil and wrap each one in foil. Bake until they're soft when pierced with a fork, at least 1 hour. When the beets are cool enough to handle, remove the skins and cut the beets into wedges.
3 tablespoons plus about 1 tablespoon extra-virgin olive oil	
1 head red lettuce (or a small bag of mesclun)	
4 blood oranges	**2** Meanwhile, wash and dry the lettuce and place it in a large bowl.
2 avocados	
¼ cup shelled pistachios or toasted pine nuts	**3** Cut both ends off the oranges, lay them on a cut side, and with a knife, remove the rind in 1-inch strips around the orange, cutting down to the flesh. Squeeze any excess juice from the cuttings over the lettuce. Cut the skinned oranges into rounds.
½ teaspoon coarse salt	
1½ tablespoons red wine vinegar	
Freshly ground black pepper, to taste	**4** Cut each avocado in half, and cut the flesh of each half into slices. Arrange the blood orange slices, the avocado slices, and the beets over the lettuce. Sprinkle with pistachios or pine nuts.
	5 When ready to serve, mix salt in the bowl of a spoon with the vinegar. Toss vinegar mixture over the salad, and then add 3 tablespoons of olive oil and black pepper to taste. Toss salad gently so that all the ingredients are lightly coated with dressing. Arrange salad on individual salad plates.

Per serving: Calories 245; Fat 18g (Saturated 3g); Cholesterol 0mg; Sodium 159mg; Carbohydrate 21g (Dietary Fiber 9g); Protein 5g.

Shrimp Salad

Prep time: 15 min • **Cook time:** 0 min • **Yield:** 4 servings

Ingredients	*Directions*
1 pound medium shrimp, cooked	**1** In a bowl, combine the shrimp, the red and yellow peppers, half of the cilantro, and the chives.
¼ cup chopped red pepper	
¼ cup chopped yellow pepper	**2** In another bowl, whisk together the mayonnaise, mustard, lemon juice, and white pepper. Spoon over the shrimp mixture and toss together.
1 tablespoon chopped fresh cilantro, divided	
¼ cup chopped fresh chives	**3** Arrange the salad greens on 4 large plates. Top the greens with equal portions of the shrimp mixture. Sprinkle with the remaining cilantro.
¼ cup low-fat mayonnaise	
1 teaspoon Dijon mustard	
1 teaspoon lemon juice	
¼ teaspoon white pepper	
4 cups fresh mixed salad greens	

Per serving: Calories 154; Fat 3g (Saturated 0g); Cholesterol 221mg; Sodium 440mg; Carbohydrate 7g (Dietary Fiber 2g); Protein 25g.

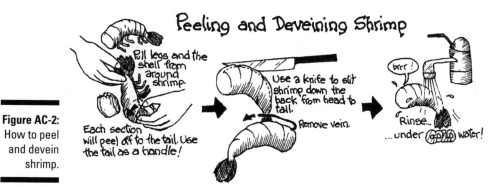

Figure AC-2: How to peel and devein shrimp.

Illustration by Liz Kurtzman

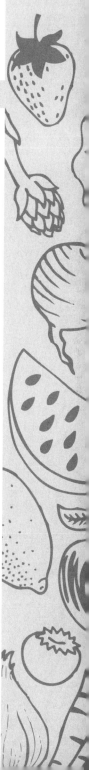

Teriyaki Salmon Salad

Prep time: 15 min • **Cook time:** 10 to 12 min • **Yield:** 2 servings

Ingredients	*Directions*
1 tablespoon Dijon mustard 1 tablespoon dry white cooking wine 1 tablespoon low-sodium teriyaki sauce 1 teaspoon low-sodium soy sauce 1 teaspoon honey 1 teaspoon lemon juice ½ teaspoon garlic powder ¼ teaspoon white pepper 2 skinless salmon fillets, 6 ounces each 2 cups field salad greens ¼ small red onion, thinly sliced	**1** Preheat the oven to 350 degrees. In a medium bowl, combine the mustard, wine, teriyaki sauce, soy sauce, honey, lemon juice, garlic powder, and white pepper. Place the salmon in the bowl and coat thoroughly. **2** Place the salmon in a baking dish, pour the remaining liquid over the salmon, and place the dish in the oven. Bake for 10 to 12 minutes. **3** Arrange 1 cup of greens on each plate and place a salmon fillet on top. Sprinkle the red onion over the plate.

Per serving: *Calories 256; Fat 7g (Saturated 1g); Cholesterol 97mg; Sodium 559mg; Carbohydrate 8g (Dietary Fiber 2g); Protein 39g.*

Border Grill's Cinnamon-Brandy Chicken

Prep time: 30 min plus marinating time • **Cook time:** 40 min • **Yield:** 6 servings

Ingredients	*Directions*
½ **cup brandy**	**1** In a medium bowl, mix the brandy, cinnamon, honey, lemon and orange juices, garlic, salt, and pepper. Add the seasoned chicken and toss to evenly coat. Cover and marinate in the refrigerator 8 hours or overnight.
1 tablespoon cinnamon	
¼ **cup honey**	
½ **cup lemon juice**	**2** Preheat the oven to 350 degrees. Remove the chicken from the bowl and shake off excess marinade. Pour the marinade into a small saucepan and bring to a boil. Boil until it begins to thicken and about 1 cup remains, 5 to 10 minutes.
½ **cup orange juice**	
4 garlic cloves, minced	
1 teaspoon salt	
½ **teaspoon freshly ground black pepper**	**3** Heat the oil in an ovenproof skillet over medium-high heat. Sear the chicken until golden on both sides. Pour the reduced marinade over the chicken and place in the oven. Bake about 20 minutes and serve.
1 frying chicken (2½ to 3 pounds), cut into pieces and seasoned	
2 tablespoons vegetable oil	

Per serving: *Calories 506; Fat 25g (Saturated 7g); Cholesterol 134mg; Sodium 502mg; Carbohydrate 16g (Dietary Fiber 0g); Protein 42g.*

Note: Serve with the rice pilaf and roasted vegetable dishes, later in this section.

MINCING GARLIC

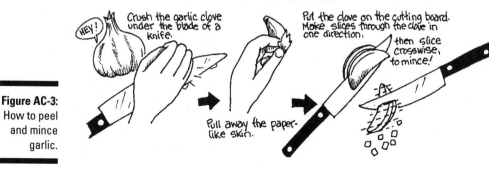

Figure AC-3: How to peel and mince garlic.

Illustration by Liz Kurtzman

Border Grill's Green Rice Pilaf

Prep time: 40 min • **Cook time:** 25 min • **Yield:** 6 servings

Ingredients

1½ tablespoons vegetable oil

1 small onion, finely diced

1 cup long-grain white rice

2 cups hot vegetable or chicken broth, preferably homemade

½ teaspoon salt

3 medium poblano chilies, roasted, peeled, seeded, and cut into strips

1 cup fresh or frozen peas

½ cup crumbled Mexican queso fresco or feta cheese

½ bunch Italian parsley leaves, finely chopped

½ bunch cilantro, finely chopped

Directions

1 Heat the oil in a heavy saucepan over medium heat. Add the onion and rice and cook, stirring frequently, for about 7 minutes, until the onion is softened but not browned.

2 Add the hot broth, salt, and chilies and bring to a boil. Reduce to a simmer and cook, covered, for about 10 minutes.

3 Add the peas and simmer 5 minutes longer. Remove from heat and let stand, covered, for about 10 minutes.

4 Add the cheese, parsley, and cilantro. Evenly mix and fluff with a fork, and serve immediately.

Per serving: Calories 202; Fat 7g (Saturated Fat 3g); Cholesterol 1mg; Sodium 948mg; Carbohydrate 28g (Dietary Fiber 2g); Protein 12g.

Note: This dish can accompany the chicken in the preceding recipe, or it can be served with meat or fish.

Border Grill's Red Roasted Root Vegetables

Prep time: 35 min • **Cook time:** 40 min • **Yield:** 6 servings

Ingredients	*Directions*
½ **pound turnips, peeled and cut into 1-inch chunks**	*1* Preheat the oven to 450 degrees. In a large bowl, toss together all the ingredients until well mixed. Arrange the mixture in a single layer in an enamel cast-iron casserole or baking dish.
½ **pound beets, peeled and cut into 1-inch chunks**	
½ **pound carrots, peeled and cut into 1-inch chunks**	*2* Cover the casserole dish and roast for 30 to 40 minutes, stirring every 10 minutes. The vegetables are done when they're golden, lightly caramelized on the edges, and easily pierced with the tip of a knife.
½ **pound butternut or other firm squash, peeled and cut into 1-inch chunks**	
1 onion, coarsely chopped	
2 garlic cloves, minced	
½ **bunch fresh oregano leaves, coarsely chopped**	
⅓ **cup olive oil**	
1 teaspoon salt	
½ **teaspoon freshly ground pepper**	

Per serving: *Calories 171; Fat 11g (Saturated Fat 2g); Cholesterol 0mg; Sodium 432mg; Carbohydrate 15g (Dietary Fiber 4g); Protein 2g.*

Vary It! You can substitute any of your favorite root vegetables in this dish.

Border Grill's Baked Apples

Prep time: 35 min • **Cook time:** 1 hr • **Yield:** 6 servings

Ingredients	Directions
1 cup plus 2 tablespoons apple juice	**1** In a small saucepan, bring 2 tablespoons apple juice and the raisins to a simmer and remove from heat. Let them sit for 10 minutes.
¼ cup raisins	
¼ cup apple butter	**2** Preheat the oven to 350 degrees. In a bowl, stir together the apple butter, walnuts, maple syrup, brandy, and raisins with their juice and mix well.
¼ cup toasted chopped walnuts	
2 tablespoons maple syrup	
2 tablespoons brandy	**3** Stuff the apples with the raisin mixture. Place the apples in a small roasting pan and top each with a dab of butter. Pour the remaining cup of apple juice into the pan and bake 50 to 60 minutes, or until the apples are tender but not split or mushy.
6 medium apples, cored and the top third peeled	
2 tablespoons unsalted butter	

Per serving: Calories 218; Fat 8g (Saturated Fat 3g); Cholesterol 11mg; Sodium 2mg; Carbohydrate 38g (Dietary Fiber 4g); Protein 2g.

CHOPPING NUTS

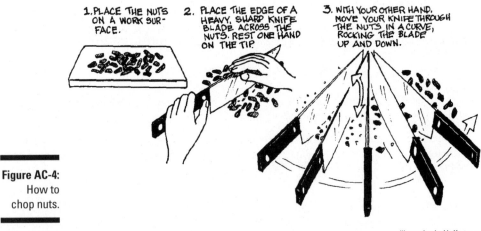

1. PLACE THE NUTS ON A WORK SURFACE.

2. PLACE THE EDGE OF A HEAVY, SHARP KNIFE BLADE ACROSS THE NUTS. REST ONE HAND ON THE TIP.

3. WITH YOUR OTHER HAND, MOVE YOUR KNIFE THROUGH THE NUTS IN A CURVE, ROCKING THE BLADE UP AND DOWN.

Figure AC-4:
How to chop nuts.

Illustration by Liz Kurtzman

Gaylord India's Seekh Kabab (Barbecued Lamb on Skewer)

Prep time: 30 min plus marinating time • **Cook time:** 15 min • **Yield:** 6 servings

Ingredients	*Directions*
1 medium onion	*1* In a blender or mini food processor, puree onion, ginger, and garlic with 2 teaspoons of water. Transfer the mix to a medium bowl and mix in salt, cayenne pepper, coriander powder, cumin powder, and garam masala.
1 inch fresh ginger, peeled	
2 garlic cloves	
2 teaspoons water	
1 teaspoon salt	*2* Add the ground lamb and mix until thoroughly combined. Let stand for 20 to 30 minutes in the refrigerator.
¼ teaspoon cayenne pepper	
½ teaspoon coriander powder	
½ teaspoon cumin powder	*3* Preheat the oven to 375 degrees. Divide the mixture into 6 equal portions. Lightly oil 6 skewers. Shape the lamb mixture into sausage shapes on the skewers, about 1 inch thick.
¾ teaspoon garam masala (available in Indian food stores)	
1 pound lean ground lamb	*4* Place skewers on a rack over a pan and bake for 15 to 20 minutes or until done. To broil, place skewers 3 to 4 inches from heat and cook approximately 7 minutes per side. Serve hot with lemon garnish.

Per serving: *Calories 123; Fat 6g (Saturated 2g); Cholesterol 42mg; Sodium 422mg; Carbohydrate 2g; Dietary Fiber 1g; Protein 14g.*

Tip: If using wood or bamboo skewers, soak them overnight in water and oil them lightly. This step prevents the skewers from burning while cooking.

Note: This dish can be served as an entree or as an appetizer. Combine this recipe with 1 cup rice to provide the necessary carbohydrate. Two servings of vegetables, one of which could be the Saag (later in this chapter), round out the meal.

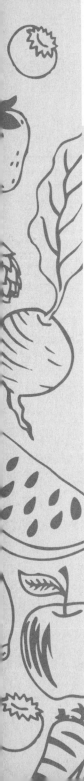

Gaylord India's Chicken Tikka Kabab (Barbecued Chicken Kebab)

Prep time: 30 min plus marinating time • **Cook time:** 10 min • **Yield:** 6 servings

Ingredients	*Directions*
2 tablespoons chopped ginger	*1* Combine the ginger, garlic, yogurt, white pepper, cumin, nutmeg, cardamom, red pepper, turmeric, lemon juice, and salt in a blender or food processor. With the motor running, drizzle in the oil.
2 tablespoons chopped garlic	
¼ cup nonfat yogurt	
½ teaspoon ground white pepper	*2* Add the chicken pieces to the marinade. Mix thoroughly to coat. Cover and let marinate for 3 to 4 hours in the refrigerator.
½ teaspoon ground cumin	
¼ teaspoon ground nutmeg	
¼ teaspoon cardamom	*3* Preheat the oven to 375 degrees. Place chicken breasts on a skewer about 1 inch apart.
½ teaspoon red pepper	
½ teaspoon ground turmeric	*4* Place skewers on a rack over a pan and bake for about 10 to 12 minutes or until cooked. To broil, place skewers 3 to 4 inches from the heat and broil approximately 5 minutes per side. Serve hot with lemon garnish.
¼ cup lemon juice	
Salt to taste	
2 teaspoons vegetable oil	
3 whole chicken breasts, boned, skinned, and cut into 18 pieces	

Per serving: Calories 197; Fat 6g (Saturated Fat 2g); Cholesterol 14mg; Sodium 8mg; Carbohydrate 2g (Dietary Fiber 1g); Protein 32g.

Tip: Make this dish early in the day and grill right before serving.

Note: You can combine this recipe with 1 cup rice to provide the necessary carbohydrate. Two servings of vegetables, one of which could be the Saag, round out the meal.

Gaylord India's Saag (Spinach)

Prep time: 10 min • **Cook time:** 10 min • **Yield:** 6 servings

Ingredients	Directions
Two 10-ounce bags fresh spinach, trimmed and washed	**1** In a large saucepan of boiling salted water, blanch the spinach in batches for 30 seconds or until wilted. Drain and refresh in cold water. Squeeze the moisture from leaves and chop finely.
2 teaspoons vegetable oil	
½ teaspoon cumin seeds	**2** Heat the vegetable oil over medium heat in a nonstick pan. Add the cumin seeds and stir for 5 seconds. Add garlic and fry until soft, 2 to 3 minutes.
10 garlic cloves sliced into ¼-inch slices	
2 dried red chilies	**3** Add the chilies and cook another minute. Add the spinach, toss well, and sauté until heated thoroughly and the liquid in the pan has evaporated (approximately 2 to 3 minutes). Season with salt. Serve hot.
Salt to taste	

Per serving: Calories 34; Fat 2g (Saturated Fat 0g); Cholesterol 0mg; Sodium 63mg; Carbohydrate 3g (Dietary Fiber 2g); Protein 3g.

Greens' Romaine Hearts with Sourdough Croutons and Parmesan Cheese

Prep time: 10 min • **Cook time:** 10 min • **Yield:** 4 servings

Ingredients	Directions
4 small heads of romaine lettuce	**1** Discard the outer leaves of the romaine heads and use the whole leaves and the hearts, which should be pale green or yellow and firm. Wash the leaves, dry them in a spinner, and wrap them loosely in a damp towel and refrigerate.
2 garlic cloves, finely chopped	
6 tablespoons extra-virgin olive oil, divided	
4 thick slices of sourdough bread, cut into ½-inch cubes, about 1½ cups	**2** Preheat the oven to 375 degrees. Add 1 garlic clove to 1 tablespoon olive oil and toss with the cubed bread. Spread the cubes on a baking sheet and bake for 7 to 8 minutes, until golden brown. Set aside to cool.
1¼ teaspoon minced lemon zest	**3** Make the vinaigrette by combining the lemon zest, salt, remaining garlic, and vinegar. Then whisk in 5 tablespoons olive oil.
¼ teaspoon salt	
1½ tablespoons vinegar or lemon juice	
8 Geata or Nicoise olives, pitted and coarsely chopped	**4** When you're ready to serve the salad, place the lettuce in a large bowl. Add the olives and toss with the vinaigrette, coating all the leaves. Add the croutons and Parmesan; toss again. Sprinkle with freshly ground pepper and serve.
1 ounce Parmesan cheese, grated, about ⅓ cup	
Freshly ground black pepper to taste	

Per serving: Calories 355; Fat 23g (Saturated Fat 4g); Cholesterol 6mg; Sodium 696mg; Carbohydrate 31g (Dietary Fiber 3g); Protein 9g.

Greens' Summer Minestrone

Prep time: 30 min • **Cook time:** 45 min • **Yield:** 6 servings

Ingredients	*Directions*
½ cup dried red beans, sorted and soaked overnight	**1** Drain and rinse the beans, and then place them in a 2-quart saucepan with 6 cups of cold water, 1 bay leaf, sage leaves, and oregano. Bring to a boil; reduce heat and simmer, uncovered, until the beans are tender, about 30 minutes. Remove the herbs.
2 bay leaves	
2 fresh sage leaves	
1 fresh oregano sprig	
1 tablespoon extra-virgin olive oil	**2** While the beans are cooking, heat the oil in a soup pot. Add the onion, salt, dried basil, and a few pinches of pepper. Sauté the onion over medium heat until soft, 5 to 7 minutes.
1 medium red onion, diced (about 2 cups)	
½ teaspoon salt	
¼ teaspoon dried basil	**3** Add the garlic, carrots, bell pepper, and zucchini to the soup pot and sauté for 7 to 8 minutes, stirring often. Add the wine and cook for 1 to 2 minutes, until the pan is almost dry.
Black pepper to taste	
6 garlic cloves, finely chopped	
1 small carrot, diced (about ¼ cup)	**4** Add the tomatoes and then add the pasta, spinach or chard, and beans with their broth. Season with salt and pepper to taste. Add the fresh basil just before serving. Garnish each serving with a generous tablespoon of Parmesan cheese.
1 small red bell pepper, diced (about ¾ cup)	
1 small zucchini, diced (about ¾ cup)	
¼ cup red wine	
2 pounds fresh tomatoes, peeled, seeded, and coarsely chopped (about 3 cups)	
¼ cup small pasta, cooked al dente, drained, and rinsed	
½ bunch of fresh spinach or chard, cut into thin ribbons and washed, about 2 cups packed	
2 tablespoons chopped fresh basil	
Grated Parmesan cheese	

Per serving: Calories 98; Fat 2g (Saturated Fat 0g); Cholesterol 1mg; Sodium 652mg; Carbohydrate 17g (Dietary Fiber 2g); Protein 4g.

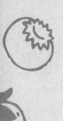

Greens' Sweet Pepper and Basil Frittata

Prep time: 30 min • **Cook time:** 30 min • **Yield:** 10 servings

Ingredients	*Directions*
2 tablespoons light olive oil 1 medium yellow onion, thinly sliced, about 2 cups ¾ teaspoon salt Freshly ground black pepper 4 medium sweet peppers, preferably a combination of red and yellow, thinly sliced (about 4 cups) 4 garlic cloves, finely chopped 1 bay leaf 6 eggs 3 ounces Fontina cheese, grated, about 1½ cups 2 ounces Parmesan cheese, grated, about ¾ cup ¼ cup fresh basil leaves, bundled and thinly sliced 3 tablespoons balsamic vinegar	**1** Preheat the oven to 475 degrees. Heat 1 tablespoon olive oil in a large skillet; add the onion, ½ teaspoon salt, and a few pinches of pepper. Sauté the onion over medium heat until it begins to soften, about 4 to 5 minutes. **2** Add the sweet peppers, garlic, and bay leaf; stew the onion and peppers together for about 15 minutes, until the peppers are tender. Set the vegetables aside to cool. Remove the bay leaf. **3** Beat the eggs in a bowl and add the onion-pepper mixture, cheeses, and basil. Season with ¼ teaspoon salt and ⅛ teaspoon pepper. **4** In a 9-inch nonstick, ovenproof sauté pan, heat the remaining tablespoon of olive oil until almost smoking. Swirl the oil around the side of the pan to coat. Turn the heat down to low and then immediately pour the egg mixture into the pan. The pan should be hot enough so that the eggs sizzle when they touch the oil. Cook the frittata over low heat for 2 to 3 minutes, until the sides begin to set. **5** Transfer the sauté pan to the oven and bake the frittata, uncovered, for 6 to 8 minutes, until firm and the eggs are completely cooked. **6** Loosen the frittata gently with a rubber spatula. Place a plate over the pan, flip it over, and put it on a plate. Brush the bottom and sides with the vinegar and cut into wedges. Serve warm or at room temperature.

Per serving: Calories 149; Fat 10g (Saturated Fat 4g); Cholesterol 159mg; Sodium 349mg; Carbohydrate 45g (Dietary Fiber 1g); Protein 10g.

Note: You can serve this dish right out of the oven as a main course or let it cool and serve as a light lunch. You can also refrigerate the dish and cut it into small squares to serve as an hors d'oeuvre.

Greens' Rhubarb-Strawberry Cobbler

Prep time: 20 min • **Cook time:** 30 min • **Yield:** 6 servings

Ingredients	Directions
Cobbler filling	**1** Preheat the oven to 375 degrees. Wash the rhubarb well, cutting off any brown spots or leaves still on the stalks. If the stalks are especially thick, cut them in half lengthwise before slicing ½-inch thick so that all the pieces are approximately the same size.
1¼ pounds rhubarb	
1 pint basket of strawberries (about 1½ cups)	
¼ cup sugar	**2** Wash the strawberries, pat them dry, and hull them. Cut them into halves or leave whole if small.
2½ tablespoons unbleached white flour	
Zest of 1 small orange	**3** Make the cobbler filling by tossing rhubarb and strawberries with sugar, flour, and zest. Place mixture in an 8-inch square baking dish, a 9-inch round cake pan, or 6 to 8 individual ovenproof dishes.
Cobbler topping	
1½ cups unbleached white flour	
¼ teaspoon salt	**4** Make the cobbler topping by combining the dry ingredients (flour, salt, baking powder, and sugar). Add the butter to the dry mix with a food processor, an electric mixer, a pastry blender, or 2 knives until it resembles coarse meal. Add the cream and mix lightly, just until the dry ingredients are moistened.
1 tablespoon baking powder	
2 tablespoons sugar	
4 tablespoons unsalted butter	
1 cup heavy cream	**5** Cover the filling with tablespoon-size dollops of cobbler topping, using all the topping. Bake for 25 to 30 minutes, until the topping is browned and cooked through and the fruit is bubbling. Individual cobblers take about 20 minutes.

Per serving: Calories 328; Fat 8g (Saturated Fat 5g); Cholesterol 21mg; Sodium 425mg; Carbohydrate 60g (Dietary Fiber 2g); Protein 5g.

Vary It! You can make this cobbler with less sugar (⅛ cup) if you omit the rhubarb and use strawberries alone. You'll need 3 baskets of berries (about 5 cups).

Gerald Hirigoyen's Lemon-Braised Sea Bass with Star Anise and Baby Spinach

Prep time: 30 min • **Cook time:** 15 min • **Yield:** 4 servings

Ingredients	Directions
4 sea bass fillets (about 4 ounces each)	**1** Preheat the oven to 475 degrees. Rub both sides of the sea bass fillets with salt and pepper and set aside.
Salt and freshly ground pepper to taste	
1 teaspoon olive oil	**2** Heat the olive oil in a large ovenproof sauté pan (preferably nonstick) over high heat. Add the celery root, fennel, carrot, garlic, and star anise and sauté until slightly caramelized, 4 to 5 minutes. Soften the caramelization with the lemon juice and cook for 1 minute.
¼ cup finely diced celery root	
⅓ cup finely diced fennel	
¼ cup finely diced carrot	
3 garlic cloves, peeled and chopped	**3** Lay the sea bass fillets on top of the sautéed vegetables, add the water, and cover the pan. Place the pan into the preheated oven just until the fish is cooked though (5 to 6 minutes). Remove the pan from oven and remove the fillets of fish and set them aside, covered to keep warm.
4 star anise	
¼ cup freshly squeezed lemon juice	
1½ cups water	
⅓ cup finely diced cucumber	**4** Add the cucumber, tomato, and apple to the vegetables in the sauté pan and place over high heat. Bring to a boil and cook for 1 to 2 minutes.
⅓ cup finely diced tomato	
⅛ cup finely diced apple	**5** Add the spinach, extra-virgin olive oil, mild cayenne, and salt and pepper to taste. Cook just until the spinach wilts (30 seconds to 1 minute).
4 cups baby spinach	
2 teaspoons extra-virgin olive oil	**6** In 4 shallow soup bowls, spread an even amount of the vegetables and juice from the pan. Lay a fillet on top of the vegetables in each bowl and place a star anise on top to garnish. Sprinkle the chives and parsley over the top of each dish and serve immediately.
Pinch of mild cayenne powder	
2 tablespoons fresh chopped chives	
2 tablespoons fresh chopped parsley	

Per serving: Calories 236; Fat 6g (Saturated Fat 1g); Cholesterol 77mg; Sodium 240mg; Carbohydrate 17g (Dietary Fiber 3g); Protein 31g.

Note: This meal is low in total carbohydrate and total fat, so you can complete the meal with a couple servings of carbohydrate (such as a serving of French bread and rice) and a tossed green salad with vinaigrette dressing.

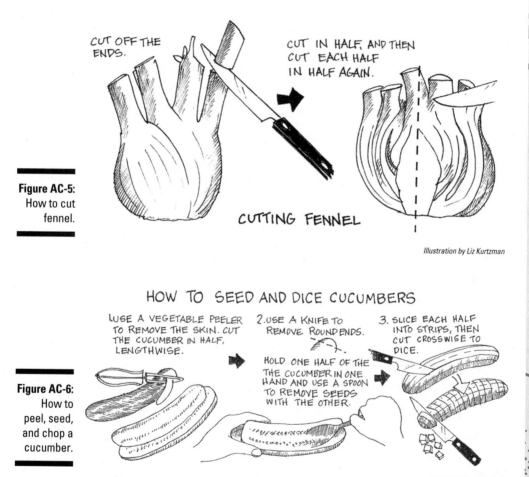

Figure AC-5: How to cut fennel.

CUT OFF THE ENDS.

CUT IN HALF, AND THEN CUT EACH HALF IN HALF AGAIN.

CUTTING FENNEL

Illustration by Liz Kurtzman

HOW TO SEED AND DICE CUCUMBERS

1. USE A VEGETABLE PEELER TO REMOVE THE SKIN. CUT THE CUCUMBER IN HALF, LENGTHWISE.

2. USE A KNIFE TO REMOVE ROUND ENDS.

HOLD ONE HALF OF THE THE CUCUMBER IN ONE HAND AND USE A SPOON TO REMOVE SEEDS WITH THE OTHER.

3. SLICE EACH HALF INTO STRIPS, THEN CUT CROSSWISE TO DICE.

Figure AC-6: How to peel, seed, and chop a cucumber.

Illustration by Liz Kurtzman

Gerald Hirigoyen's Marinated Chicken in Red Wine with Braising Greens, Parsnips, and Cippolini Onions

Prep time: 30 min plus marinating time • **Cook time:** 80 min • **Yield:** 4 servings

Ingredients	Directions
4 chicken thighs, without skin	**1** In a large bowl, combine the chicken thighs, breasts, red wine, onion, garlic, thyme, black peppercorns, and salt and pepper to season. Cover with plastic wrap and refrigerate for at least 6 hours, preferably overnight.
4 chicken breasts, split, without skin	
2 cups red wine	
1 small onion, chopped	**2** Preheat the oven to 450 degrees. Separate the chicken from the marinade and set both aside.
2 garlic cloves, chopped	
6 sprigs thyme	**3** Warm 1 tablespoon olive oil in a large casserole. Add the chicken thighs and sauté until browned, about 5 minutes.
1 tablespoon whole black peppercorns	
Kosher salt and freshly ground black pepper to taste	**4** Pour the marinade into the casserole with the thighs, add the veal stock, and bring to a boil. When it boils, reduce heat and let the ingredients simmer for 25 to 30 minutes, or until the chicken is cooked all the way through.
2 tablespoons olive oil, divided	
1 cup veal stock	
8 cippolini onions, peeled	**5** Warm 1 tablespoon olive oil in a large sauté pan over high heat. Add breasts and sauté until browned, about 3 to 4 minutes. Season with salt and pepper to taste and place in the oven until cooked, about 10 minutes.
8 baby carrots, peeled	
2 medium parsnips, peeled and cut into large matchsticks	
3 tablespoons unsalted butter, divided	**6** Place the cippolini onions in a small pan with enough water to cover, bring to a boil, and cook until soft and tender, about 20 minutes. Strain and set aside.
2 pounds braising greens, such as green chard, with stems removed and leaves torn into large pieces	**7** Fill a saucepan two-thirds full of water, bring to a boil, add baby carrots, and cook until tender, about 6 to 8 minutes. Strain and set aside.
2 tablespoons finely chopped parsley	

8 Place parsnips in a saucepan with enough water to cover, bring to a boil, and cook until tender, about 10 to 12 minutes. Strain and set aside.

9 After the chicken thighs are done, separate them from the marinade and set aside. Using a fine meshed sieve, strain the marinade into a small saucepan and discard the vegetables.

10 Bring the marinade to a boil and reduce by half. Turn off the heat, swirl in 1 tablespoon butter in a steady motion until completely incorporated, and season with salt and pepper to taste.

11 To prepare braising greens, combine ⅓ cup water, 1 tablespoon butter, the braising greens, and salt and pepper to taste in a large saucepan. Cover and cook over high heat just until wilted, about 5 minutes.

12 In a separate sauté pan, warm 1 tablespoon butter and then add the onion mixture and salt and pepper to taste and sauté until nicely caramelized, about 6 minutes. Add the parsley and set aside.

13 To assemble the dish, using a slotted spoon, place a small bed of the braising greens in the center of each plate. Lay one chicken thigh and one breast on top of the greens. Evenly scatter the cippolini onions, carrots, and parsnips on top of the chicken and spoon the sauce on top of and around the edges of the dish.

Per serving: Calories 596; Fat 25g (Saturated Fat 9g); Cholesterol 195mg; Sodium 936mg; Carbohydrate 30g (Dietary Fiber 5g); Protein 49g.

Note: This dish allows room for two additional servings of starches. You may want to include a couple servings of bread to soak up this wonderful sauce!

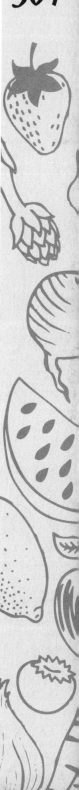

Gerald Hirigoyen's Onion Pie with Roquefort and Walnuts

Prep time: 1 hr • **Cook time:** 40 min • **Yield:** 8 servings

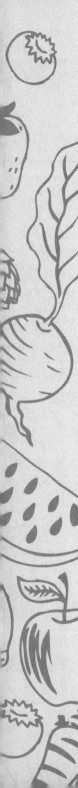

Ingredients

2 tablespoons olive oil

2 white onions, very thinly sliced

¼ cup water

3 ounces Roquefort cheese, crumbled into small pieces

Salt and freshly ground pepper to taste

½ cup walnuts, coarsely chopped

1 tablespoon melted butter

2 puff pastry sheets (11-x-15-inch sheets), fresh or thawed frozen

1 egg, lightly beaten

8 slices of prosciutto (about ½-ounce each)

Mixed greens to garnish

Directions

1 Place a baking sheet with sides in the freezer.

2 In a sauté pan over medium-high heat, warm the olive oil. Add the onions and sauté until golden brown (about 10 minutes). Add the water and continue to sauté until all the moisture evaporates, about 5 minutes.

3 Reduce heat to medium low. Add the Roquefort cheese and continue cooking, stirring occasionally, until melted, about 5 more minutes. Season lightly with salt, if needed, and add pepper to taste.

4 Stir in the walnuts and then spread the mixture out onto the chilled sheet pan. Place in the freezer until the onions cool down completely (about 10 minutes).

5 Preheat the oven to 450 degrees and evenly brush a sheet pan with melted butter.

6 Place the puff pastry on a cutting board. Using the rim of a small plate about 5 inches in diameter as a guide, cut the pastry into 8 rounds. Discard scraps.

7 Place the rounds onto the prepared baking sheet. Brush the outer rims and tops with the beaten egg. Evenly distribute the cooled onion mixture in the middle of each of the 8 rounds, leaving 1 inch uncovered all around the edges.

8 Place 1 prosciutto slice on top of each mound of the onion mixture. Fold over the pastry rounds to create half-moon shapes. Pinch down firmly around the edges to seal in the filling.

9 Brush the top of each pie with more of the beaten egg. Using a sharp knife, pierce the top of each pie with a small slit.

10 Bake until the pastry is pale golden and fully puffed, about 20 to 25 minutes.

Per serving: Calories 454; Fat 34g (Saturated Fat 7g); Cholesterol 47mg; Sodium 562mg; Carbohydrate 26g (Dietary Fiber 1g); Protein 13g.

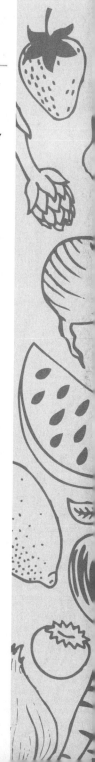

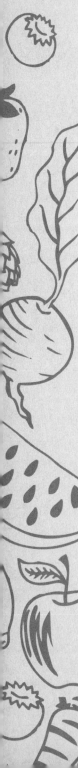

Paulette Mitchell's Beef and Broccoli Stir-Fry

Prep time: 15 min • **Cook time:** 10 min • **Yield:** 4 servings

Ingredients	Directions

Ingredients

Beef

1 tablespoon soy sauce

1 tablespoon dark (Asian) sesame oil

2 teaspoons finely chopped fresh ginger

1 teaspoon cornstarch

2 garlic cloves, minced

8 ounces boneless beef sirloin, cut into ⅛-inch slices

Sauce

¾ cup reduced-sodium beef broth

2 tablespoons Chinese oyster sauce

1 tablespoon soy sauce

¼ teaspoon red pepper flakes, or to taste

2 teaspoons cornstarch

To complete the recipe

2 tablespoons canola oil, divided

2 cups small broccoli florets

1 cup thinly sliced onion

½ red bell pepper, cut into ¼-inch strips

Directions

1 For the beef, stir together all the ingredients, except the beef, in a medium bowl. Add the beef and stir until the mixture is evenly combined.

2 Stir together the sauce ingredients in a small bowl.

3 Heat 1 tablespoon of the oil in a large sauté pan over medium-high heat. Add the beef mixture. Cook, stirring constantly, for 3 minutes or until the beef is just cooked. Use a slotted spoon to transfer the beef to a bowl and cover to keep warm.

4 Heat the remaining 1 tablespoon oil in the pan. Add the broccoli, onion, and bell pepper; cook, stirring constantly, for 3 minutes or until the broccoli is crisp-tender.

5 Add the beef and sauce. Stir gently for 1 minute or until the sauce thickens.

Per serving: Calories 243; Fat 17g (Saturated 4g); Cholesterol 37mg; Sodium 634mg; Carbohydrate 8g; Dietary Fiber 2g; Protein 15g.

Tip: To speed up preparation, you can buy precut broccoli florets. Serve this colorful stir-fry over brown basmati rice that can cook on the stove as you prepare this dish.

Paulette Mitchell's Cannellini Bean and Chicken Salad with Red-Wine Vinaigrette

Prep time: 20 min • **Cook time:** 0 min • **Yield:** 4 servings

Ingredients	*Directions*
Vinaigrette	**1** Whisk together the vinaigrette ingredients, except the basil, in a medium bowl. Stir in the basil.
¼ cup red-wine vinegar	
2 tablespoons extra-virgin olive oil	**2** Add the salad ingredients and stir gently.
1 tablespoon fresh lemon juice	
2 teaspoons Dijon mustard	
1 teaspoon minced garlic	
¼ teaspoon salt, or to taste	
¼ teaspoon pepper, or to taste	
¼ cup finely chopped fresh basil	
Salad	
2 cups coarsely chopped rotisserie chicken, skin removed, cooled	
One 15-ounce can cannellini beans, drained and rinsed	
1 tomato, coarsely chopped	
½ cup thinly sliced red onion	

Per serving: Calories 253; Fat 13g (Saturated 3g); Cholesterol 50mg; Sodium 685mg; Carbohydrate 15g; Dietary Fiber 4g; Protein 20g.

Paulette Mitchell's Chunky Gazpacho

Prep time: 20 min plus chilling time • **Cook time:** 0 min • **Yield:** 4 servings

Ingredients	*Directions*
One 15-ounce can tomato sauce	**1** Combine the tomato sauce, vinegar, oil, and honey in a medium bowl. Stir in the remaining ingredients.
2 tablespoons red-wine vinegar	
1 tablespoon extra-virgin olive oil	**2** To allow flavors to blend, refrigerate in a covered container for at least 2 hours, or until chilled.
1 tablespoon honey	
½ cucumber, seeded and coarsely chopped	
1 tomato, cut into ½-inch cubes	
½ green bell pepper, coarsely chopped	
1 rib celery, coarsely chopped	
2 tablespoons finely chopped red onion, or to taste	
1 teaspoon minced garlic, or to taste	
¼ teaspoon Tabasco sauce, or to taste	
¼ teaspoon pepper, or to taste	
Salt to taste	

Per serving: Calories 118; Fat 4g (Saturated 1g); Cholesterol 0mg; Sodium 495mg; Carbohydrate 23g; Dietary Fiber 4g; Protein 2g.

Tip: This gazpacho is best served in chilled bowls on a blistering-hot day, topped with whole-grain croutons.

Note: This soup will keep for up to 5 days in a covered container in the refrigerator. After storage, thin the soup with water or tomato juice to the desired consistency. You can spoon the thickened gazpacho over chilled grilled fish or chicken, or bring it to room temperature to serve over polenta or baked potatoes.

Paulette Mitchell's Jamaican Chicken with Black Beans

Prep time: 15 min • **Cook time:** 15 min • **Yield:** 4 servings

Ingredients	Directions
1 tablespoon olive oil	*1* Heat the oil in a large sauté pan over medium-high heat. Add the chicken, onion, curry powder, and garlic; cook, stirring occasionally, for 5 minutes or until the chicken is thoroughly cooked and the onions are tender.
12 ounces skinless, boneless chicken breasts, cut into 1-inch squares	
1 cup finely chopped onion	
2 teaspoons curry powder	
3 garlic cloves, minced	*2* Stir in the remaining ingredients, except cilantro. Reduce the heat to low; cover and simmer for 5 minutes or until heated through.
One 15-ounce can black beans, drained and rinsed	
One 14-ounce can diced tomatoes	*3* Garnish the servings with cilantro.
1 tablespoon finely chopped fresh thyme	
½ teaspoon ground allspice	
½ teaspoon red pepper flakes, or to taste	
½ teaspoon black pepper, or to taste	
Salt to taste	
Coarsely chopped fresh cilantro for garnish	

Per serving: Calories 224; Fat 6g (Saturated 1g); Cholesterol 47mg; Sodium 450mg; Carbohydrate 19g; Dietary Fiber 7g; Protein 23g.

Tip: Serve this aromatic dish with brown rice.

Paulette Mitchell's Shrimp Lettuce Wraps

Prep time: 20 min • **Cook time:** 10 min • **Yield:** 4 servings

Ingredients

1 teaspoon cold water

1 teaspoon cornstarch

12 ounces medium (26 to 30 count) raw shrimp, shelled, deveined, cut into ¼-inch pieces

2 tablespoons Chinese hot oil (also called chili oil)

2 tablespoons canola oil

¼ cup finely chopped onion

½ cup frozen baby peas, thawed

4 green onions, finely chopped

1 tablespoon soy sauce

1 tablespoon water

1 teaspoon dark (Asian) sesame oil

1 teaspoon finely chopped fresh ginger

8 whole iceberg lettuce leaves

Directions

1 Stir together the cold water and cornstarch in a medium bowl until smooth. Add the shrimp and stir until the mixture is evenly combined.

2 Heat the Chinese hot oil in a large skillet over medium-high heat. Add the shrimp; cook, stirring constantly, for 1 minute or until they begin to turn pink. Transfer to a bowl and cover to keep warm.

3 Heat the canola oil in the skillet over medium-high heat. Add the onion; cook, stirring occasionally, for 2 minutes or until tender.

4 Stir in the shrimp and the remaining ingredients, except the lettuce. Stir for 30 seconds or until the shrimp are completely cooked and the peas are warm. Remove from the heat.

5 Spoon a scant ¼ cup of the shrimp mixture into each lettuce leaf and roll.

Per serving: Calories 244; Fat 18g (Saturated 2g); Cholesterol 126mg; Sodium 420mg; Carbohydrate 5g; Dietary Fiber 2g; Protein 15g.

Index

Notes

Notes

Apple & Mac

iPad 2 For Dummies,
3rd Edition
978-1-118-17679-5

iPhone 4S For Dummies,
5th Edition
978-1-118-03671-6

iPod touch For Dummies,
3rd Edition
978-1-118-12960-9

Mac OS X Lion
For Dummies
978-1-118-02205-4

Blogging & Social Media

CityVille For Dummies
978-1-118-08337-6

Facebook For Dummies,
4th Edition
978-1-118-09562-1

Mom Blogging
For Dummies
978-1-118-03843-7

Twitter For Dummies,
2nd Edition
978-0-470-76879-2

WordPress For Dummies,
4th Edition
978-1-118-07342-1

Business

Cash Flow For Dummies
978-1-118-01850-7

Investing For Dummies,
6th Edition
978-0-470-90545-6

Job Searching with Social
Media For Dummies
978-0-470-93072-4

QuickBooks 2012
For Dummies
978-1-118-09120-3

Resumes For Dummies,
6th Edition
978-0-470-87361-8

Starting an Etsy Business
For Dummies
978-0-470-93067-0

Cooking & Entertaining

Cooking Basics
For Dummies, 4th Edition
978-0-470-91388-8

Wine For Dummies,
4th Edition
978-0-470-04579-4

Diet & Nutrition

Kettlebells For Dummies
978-0-470-59929-7

Nutrition For Dummies,
5th Edition
978-0-470-93231-5

Restaurant Calorie Counter
For Dummies,
2nd Edition
978-0-470-64405-8

Digital Photography

Digital SLR Cameras &
Photography For Dummies,
4th Edition
978-1-118-14489-3

Digital SLR Settings
& Shortcuts
For Dummies
978-0-470-91763-3

Photoshop Elements 10
For Dummies
978-1-118-10742-3

Gardening

Gardening Basics
For Dummies
978-0-470-03749-2

Vegetable Gardening
For Dummies,
2nd Edition
978-0-470-49870-5

Green/Sustainable

Raising Chickens
For Dummies
978-0-470-46544-8

Green Cleaning
For Dummies
978-0-470-39106-8

Health

Diabetes For Dummies,
3rd Edition
978-0-470-27086-8

Food Allergies
For Dummies
978-0-470-09584-3

Living Gluten-Free
For Dummies,
2nd Edition
978-0-470-58589-4

Hobbies

Beekeeping
For Dummies,
2nd Edition
978-0-470-43065-1

Chess For Dummies,
3rd Edition
978-1-118-01695-4

Drawing For Dummies,
2nd Edition
978-0-470-61842-4

eBay For Dummies,
7th Edition
978-1-118-09806-6

Knitting For Dummies,
2nd Edition
978-0-470-28747-7

Language &
Foreign Language

English Grammar
For Dummies,
2nd Edition
978-0-470-54664-2

French For Dummies,
2nd Edition
978-1-118-00464-7

German For Dummies,
2nd Edition
978-0-470-90101-4

Spanish Essentials
For Dummies
978-0-470-63751-7

Spanish For Dummies,
2nd Edition
978-0-470-87855-2

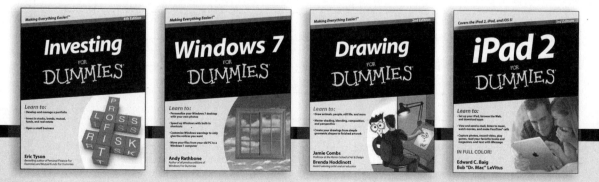

Available wherever books are sold. For more information or to order direct: U.S. customers visit www.dummies.com or call 1-877-762-2974.
U.K. customers visit www.wileyeurope.com or call (0) 1243 843291. Canadian customers visit www.wiley.ca or call 1-800-567-4797.

Connect with us online at www.facebook.com/fordummies or @fordummies

Math & Science

Algebra I For Dummies,
2nd Edition
978-0-470-55964-2

Biology For Dummies,
2nd Edition
978-0-470-59875-7

Chemistry For Dummies,
2nd Edition
978-1-1180-0730-3

Geometry For Dummies,
2nd Edition
978-0-470-08946-0

Pre-Algebra Essentials
For Dummies
978-0-470-61838-7

Microsoft Office

Excel 2010 For Dummies
978-0-470-48953-6

Office 2010 All-in-One
For Dummies
978-0-470-49748-7

Office 2011 for Mac
For Dummies
978-0-470-87869-9

Word 2010
For Dummies
978-0-470-48772-3

Music

Guitar For Dummies,
2nd Edition
978-0-7645-9904-0

Clarinet For Dummies
978-0-470-58477-4

iPod & iTunes
For Dummies,
9th Edition
978-1-118-13060-5

Pets

Cats For Dummies,
2nd Edition
978-0-7645-5275-5

Dogs All-in One
For Dummies
978-0470-52978-2

Saltwater Aquariums
For Dummies
978-0-470-06805-2

Religion & Inspiration

The Bible For Dummies
978-0-7645-5296-0

Catholicism For Dummies,
2nd Edition
978-1-118-07778-8

Spirituality For Dummies,
2nd Edition
978-0-470-19142-2

Self-Help & Relationships

Happiness For Dummies
978-0-470-28171-0

Overcoming Anxiety
For Dummies,
2nd Edition
978-0-470-57441-6

Seniors

Crosswords For Seniors
For Dummies
978-0-470-49157-7

iPad 2 For Seniors
For Dummies, 3rd Edition
978-1-118-17678-8

Laptops & Tablets
For Seniors For Dummies,
2nd Edition
978-1-118-09596-6

Smartphones & Tablets

BlackBerry For Dummies,
5th Edition
978-1-118-10035-6

Droid X2 For Dummies
978-1-118-14864-8

HTC ThunderBolt
For Dummies
978-1-118-07601-9

MOTOROLA XOOM
For Dummies
978-1-118-08835-7

Sports

Basketball For Dummies,
3rd Edition
978-1-118-07374-2

Football For Dummies,
2nd Edition
978-1-118-01261-1

Golf For Dummies,
4th Edition
978-0-470-88279-5

Test Prep

ACT For Dummies,
5th Edition
978-1-118-01259-8

ASVAB For Dummies,
3rd Edition
978-0-470-63760-9

The GRE Test For
Dummies, 7th Edition
978-0-470-00919-2

Police Officer Exam
For Dummies
978-0-470-88724-0

Series 7 Exam
For Dummies
978-0-470-09932-2

Web Development

HTML, CSS, & XHTML
For Dummies, 7th Edition
978-0-470-91659-9

Drupal For Dummies,
2nd Edition
978-1-118-08348-2

Windows 7

Windows 7
For Dummies
978-0-470-49743-2

Windows 7
For Dummies,
Book + DVD Bundle
978-0-470-52398-8

Windows 7 All-in-One
For Dummies
978-0-470-48763-1

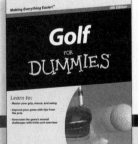
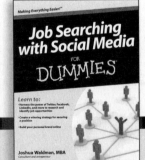
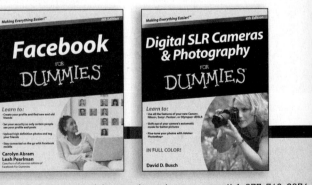

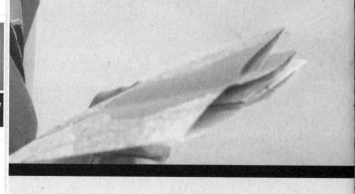

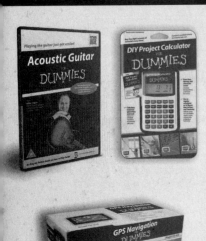
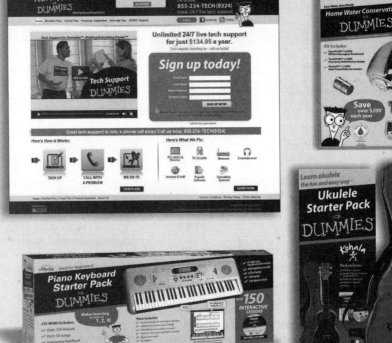
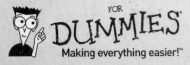